SKILLS PERFORMANCE CHECKLISTS

to accompany

Perry • Potter

CLINICAL NURSING SKILLS & TECHNIQUES

FIFTH EDITION

PATRICIA A. CASTALDI, RN, BSN, MSN
Associate Dean
Trinitas School of Nursing
Elizabeth, New Jersey
A Cooperative Program with Union County College
Cranford, New Jersey

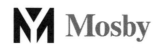

Mosby

A Harcourt Health Sciences Company

St. Louis   London   Philadelphia   Sydney   Toronto

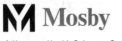

A Harcourt Health Sciences Company

Vice President and Publishing Director, Nursing: Sally Schrefer
Executive Editor: Susan Epstein
Senior Developmental Editor: Sharon Malchow
Project Manager: Gayle Morris
Production Editor: Jennifer Etling
Designer: Kathi Gosche

Mosby, Inc.
A Harcourt Health Sciences Company
11830 Westline Industrial Drive
St. Louis, Missouri 63146

Printed in the United States of America

International Standard Book Number: 0-323-01493-3

01 02 03 04 05 GW/EB 9 8 7 6 5 4 3 2 1

The checklists in this book were developed to provide an evaluation tool to determine your competence at performing the skills presented in *Clinical Nursing Skills and Techniques.* Instructors can check "Satisfactory," "Unsatisfactory," or "Needs Practice" for each step. Specific instructions or feedback can be provided in the "Comments" column or at the end of the checklist. These checklists can also be used for the independent self-evaluation of competency.

Although we understand that each instructor may require slightly different steps in the evaluation of the performance of a specific skill, these checklists have been streamlined to include only the critical steps needed to satisfactorily master the skill. They are not intended to replace the text, which describes and illustrates in detail each step of the nursing skill.

These checklists will be a valuable time-saver for instructors or a handy tool for self-evaluation. Each checklist begins on a separate page and is perforated for easy removal.

SKILLS PERFORMANCE CHECKLISTS

Student _____   Date _____

Instructor _____   Date _____

PERFORMANCE CHECKLIST 1-1 **ADMITTING CLIENTS**

	S	U	NP	Comments
ROOM PREPARATION				
1. Washed hands before preparing room equipment, furniture, and bed.	___	___	___	_____
2. Assembled special equipment. Checked that all equipment operated correctly.	___	___	___	_____
ASSESSMENT				
1. Greeted client and family cordially and introduced self by name and job title.	___	___	___	_____
2. Arranged for translation service, if necessary.	___	___	___	_____
3. Escorted client and family members to room and introduced roommate.	___	___	___	_____
4. Assessed client's general appearance and condition before beginning admitting procedures (postponed routine procedures when client presented acute physical or psychologic problems).	___	___	___	_____
5. Assessed client's and family members' psychologic response to admitting procedures.	___	___	___	_____
6. Assessed client's vital signs.	___	___	___	_____
7. Provided for privacy and prepared client for examination.	___	___	___	_____
8. Obtained a complete nursing history. Identified food, drug, and other substance allergies.	___	___	___	_____
9. Conducted physical assessment of appropriate body systems.	___	___	___	_____
10. Checked physician's admitting orders.	___	___	___	_____
11. Oriented client and family to nursing division.	___	___	___	_____
NURSING DIAGNOSIS				
1. Developed appropriate nursing diagnoses based on assessment data.	___	___	___	_____
PLANNING				
1. Identified expected outcomes.	___	___	___	_____
2. Informed client of planned procedures or treatments.	___	___	___	_____

	S	U	NP	Comments

IMPLEMENTATION

1. Allowed client and family opportunity to ask questions about admission procedures or therapies. ___ ___ ___ _____

2. Collected client's valuables and explained policy for ensuring safekeeping. ___ ___ ___ _____

3. Allowed client and family time alone. ___ ___ ___ _____

4. Placed call light within client's reach; placed bed in low position; raised side rails as needed. ___ ___ ___ _____

5. Washed hands after assessment. ___ ___ ___ _____

EVALUATION

1. Confirmed client's understanding of tests and procedures. ___ ___ ___ _____

2. Observed client for nonverbal signs. ___ ___ ___ _____

3. Monitored client's ability to ambulate independently. ___ ___ ___ _____

4. Checked client's room setup regularly. ___ ___ ___ _____

5. Assessed for unexpected outcomes. ___ ___ ___ _____

RECORDING AND REPORTING

1. Recorded history and assessment findings. Included information about advance directive. ___ ___ ___ _____

2. Notified physician of client's admission; reported unusual assessment findings; obtained admission orders, if necessary. ___ ___ ___ _____

3. Began to develop nursing plan of care. ___ ___ ___ _____

Student _____   Date _____

Instructor _____   Date _____

PERFORMANCE CHECKLIST 1-2 **TRANSFERRING CLIENTS**

	S	U	NP	Comments
ASSESSMENT				
1. Assessed reason for client's transfer.	___	___	___	_____
2. Determined client's and family's consent for transfer.	___	___	___	_____
3. Assessed client's physical condition and determined method and vehicle for transport.	___	___	___	_____
4. Assessed client's need for analgesic or antiemetic prior to transfer.	___	___	___	_____
5. Assessed if client's family or significant others had been notified of transfer.	___	___	___	_____
NURSING DIAGNOSIS				
1. Developed appropriate nursing diagnoses based on assessment data.	___	___	___	_____
PLANNING				
1. Identified expected outcomes for transfer.	___	___	___	_____
2. Arranged for transport vehicle.	___	___	___	_____
3. Obtained transfer order.	___	___	___	_____
4. Arranged for placement in new agency.	___	___	___	_____
IMPLEMENTATION				
1. Explained transfer reason and procedure to client or family.	___	___	___	_____
2. Checked accuracy and completeness of client's record.	___	___	___	_____
3. Obtained signed release from client giving permission to copy necessary part of record.	___	___	___	_____
4. Completed nursing care transfer form.	___	___	___	_____
5. Gathered and secured client's personal items.	___	___	___	_____
6. Attended to any last-minute physical needs of client.	___	___	___	_____
7. Transferred client to stretcher or wheelchair.	___	___	___	_____
8. Performed final assessment of client's physical stability.	___	___	___	_____
9. Accompanied client to transport vehicle.	___	___	___	_____

	S	U	NP	Comments
10. Notified receiving agency of impending transfer and client's status.	___	___	___	_____

EVALUATION

	S	U	NP	Comments
1. Compared final assessment data with previous finding.	___	___	___	_____
2. Inspected client's alignment and positioning in transport vehicle.	___	___	___	_____
3. Confirmed client's understanding of transfer and procedures.	___	___	___	_____
4. Determined if receiving agency had questions regarding client's care.	___	___	___	_____
5. Identified unexpected outcomes.	___	___	___	_____

RECORDING AND REPORTING

	S	U	NP	Comments
1. Documented client's status and method of transfer.	___	___	___	_____

Student _____ Date _____

Instructor _____ Date _____

PERFORMANCE CHECKLIST 1-3 **DISCHARGING CLIENTS**

	S	U	NP	Comments
ASSESSMENT				
1. Began assessing client's discharge needs upon admission.	___	___	___	_____
2. Assessed client's and family members' need for health teaching.	___	___	___	_____
3. Assessed existence of environmental barriers in client's home setting.	___	___	___	_____
4. Collaborated with physician and staff in other disciplines about client's need for referral for home health care services or an extended care facility.	___	___	___	_____
5. Assessed client's and family's perceptions of continued health care needs outside the hospital.	___	___	___	_____
6. Assessed client's acceptance of health problems.	___	___	___	_____
7. Consulted other health team members to determine client's discharge needs; made appropriate referrals.	___	___	___	_____
NURSING DIAGNOSIS				
1. Developed appropriate nursing diagnoses based on assessment data.	___	___	___	_____
PLANNING				
1. Identified expected outcomes for client's discharge.	___	___	___	_____
IMPLEMENTATION				
Before Day of Discharge				
1. Suggested ways to change physical arrangement of home environment to meet client's needs.	___	___	___	_____
2. Provided client and family with information about community health care resources.	___	___	___	_____
3. Conducted teaching sessions related to health care needs.	___	___	___	_____
4. Communicated client's/family's response to teaching and proposed discharge plan to other health care team members.	___	___	___	_____

	S	U	NP	Comments

Day of Discharge

1. Completed any of the following activities prior to discharge, if possible.   ___ ___ ___ _____

2. Allowed client and family opportunity to ask questions and discuss issues related to home health care; considered variations in the home setting for skill performance.   ___ ___ ___ _____

3. Checked physician's discharge orders.   ___ ___ ___ _____

4. Determined if transportation had been arranged for client.   ___ ___ ___ _____

5. Assisted client with dressing and packing personal items.   ___ ___ ___ _____

6. Checked all closets and drawers for belongings; obtained copy of valuables list and had valuables delivered to client; accounted for all valuables.   ___ ___ ___ _____

7. Gave client prescriptions or medications and reviewed drug information.   ___ ___ ___ _____

8. Provided information about follow-up with physician.   ___ ___ ___ _____

9. Assisted client in arranging with business office for bill payment.   ___ ___ ___ _____

10. Transported client and belongings to source of transportation.   ___ ___ ___ _____

11. Assisted client to wheelchair or stretcher; escorted client to agency entrance; safely assisted client into transport vehicle with personal belongings.   ___ ___ ___ _____

12. Notified admitting or appropriate department of discharge time.   ___ ___ ___ _____

EVALUATION

1. Asked client to describe nature of illness, treatment regimens, and signs and symptoms to be reported.   ___ ___ ___ _____

2. Had client or family member perform treatments to be continued at home.   ___ ___ ___ _____

3. Inspected home environment for risks.   ___ ___ ___ _____

4. Identified unexpected outcomes.   ___ ___ ___ _____

RECORDING AND REPORTING

1. Documented client's discharge.   ___ ___ ___ _____

2. Documented status of client's health problems at time of discharge.   ___ ___ ___ _____

Student _____   Date _____

Instructor _____   Date _____

PERFORMANCE CHECKLIST 2-1   **ESTABLISHING THE NURSE-CLIENT RELATIONSHIP**

	S	U	NP	Comments
ASSESSMENT				
1. Assessed client's behaviors and needs.	___	___	___	_____
2. Determined client's specific need to communicate.	___	___	___	_____
3. Assessed client's reason for need of health care.	___	___	___	_____
4. Assessed factors about self and client that influence communication.	___	___	___	_____
5. Assessed own barriers to communication with client.	___	___	___	_____
6. Assessed client's language and ability to speak.	___	___	___	_____
7. Observed client's pattern of communication and verbal and nonverbal behavior.	___	___	___	_____
8. Determined available resources for selection of communication methods.	___	___	___	_____
9. Assessed client's readiness to work toward goals.	___	___	___	_____
10. Considered time of client's discharge/transfer.	___	___	___	_____
NURSING DIAGNOSIS				
1. Developed appropriate nursing diagnoses based on assessment data.	___	___	___	_____
PLANNING				
1. Identified expected outcomes for communication goals.	___	___	___	_____
2. Prepared client and physical environment.	___	___	___	_____
3. Identified strategies to achieve goals and summarized pertinent information.	___	___	___	_____
IMPLEMENTATION				
Orientation Phase				
1. Created a climate of warmth and acceptance, with consideration of environment and client's status.	___	___	___	_____
2. Addressed client by name and introduced self by name and role.	___	___	___	_____
3. Used appropriate nonverbal behaviors.	___	___	___	_____
4. Observed client's nonverbal behaviors and actively listened to client.	___	___	___	_____

	S	U	NP	Comments

5. Explained the purpose of the interaction and if the information is to be shared. ___ ___ ___ _____

6. Identified client's expectations. ___ ___ ___ _____

7. Encouraged client to seek clarification during the interaction. ___ ___ ___ _____

8. Used therapeutic communication techniques during the interaction. ___ ___ ___ _____

Working Phase

1. Used effective communication skills. ___ ___ ___ _____

2. Discussed and prioritized problem areas. ___ ___ ___ _____

3. Provided information to client and assisted client with expressing feelings. ___ ___ ___ _____

4. Avoided barriers to communication. ___ ___ ___ _____

Termination Phase

1. Used effective communication skills to discuss discharge/termination issues. ___ ___ ___ _____

2. Summarized what was discussed with client. ___ ___ ___ _____

EVALUATION

1. Observed client's verbal and nonverbal responses. ___ ___ ___ _____

2. Noted nurse's responses and effectiveness of therapeutic techniques. ___ ___ ___ _____

3. Requested feedback from client on information that was communicated. ___ ___ ___ _____

4. Assessed for unexpected outcomes. ___ ___ ___ _____

5. Reinforced client's strengths; developed action plan. ___ ___ ___ _____

RECORDING AND REPORTING

1. Reported pertinent information to health care team members. ___ ___ ___ _____

2. Recorded communication pertinent to client's status and level of understanding. ___ ___ ___ _____

Student _____ Date _____

Instructor _____ Date _____

PERFORMANCE CHECKLIST 2-2 **COMMUNICATING WITH THE ANXIOUS CLIENT**

	S	U	NP	Comments
ASSESSMENT				
1. Assessed client for physical, behavioral, and verbal cues indicating anxiety.	—	—	—	_____
2. Assessed for possible factors causing client anxiety.	—	—	—	_____
3. Assessed factors influencing communication with client.	—	—	—	_____
4. Assessed own level of anxiety; made conscious effort to remain calm.	—	—	—	_____
5. Discussed possible causes of client anxiety with family.	—	—	—	_____
NURSING DIAGNOSIS				
1. Developed appropriate nursing diagnoses based on assessment data.	—	—	—	_____
PLANNING				
1. Identified expected outcomes.	—	—	—	_____
2. Recognized and controlled own anxiety.	—	—	—	_____
3. Prepared physical environment to provide quiet, calm area with ample personal space.	—	—	—	_____
IMPLEMENTATION				
1. Provided brief, simple introduction of self and role.	—	—	—	_____
2. Used appropriate nonverbal behaviors and active listening skills.	—	—	—	_____
3. Used clear and concise verbal techniques.	—	—	—	_____
4. Helped client acquire alternate coping strategies.	—	—	—	_____
5. Minimized noise in physical setting.	—	—	—	_____
6. Provided necessary comfort measures.	—	—	—	_____
EVALUATION				
1. Observed client for continuing presence of signs and symptoms and behaviors reflecting anxiety.	—	—	—	_____
2. Had client discuss ways to cope with anxiety in the future.	—	—	—	_____

	S	U	NP	Comments
3. Evaluated client's ability to discuss factors causing anxiety.	—	—	—	_____
4. Identified unexpected outcomes.	—	—	—	_____

RECORDING AND REPORTING

	S	U	NP	Comments
1. Recorded cause of client's anxiety and exhibited signs and symptoms and behaviors.	—	—	—	_____
2. Recorded and reported methods used to relieve anxiety and client's response.	—	—	—	_____

Student _____   Date _____

Instructor _____   Date _____

PERFORMANCE CHECKLIST 2-3 **VERBALLY DE-ESCALATING THE POTENTIALLY VIOLENT CLIENT**

	S	U	NP	Comments
ASSESSMENT				
1. Observed client for behaviors or expressions that indicate anger.	—	—	—	_____
2. Assessed factors that influence communication of the angry client.	—	—	—	_____
3. Considered available resources to assist in communication with the angry client.	—	—	—	_____
NURSING DIAGNOSIS				
1. Developed appropriate nursing diagnoses based on assessment data.	—	—	—	_____
PLANNING				
1. Identified expected outcomes.	—	—	—	_____
2. Prepared self for interaction with the angry client.	—	—	—	_____
3. Prepared environment to deescalate the potentially violent client.	—	—	—	_____
IMPLEMENTATION				
1. Created climate of acceptance for client; maintained nonthreatening communication skills.	—	—	—	_____
2. Responded appropriately to the potentially violent client by using therapeutic silence, answering questions, remaining calm, maintaining personal space and safety, and exploring alternatives to situation.	—	—	—	_____
EVALUATION				
1. Observed for continuing behaviors or expressions of anger.	—	—	—	_____
2. Noted client's ability to answer questions and problem solve.	—	—	—	_____
3. Identified unexpected outcomes.	—	—	—	_____
RECORDING AND REPORTING				
1. Recorded observations related to anger; reported verbal threats to appropriate agency personnel.	—	—	—	_____
2. Recorded and reported nursing interventions used and client's responses.	—	—	—	_____

Student _____   Date _____

Instructor _____   Date _____

PERFORMANCE CHECKLIST 3-1   **GIVING A CHANGE-OF-SHIFT REPORT**

	S	U	NP	Comments

ASSESSMENT
1. Gathered pertinent client information from available sources.   ___ ___ ___ _____

PLANNING
1. Prioritized information.   ___ ___ ___ _____

IMPLEMENTATION
1. Provided a detailed description of the client's current status and progress, including background information, assessment data, nursing diagnoses, interventions, and evaluation.   ___ ___ ___ _____

   a. Described treatment given and client's response.   ___ ___ ___ _____

   b. Described instructions given and client's progress in discharge plan. Included family information and explanation of current priorities.   ___ ___ ___ _____

2. Clarified report with oncoming shift.   ___ ___ ___ _____

Student _____   Date _____

Instructor _____   Date _____

PERFORMANCE CHECKLIST 3-2   **DOCUMENTING NURSES' PROGRESS NOTES**

	S	U	NP	Comments
ASSESSMENT				
1. Completed assessments and interventions and noted responses.	___	___	___	_____
IMPLEMENTATION				
1. Identified forms to be maintained and their location.	___	___	___	_____
2. Determined information to be documented.	___	___	___	_____
3. Documented information in a timely manner using appropriate agency format.	___	___	___	_____

Student _____   Date _____

Instructor _____   Date _____

PERFORMANCE CHECKLIST 3-3 **INCIDENT REPORTING**

	S	U	NP	Comments
ASSESSMENT				
1. Reported accurate, objective, chronological information.	___	___	___	_____
2. Assessed the extent of injury to client or others.	___	___	___	_____
IMPLEMENTATION				
1. Restored individual's safety, if injured.	___	___	___	_____
2. Notified physician if injury occurred.	___	___	___	_____
3. Referred nonclient injury to appropriate setting.	___	___	___	_____
4. Completed incident report correctly and promptly.	___	___	___	_____
5. Documented events of incident in client's chart correctly.	___	___	___	_____
6. Assessed and implemented ordered therapies in case of injured client.	___	___	___	_____

Student _____   Date _____

Instructor _____   Date _____

PERFORMANCE CHECKLIST 4-1 **FALL PREVENTION**

	S	U	NP	Comments

ASSESSMENT
1. Observed older adult for physiologic changes common to aging process. ___ ___ ___ _____
2. Reviewed client's medication history. ___ ___ ___ _____
3. Assessed risk factors in home and community. ___ ___ ___ _____
4. Determined potential risk of injury caused by motor-sensory or cognitive changes. ___ ___ ___ _____

NURSING DIAGNOSIS
1. Developed appropriate nursing diagnoses based on assessment data. ___ ___ ___ _____

PLANNING
1. Identified expected outcomes. ___ ___ ___ _____

IMPLEMENTATION
Home or Health Care Facility
1. Provided adequate, nonglare lighting. ___ ___ ___ _____
2. Removed unnecessary objects from walkways and stairs. ___ ___ ___ _____
3. Arranged necessary objects in a logical way in easy-to-reach locations. ___ ___ ___ _____
4. Installed grip bars or handrails in hallways and bathrooms, and provided raised toilet seats. ___ ___ ___ _____
5. Stairs:
   a. Installed appropriately colored and textured treads. ___ ___ ___ _____
   b. Ensured proper lighting and room for mobility. ___ ___ ___ _____
   c. Removed protrusions from stairway walls. ___ ___ ___ _____
   d. Kept stairs and walkways in good condition. ___ ___ ___ _____
6. Secured all carpeting, mats, and tile. ___ ___ ___ _____
7. Kept floors clean and dry. ___ ___ ___ _____

In a Health Care Facility
1. Identified client correctly. ___ ___ ___ _____
2. Introduced self by name and role to client. ___ ___ ___ _____
3. Gathered equipment. ___ ___ ___ _____

	S	U	NP	Comments
4. Washed hands correctly.	___	___	___	_____
5. Provided privacy. Positioned and draped client as needed.	___	___	___	_____
6. Adjusted bed and side rails properly.	___	___	___	_____
7. Explained and demonstrated use of call bell/ intercom system. Placed call bell within client's reach.	___	___	___	_____
8. Side rails:				
a. Explained use to client and family.	___	___	___	_____
b. Checked agency policy for use.	___	___	___	_____
c. Kept side rails up and bed in lowest position with wheels locked, as indicated.	___	___	___	_____
d. Left one side rail down for oriented, ambulatory client.	___	___	___	_____
9. Explained safety measures to client and family.	___	___	___	_____
10. Cleared pathway to bathroom.	___	___	___	_____

EVALUATION

1. Observed modification of client's environment for safety needs.	___	___	___	_____
2. Evaluated need for assistive devices.	___	___	___	_____
3. Asked client to identify safety risks.	___	___	___	_____
4. Reassessed motor, sensory, and cognitive status.	___	___	___	_____
5. Identified unexpected outcomes.	___	___	___	_____

RECORDING AND REPORTING

1. Recorded specific interventions to promote safety.	___	___	___	_____
2. Reported specific threats to safety and measures taken to reduce threats to all health care providers.	___	___	___	_____
3. Documented instructions given to client and family.	___	___	___	_____
4. Documented client falls and follow-up.	___	___	___	_____

Student _____   Date _____

Instructor _____   Date _____

PERFORMANCE CHECKLIST 4-2   **DESIGNING A RESTRAINT-FREE ENVIRONMENT**

	S	U	NP	Comments

ASSESSMENT

1. Assessed client's physical and mental status.   ___ ___ ___ _____

2. Reviewed prescribed medications.   ___ ___ ___ _____

3. Assessed client's knowledge of medical condition and treatment.   ___ ___ ___ _____

NURSING DIAGNOSIS

1. Developed appropriate nursing diagnoses based on assessment data.   ___ ___ ___ _____

PLANNING

1. Identified expected outcomes.   ___ ___ ___ _____

IMPLEMENTATION

1. Oriented client and family to surroundings, introduced to staff, and explained all treatments and procedures.   ___ ___ ___ _____

2. Encouraged family and friends to stay with client.   ___ ___ ___ _____

3. Placed client in room close to staff.   ___ ___ ___ _____

4. Provided appropriate visual and auditory stimuli.   ___ ___ ___ _____

5. Met client needs as quickly as possible.   ___ ___ ___ _____

6. Approached client in calm, nonthreatening, professional manner.   ___ ___ ___ _____

7. Limited number of caregivers interacting with client.   ___ ___ ___ _____

8. Organized treatments to allow for long, uninterrupted periods.   ___ ___ ___ _____

9. Reduced client's access to tubes and lines.   ___ ___ ___ _____

10. Employed stress reduction techniques.   ___ ___ ___ _____

11. Made use of diversional activities.   ___ ___ ___ _____

12. Used various disciplines (e.g., physical therapy).   ___ ___ ___ _____

13. Reviewed medications frequently.   ___ ___ ___ _____

	S	U	NP	Comments

EVALUATION

1. Observed client for injuries.

2. Avoided injury to others by client.

3. Determined the need for continuation of invasive treatments.

4. Identified unexpected outcomes.

RECORDING AND REPORTING

1. Recorded and reported client behaviors and nursing interventions.

Student _____   Date _____

Instructor _____   Date _____

PERFORMANCE CHECKLIST 4-3   **APPLYING PHYSICAL RESTRAINTS**

	S	U	NP	Comments
ASSESSMENT				
1. Determined if client required restraint.	—	—	—	_____
2. Assessed client's behavior and ability to follow directions.	—	—	—	_____
3. Reviewed agency policy and medical orders.	—	—	—	_____
4. Reviewed manufacturer's instructions for restraint use.	—	—	—	_____
5. Inspected site for restraint placement.	—	—	—	_____
NURSING DIAGNOSIS				
1. Developed appropriate nursing diagnoses based on assessment data.	—	—	—	_____
PLANNING				
1. Identified expected outcomes.	—	—	—	_____
IMPLEMENTATION				
1. Identified client.	—	—	—	_____
2. Introduced self by name and role; explained procedure.	—	—	—	_____
3. Gathered equipment.	—	—	—	_____
4. Washed hands.	—	—	—	_____
5. Provided privacy; draped client.	—	—	—	_____
6. Adjusted bed to working height.	—	—	—	_____
7. Positioned client appropriately.	—	—	—	_____
8. Padded skin and bony prominences beneath restraint.	—	—	—	_____
9. Applied selected restraint correctly:	—	—	—	_____
a. Jacket restraint	—	—	—	_____
b. Belt restraint	—	—	—	_____
c. Extremity restraint	—	—	—	_____
d. Mitten restraint	—	—	—	_____
10. Attached restraint appropriately to bed frame or wheelchair.	—	—	—	_____
11. Secured restraints with quick-release ties.	—	—	—	_____

	S	U	NP	Comments
12. Inserted two fingers under restraint to check for constriction.	___	___	___	_____
13. Checked placement of restraint and status of site/extremity every 30 to 60 minutes.	___	___	___	_____
14. Removed restraint every 2 hours. Obtained assistance, if necessary, for client safety.	___	___	___	_____
15. Secured call bell/intercom within client's reach.	___	___	___	_____
16. Left bed in lowest position; locked wheels of bed or chair.	___	___	___	_____
17. Washed hands.	___	___	___	_____

EVALUATION

	S	U	NP	Comments
1. Inspected client for injury.	___	___	___	_____
2. Observed IV and urinary catheters for positioning and functioning.	___	___	___	_____
3. Reassessed need for continued use of restraint.	___	___	___	_____
4. Identified unexpected outcomes.	___	___	___	_____

RECORDING AND REPORTING

	S	U	NP	Comments
1. Recorded client's prior behavior and status; type and specific use of restraint; nursing interventions to promote client safety; and client's response to restraint.	___	___	___	_____

Student _____   Date _____

Instructor _____   Date _____

PERFORMANCE CHECKLIST 4-4 **SEIZURE PRECAUTIONS**

	S	U	NP	Comments
ASSESSMENT				
1. Assessed client's seizure history.	___	___	___	_____
2. Assessed client for medical and surgical conditions that may lead to or exacerbate existing seizure condition.	___	___	___	_____
3. Assessed client's medication history.	___	___	___	_____
4. Inspected client's environment for potential safety hazards.	___	___	___	_____
NURSING DIAGNOSIS				
1. Developed appropriate nursing diagnoses based on assessment data.	___	___	___	_____
PLANNING				
1. Identified expected outcomes.	___	___	___	_____
IMPLEMENTATION				
1. Positioned client safely prior to and during a seizure.	___	___	___	_____
2. Provided privacy.	___	___	___	_____
3. Turned client on side with head flexed slightly forward, if possible.	___	___	___	_____
4. Did not restrain client; loosened clothing.	___	___	___	_____
5. Did not force objects into client's mouth.	___	___	___	_____
6. Remained with client, observing sequence and timing of seizure activity.	___	___	___	_____
7. Explained event and answered client's questions after seizure.	___	___	___	_____
8. Applied clean gloves and inspected oral airway when jaw relaxed for client with status epilepticus; kept own fingers away from client's mouth.	___	___	___	_____
9. Padded side rails and headboard.	___	___	___	_____
10. Assisted client to position of comfort and safety in bed following seizure.	___	___	___	_____
11. Offered psychosocial support to client.	___	___	___	_____
12. Washed hands.	___	___	___	_____

	S	U	NP	Comments

EVALUATION

1. Assessed client for traumatic injury during and after seizure. ____ ____ ____ _____

2. Determined client's mental status after seizure. ____ ____ ____ _____

3. Observed client's color and respiratory status during and after seizure. ____ ____ ____ _____

4. Assessed for bowel and bladder incontinence. ____ ____ ____ _____

5. Asked client to verbalize feelings after seizure. ____ ____ ____ _____

6. Identified unexpected outcomes. ____ ____ ____ _____

RECORDING AND REPORTING

1. Recorded the timing of seizure activity and sequence of events, including presence of aura, level of consciousness, and client status following seizure. ____ ____ ____ _____

2. Reported seizure episode immediately to nurse in charge or physician. ____ ____ ____ _____

Student _____ Date _____

Instructor _____ Date _____

PERFORMANCE CHECKLIST 5-1   **REMOVING PAINFUL STIMULI**

	S	U	NP	Comments

ASSESSMENT

1. Assessed client's risk for pain or discomfort. ___ ___ ___ _____

2. Assessed physical, behavioral, and emotional signs and symptoms of acute pain or discomfort. ___ ___ ___ _____

3. Assessed physical, behavioral, and emotional signs and symptoms of chronic pain. ___ ___ ___ _____

4. Assessed characteristics of pain. ___ ___ ___ _____

5. Examined area of pain or discomfort. ___ ___ ___ _____

6. Checked physician's orders for position restrictions. ___ ___ ___ _____

NURSING DIAGNOSIS

1. Developed appropriate nursing diagnoses based on assessment data. ___ ___ ___ _____

PLANNING

1. Identified expected outcomes. ___ ___ ___ _____

2. Adjusted environmental factors affecting client's comfort and provided privacy. ___ ___ ___ _____

3. Explained to client that splinting with pillows and positioning can reduce pain. ___ ___ ___ _____

4. Explained steps to be taken to minimize pain stimuli. ___ ___ ___ _____

IMPLEMENTATION

1. Washed hands and applied gloves. ___ ___ ___ _____

2. Removed any painful stimuli: ___ ___ ___ _____

    a. Positioned client so that area of discomfort is accessible. ___ ___ ___ _____

    b. Kept client draped properly. ___ ___ ___ _____

    c. Removed soiled dressings. ___ ___ ___ _____

    d. Smoothed wrinkled bed linen. ___ ___ ___ _____

    e. Loosened constrictive bandages or devices. ___ ___ ___ _____

    f. Removed underlying tubes, wires, or equipment. ___ ___ ___ _____

	S	U	NP	Comments
3. Splinted area of discomfort:	___	___	___	_____
a. Explained purpose of splinting.	___	___	___	_____
b. Assisted client in placement of hands over painful body part.	___	___	___	_____
c. Assisted client to splint during coughing, deep breathing, and turning.	___	___	___	_____
4. Positioned client comfortably, using pillows to support body position.	___	___	___	_____
5. Removed and disposed of gloves and washed hands.	___	___	___	_____

EVALUATION

	S	U	NP	Comments
1. Evaluated client's level of comfort.	___	___	___	_____
2. Identified unexpected outcomes.	___	___	___	_____

RECORDING AND REPORTING

	S	U	NP	Comments
1. Reported changes in character of pain or client status to nurse in charge or physician.	___	___	___	_____
2. Recorded assessment, interventions, and client's response.	___	___	___	_____

Student _____   Date _____

Instructor _____   Date _____

PERFORMANCE CHECKLIST 5-2   **PATIENT-CONTROLLED ANALGESIA**

	S	U	NP	Comments
ASSESSMENT				
1. Assessed client's comfort level.	___	___	___	_____
2. Assessed client for physical, behavioral, and emotional signs and symptoms of pain or discomfort.	___	___	___	_____
3. Assessed characteristics of pain.	___	___	___	_____
4. Assessed environment for factors that contribute to pain.	___	___	___	_____
5. Inspected incision on postoperative client.	___	___	___	_____
6. Assessed patency of existing IV infusion line.	___	___	___	_____
7. Assessed venipuncture site for signs of infiltration or inflammation.	___	___	___	_____
8. Assessed response to previous pain management strategies.	___	___	___	_____
9. Checked physician's orders for dose and frequency of PCA-delivered medication.	___	___	___	_____
10. Determined client's history of drug allergies.	___	___	___	_____
NURSING DIAGNOSIS				
1. Developed appropriate nursing diagnoses based on assessment data.	___	___	___	_____
PLANNING				
1. Identified expected outcomes.	___	___	___	_____
2. Explained purpose and demonstrated functioning of PCA.	___	___	___	_____
3. Checked infusor and patient-control module for accurate labeling or evidence of leaking.	___	___	___	_____
4. Set the PCA pump to deliver prescribed dosage and lockout interval.	___	___	___	_____
5. Maintained client's privacy.	___	___	___	_____
6. Positioned client comfortably.	___	___	___	_____
IMPLEMENTATION				
1. Washed hands.	___	___	___	_____
2. Followed the "five rights" to ensure correct medication; checked client's ID.	___	___	___	_____

	S	U	NP	Comments

3. Applied gloves.

4. Attached 18- or 19-gauge needle to adapter of exit tubing of patient-control module.

5. Cleansed injection port of IV line with alcohol.

6. Inserted needle into injection port nearest IV site. For needleless system, connected exit tubing adapter to port nearest IV site.

7. Secured connection and immobilized PCA tubing with tape.

8. Administered loading dose of analgesia as prescribed.

9. Disposed of gloves and supplies.

10. Determined client's understanding of PCA system through return demonstration or repeating instructions.

11. Disposed of empty cassette or syringe per agency policy.

EVALUATION

1. Used pain rating scale to evaluate comfort level.

2. Observed for signs of adverse reactions.

3. Periodically checked infusion rate and site.

4. Had client demonstrate a dose delivery.

5. Assessed for unexpected outcomes.

RECORDING AND REPORTING

1. Recorded drug, dose, and time begun on medication record; included concentration and diluent.

2. Recorded periodic assessment of client status on PCA medication record.

3. Reported adverse reactions and pain status to appropriate staff.

Student _____ Date _____

Instructor _____ Date _____

PERFORMANCE CHECKLIST 5-3 **INTRASPINAL ANALGESIA**

	S	U	NP	Comments
ASSESSMENT				
1. Assessed client's comfort level and current medical condition.	___	___	___	_____
2. Assessed client for physical, behavioral, and emotional signs and symptoms of pain or discomfort.	___	___	___	_____
3. Assessed characteristics of pain.	___	___	___	_____
4. Assessed environmental factors.	___	___	___	_____
5. Assessed client's sedation level.	___	___	___	_____
6. Checked client's history of drug allergies.	___	___	___	_____
7. Checked rate, pattern, and depth of respirations.	___	___	___	_____
8. Checked blood pressure.	___	___	___	_____
9. Assessed mobility and motor and sensory function before getting client into or out of bed.	___	___	___	_____
10. Determined if epidural catheter was secured to client's skin.	___	___	___	_____
11. Assessed catheter insertion site for signs of inflammation or infection.	___	___	___	_____
12. Checked physician's order for medication and dosage.	___	___	___	_____
13. If continuous infusion, checked infusion pump for proper calibration and operation.	___	___	___	_____
14. If continuous infusion, checked patency of tubing.	___	___	___	_____
15. Kept patient IV intact for 24 hours after analgesia ended.	___	___	___	_____
NURSING DIAGNOSIS				
1. Developed appropriate nursing diagnoses based on assessment data.	___	___	___	_____
PLANNING				
1. Identified expected outcomes.	___	___	___	_____
2. Identified client ID.	___	___	___	_____
3. Explained purpose and function of epidural analgesia and expectations of client during procedure.	___	___	___	_____

	S	U	NP	Comments

4. Attached "epidural line" label for intermittent bolus or continuous infusion.   ___ ___ ___ _____

5. Used tubing without Y-port for continuous infusions.   ___ ___ ___ _____

6. Provided for client's privacy.   ___ ___ ___ _____

IMPLEMENTATION

1. Washed hands and applied gloves.   ___ ___ ___ _____

2. Followed the "five rights" in preparing medication.   ___ ___ ___ _____

3. Administered continuous infusion: ___ ___ ___ _____

   a. Attached medication container to infusion pump tubing and primed.   ___ ___ ___ _____

   b. Attached proximal end of tubing to pump and distal end to catheter.   ___ ___ ___ _____

   c. Checked pump for calibration and operation.   ___ ___ ___ _____

4. Removed and disposed of gloves.   ___ ___ ___ _____

5. Washed hands.   ___ ___ ___ _____

EVALUATION

1. Evaluated comfort level and compared with original assessment data.   ___ ___ ___ _____

2. Observed for signs of adverse reactions to epidurally administered narcotic.   ___ ___ ___ _____

3. Assessed respiratory status.   ___ ___ ___ _____

4. Monitored blood pressure and pulse.   ___ ___ ___ _____

5. Monitored intake and output (I&O).   ___ ___ ___ _____

6. Observed for pruritus.   ___ ___ ___ _____

7. Observed for nausea and vomiting.   ___ ___ ___ _____

8. Checked insertion site for clear or bloody drainage. Listened for complaints of headache.   ___ ___ ___ _____

9. Monitored temperature. Observed for signs of inflammation.   ___ ___ ___ _____

10. Evaluated for paresthesias.   ___ ___ ___ _____

11. Identified unexpected outcomes.   ___ ___ ___ _____

RECORDING AND REPORTING

1. Recorded drug, dose, and time given (if injection) or time begun and ended (if infusion). Specified concentration and diluent.   ___ ___ ___ _____

2. Recorded any supplemental analgesic requirements.   ___ ___ ___ _____

	S	U	NP	Comments
3. If continuous infusion, obtained and recorded pump settings and usage at required time intervals.	——	——	——	_____
4. Recorded regular periodic assessment of client's status.	——	——	——	_____
5. Reported any adverse reactions or complications to physician.	——	——	——	_____

Student _____ Date _____

Instructor _____ Date _____

PERFORMANCE CHECKLIST 5-4 **NONPHARMACOLOGIC AIDS TO PROMOTE COMFORT**

	S	U	NP	Comments
ASSESSMENT				
1. Had client identify level of pain or comfort.	—	—	—	_____
2. Assessed client for physiologic, behavioral, and emotional signs and symptoms of pain or discomfort.	—	—	—	_____
3. Assessed characteristics of client's pain.	—	—	—	_____
4. Examined site of client's pain.	—	—	—	_____
5. Assessed client's willingness to participate in pain-relief program.	—	—	—	_____
6. Assessed potential types of distraction activities.	—	—	—	_____
7. Assessed client's language level and identified terms to be used.	—	—	—	_____
NURSING DIAGNOSIS				
1. Developed appropriate nursing diagnoses based on assessment data.	—	—	—	_____
PLANNING				
1. Identified expected outcomes.	—	—	—	_____
2. Explained purpose of technique and expectations of client during procedure.	—	—	—	_____
3. Planned to explain procedures in advance.	—	—	—	_____
4. Planned to perform technique before or after client's rest period.	—	—	—	_____
5. Assisted client to bathroom, if needed.	—	—	—	_____
6. Prepared environment conducive to relaxation.	—	—	—	_____
7. Closed room curtains or door for privacy.	—	—	—	_____
8. Assisted client to comfortable position.	—	—	—	_____
IMPLEMENTATION				
Anticipatory Guidance				
1. Explained procedure to client.	—	—	—	_____
2. Explained anticipated length of time.	—	—	—	_____
3. Described sensory experiences connected with procedural steps.	—	—	—	_____

	S	U	NP	Comments

4. Guided client verbally through procedure.

5. Assisted client in returning to comfortable position.

Massage

1. Washed hands.

2. Adjusted bed to high position and lowered side rail.

3. Assisted client to comfortable position, such as prone or side-lying.

4. Exposed only area to be massaged.

5. Warmed lotion in hands.

6. Used techniques of effleurage, petrissage, and friction on muscle groups.

7. Encouraged client to breathe deeply and relax during massage.

8. Massaged muscles at base of client's head.

9. Massaged client's scalp and temples.

10. Massaged client's hands and arms.

11. Placed client in prone position, unless contraindicated.

12. Massaged client's neck, as appropriate.

13. Massaged client's back, keeping hands in contact with skin.

14. Massaged client's feet, as appropriate, with client in supine position.

15. Told client when massage completed.

16. Completed procedure by having client breathe deeply and slowly resume activity.

17. Removed excess lotion from client's body.

18. Washed hands.

Relaxation

1. Instructed client to breathe slowly and deeply.

2. Instructed client to close eyes, if desired.

3. Provided verbal clues for client to follow during muscle relaxation procedure.

4. Instructed client on alternating tightening and relaxation of muscle groups.

	S	U	NP	Comments

5. Asked client to relax and breathe deeply after each muscle group completed. ___ ___ ___ _____

6. Had client repeat each step two times. ___ ___ ___ _____

7. Explained expected sensations. ___ ___ ___ _____

8. Instructed client to breathe deeply and move around slowly after a few minutes of rest after completion of exercise. ___ ___ ___ _____

Guided Imagery

1. Directed client through exercise. ___ ___ ___ _____

2. Directed client imagery with suggestions for pleasant and relaxing sensory experiences. ___ ___ ___ _____

3. On completion, instructed client to breathe deeply, open eyes, and move around slowly. ___ ___ ___ _____

4. Provided uninterrupted practice time for client. ___ ___ ___ _____

Distraction

1. Directed client's attention from pain. ___ ___ ___ _____

2. Asked client to close eyes or focus on a single object. ___ ___ ___ _____

3. Instructed/guided client in slow rhythmic breathing. ___ ___ ___ _____

4. Continued skill with method of choice (e.g., music, conversation). ___ ___ ___ _____

EVALUATION

1. Determined client's physiologic and behavioral response to technique. ___ ___ ___ _____

2. Used pain rating scale to evaluate client's comfort level. ___ ___ ___ _____

3. Observed client's performance of techniques. ___ ___ ___ _____

4. Identified unexpected outcomes. ___ ___ ___ _____

REPORTING AND RECORDING

1. Recorded procedure, technique, preparation given to client, and client's response. ___ ___ ___ _____

2. Recorded alterations in client's condition (e.g., vital signs). ___ ___ ___ _____

3. Reported client's response to techniques to nurse in charge. ___ ___ ___ _____

4. Reported any unusual responses to techniques. ___ ___ ___ _____

Student _____   Date _____

Instructor _____   Date _____

PERFORMANCE CHECKLIST 6-1 **BATHING A CLIENT**

	S	U	NP	Comments
ASSESSMENT				
1. Determined client's ability to participate in bathing.	—	—	—	_____
2. Determined client's preferences for bathing practices.	—	—	—	_____
3. Noted client's awareness of existing skin problems.	—	—	—	_____
4. Identified risks for skin impairment.	—	—	—	_____
5. Assessed client's knowledge of skin hygiene.	—	—	—	_____
6. Checked physician's order for therapeutic bath.	—	—	—	_____
7. Reviewed restrictions affecting client's movement or positioning during bath.	—	—	—	_____
NURSING DIAGNOSIS				
1. Developed appropriate nursing diagnoses based on assessment data.	—	—	—	_____
PLANNING				
1. Identified expected outcomes.	—	—	—	_____
2. Explained procedure to client and asked for client's suggestions.	—	—	—	_____
3. Adjusted room temperature and ventilation for client's comfort and provided for client's privacy during bath.	—	—	—	_____
4. Prepared necessary equipment and supplies.	—	—	—	_____
IMPLEMENTATION				
Complete or Partial Bed Bath				
1. Offered bedpan or urinal before bath.	—	—	—	_____
2. Washed hands and applied gloves if needed.	—	—	—	_____
3. Lowered side rail, assisted client in assuming comfortable position, and positioned client to avoid strain on nurse.	—	—	—	_____
4. Used bath blanket properly while removing top linens of bed.	—	—	—	_____
5. Disposed of soiled linen correctly.	—	—	—	_____
6. Removed client's gown correctly.	—	—	—	_____

	S	U	NP	Comments

7. Raised side rail and filled washbasin two-thirds full; checked temperature of bathwater and client's tolerance. Warmed bath lotion, if desired.   ____ ____ ____ _____

8. Removed pillow if allowed and raised head of bed; placed a towel under client's head and a towel over client's chest.   ____ ____ ____ _____

9. Folded washcloth into mitt.   ____ ____ ____ _____

10. Washed and dried client's eyes correctly (without using soap).   ____ ____ ____ _____

11. Washed, rinsed, and dried client's forehead, cheeks, nose, neck, and ears, using or avoiding soap as appropriate.   ____ ____ ____ _____

12. Removed bath blanket from client's far arm and placed bath towel under arm.   ____ ____ ____ _____

13. Bathed client's far arm and axilla.   ____ ____ ____ _____

14. Rinsed and dried arm and axilla thoroughly; provided deodorant (or talcum powder if used by client).   ____ ____ ____ _____

15. Followed procedure for soaking and drying client's hand.   ____ ____ ____ _____

16. Repeated Steps 12-15 for other arm.   ____ ____ ____ _____

17. Checked temperature of bathwater and changed water if necessary.   ____ ____ ____ _____

18. Placed bath towel and blanket correctly for washing client's chest; washed, rinsed, and dried chest correctly.   ____ ____ ____ _____

19. Placed bath towel and blanket correctly for washing client's abdomen.   ____ ____ ____ _____

20. Washed, rinsed, and dried abdomen correctly.   ____ ____ ____ _____

21. Applied clothing if appropriate to maintain client's warmth and comfort.   ____ ____ ____ _____

22. Draped client correctly for washing far leg.   ____ ____ ____ _____

23. Followed procedure for placing towel under client's leg and asked client to hold foot still while positioning basin near foot.   ____ ____ ____ _____

24. Placed client's foot in basin and allowed it to soak (if appropriate) while washing leg.   ____ ____ ____ _____

25. Washed client's leg from ankle to knee and from knee to thigh. Dried well.   ____ ____ ____ _____

26. Washed and dried foot correctly. Provided nail care.   ____ ____ ____ _____

	S	U	NP	Comments

27. Raised side rail and moved to other side of bed. Repeated Steps 22-26 for other leg and foot.   —— —— —— _____

28. Covered client with bath blanket and changed bathwater.   —— —— —— _____

29. Positioned client correctly for bathing back and buttocks.   —— —— —— _____

30. Kept client properly draped for bathing back and buttocks.   —— —— —— _____

31. Washed, rinsed, and dried client's back from neck to buttocks.   —— —— —— _____

32. Changed bathwater and washcloth. Applied gloves, if not done before.   —— —— —— _____

33. Positioned and draped client in correct position for washing genitalia; washed, rinsed, and dried perineum or allowed client to do so.   —— —— —— _____

34. Disposed of gloves.   —— —— —— _____

35. Applied moisturizing lotion to skin.   —— —— —— _____

36. Assisted client in dressing; combed client's hair.   —— —— —— _____

37. Made client's bed.   —— —— —— _____

38. Disposed of soiled linen properly; cleaned and replaced bathing equipment; replaced call light and personal possessions.   —— —— —— _____

39. Washed hands.   —— —— —— _____

Tub Bath or Shower

1. Considered client's condition and reviewed medical orders.   —— —— —— _____

2. Scheduled use of shower or tub.   —— —— —— _____

3. Cleaned tub or shower according to agency policy; provided rubber bath mat or disposable mat to prevent slipping.   —— —— —— _____

4. Arranged all hygienic aids, toilet items, and linen within reach of client.   —— —— —— _____

5. Assisted client into tub or shower.   —— —— —— _____

6. Instructed client on use of call signal.   —— —— —— _____

7. Placed "Occupied" sign on bathroom door.   —— —— —— _____

8. Filled tub halfway, adjusted water temperature, and instructed client on use of faucets. If client was taking a shower, turned shower on and adjusted water temperature before client entered shower stall. Used shower seat or chair, if necessary.   —— —— —— _____

	S	U	NP	Comments

9. Instructed client on use of safety bars and cautioned client against use of bath oil in tub water.   ___ ___ ___ _____

10. Cautioned client against remaining in tub for more than 20 minutes and checked on client every 5 minutes.   ___ ___ ___ _____

11. Returned to bathroom when client signaled, and knocked before entering.   ___ ___ ___ _____

12. Drained water from tub; placed bath towel over client's shoulders; assisted client in getting out of tub and with drying.   ___ ___ ___ _____

13. Assisted client with dressing.   ___ ___ ___ _____

14. Assisted client in returning to room.   ___ ___ ___ _____

15. Prepared bathroom for next use.   ___ ___ ___ _____

16. Washed hands.   ___ ___ ___ _____

EVALUATION

1. Assessed skin for signs of breakdown or irritation.   ___ ___ ___ _____

2. Assessed extent of range of motion (ROM) during bath.   ___ ___ ___ _____

3. Determined client's comfort and level of fatigue.   ___ ___ ___ _____

4. Assessed vital signs if necessary.   ___ ___ ___ _____

5. Assessed client's knowledge of proper hygiene techniques.   ___ ___ ___ _____

6. Identified unexpected outcomes.   ___ ___ ___ _____

RECORDING AND REPORTING

1. Recorded bath on flowsheet and noted level of assistance required.   ___ ___ ___ _____

2. Recorded condition of skin and significant findings.   ___ ___ ___ _____

3. Reported evidence of alterations in skin integrity to nurse in charge or physician.   ___ ___ ___ _____

Student _____ Date _____

Instructor _____ Date _____

PERFORMANCE CHECKLIST 6-2 **PROVIDING PERINEAL CARE**

	S	U	NP	Comments
ASSESSMENT				
1. Identified client's risk for developing infection of genitalia, urinary tract, or reproductive tract.	___	___	___	_____
2. Assessed client's ability to perform own perineal care.	___	___	___	_____
3. Assessed condition of client's genitalia.	___	___	___	_____
4. Assessed client's knowledge of importance of perineal hygiene.	___	___	___	_____
NURSING DIAGNOSIS				
1. Developed appropriate nursing diagnoses based on assessment data.	___	___	___	_____
PLANNING				
1. Identified expected outcomes.	___	___	___	_____
2. Explained procedure and its purpose to client.	___	___	___	_____
3. Prepared necessary equipment and supplies.	___	___	___	_____
IMPLEMENTATION				
1. Provided for client's privacy during perineal care; assembled supplies at bedside.	___	___	___	_____
2. Raised client's bed to comfortable working position; lowered side rail and assisted client in assuming proper position.	___	___	___	_____
3. Applied disposable gloves.	___	___	___	_____
4. Removed fecal material, if present. Cleansed, rinsed, and dried buttocks and anus thoroughly.	___	___	___	_____
5. Changed soiled gloves.	___	___	___	_____
6. Folded top bed linen down and raised client's gown.	___	___	___	_____
7. Applied "diamond" drape correctly.	___	___	___	_____
8. Raised side rail. Filled washbasin with water and tested temperature.	___	___	___	_____
9. Placed washbasin and tissue on overbed table. Placed washcloths in basin.	___	___	___	_____
10. Provided perineal care.	___	___	___	_____

	S	U	NP	Comments

Female Perineal Care

a. Lowered side rail and positioned client for full exposure of genitalia.   ___ ___ ___ _____

b. Uncovered client's genitalia. Washed and dried client's upper thighs.   ___ ___ ___ _____

c. Retracted labia and correctly cleansed, rinsed, and dried skinfolds.   ___ ___ ___ _____

d. Separated labia to expose urethral meatus and vaginal orifice and correctly cleaned area.   ___ ___ ___ _____

e. Poured warm water over perineal area if client was on bedpan and dried perineal area thoroughly.   ___ ___ ___ _____

f. Covered client with bath blanket and positioned comfortably.   ___ ___ ___ _____

Male Perineal Care

a. Lowered side rail. Noted any mobility restrictions.   ___ ___ ___ _____

b. Uncovered client's perineum. Washed and dried client's upper thighs.   ___ ___ ___ _____

c. Positioned towel under penis; gently grasped shaft of penis; retracted foreskin if client uncircumcised.   ___ ___ ___ _____

d. Cleansed, rinsed, and dried glans penis correctly. Deferred procedure if client had an erection.   ___ ___ ___ _____

e. Returned foreskin to natural position after cleansing.   ___ ___ ___ _____

f. Gently washed, rinsed, and dried shaft of penis on all surfaces; rinsed and dried penis thoroughly; instructed client to abduct legs for washing of scrotum.   ___ ___ ___ _____

g. Gently washed, rinsed, and dried scrotum, including underlying skinfolds.   ___ ___ ___ _____

h. Covered perineum and positioned client on side.   ___ ___ ___ _____

11. Applied thin layer of skin barrier over anal and perineal area if client has had bladder or bowel incontinence.   ___ ___ ___ _____

12. Removed and disposed of gloves.   ___ ___ ___ _____

13. Assisted client to comfortable position and returned covers.   ___ ___ ___ _____

14. Removed bath blanket and disposed of soiled linen. Returned unused equipment.   ___ ___ ___ _____

	S	U	NP	Comments

EVALUATION

1. Inspected surface of external genitalia and surrounding skin after cleansing.

2. Assessed client's level of comfort and cleanliness.

3. Evaluated client's ability to perform hygiene.

4. Identified unexpected outcomes.

RECORDING AND REPORTING

1. Recorded procedure and presence of any abnormal findings.

2. Recorded appearance of suture line, if present.

3. Reported any break in suture line or presence of abnormalities to nurse in charge or physician.

Student _____   Date _____

Instructor _____   Date _____

PERFORMANCE CHECKLIST 6-3 **ORAL CARE PART I—BRUSHING TEETH**

	S	U	NP	Comments

ASSESSMENT

1. Washed hands. Applied disposable gloves.   ___ ___ ___ _____

2. Performed physical assessment of oral cavity.   ___ ___ ___ _____

3. Identified presence of common oral problems.   ___ ___ ___ _____

4. Removed gloves and washed hands.   ___ ___ ___ _____

5. Assessed client's risk for oral hygiene problems.   ___ ___ ___ _____

6. Determined client's oral hygiene practices.   ___ ___ ___ _____

7. Assessed client's ability to grasp and manipulate toothbrush.   ___ ___ ___ _____

NURSING DIAGNOSIS

1. Developed appropriate nursing diagnoses based on assessment data.   ___ ___ ___ _____

PLANNING

1. Identified expected outcomes.   ___ ___ ___ _____

2. Prepared equipment at bedside.   ___ ___ ___ _____

3. Explained procedure to client and discussed preferences.   ___ ___ ___ _____

IMPLEMENTATION

1. Arranged equipment on paper towels on bedside table.   ___ ___ ___ _____

2. Raised bed to comfortable working position, lowered side rail, positioned client on side near nurse in semi-Fowler's position to avoid aspiration.   ___ ___ ___ _____

3. Placed towel over client's chest to prevent soiling gown and bed linen.   ___ ___ ___ _____

4. Applied gloves.   ___ ___ ___ _____

5. Applied toothpaste to brush and moistened paste.   ___ ___ ___ _____

6. Held or had client hold toothbrush at 45-degree angle to gum line and used short strokes to brush tooth surfaces from gum to crown; held brush parallel to teeth to clean biting surfaces; brushed sides of teeth, moving bristles back and forth.   ___ ___ ___ _____

	S	U	NP	Comments

7. Held or had client hold brush at 45-degree angle and lightly brushed tongue surface without stimulating gag reflex. ___ ___ ___ _____

8. Provided water for client to rinse mouth thoroughly. ___ ___ ___ _____

9. Offered mouthwash for gargling and rinsing. ___ ___ ___ _____

10. Assisted in wiping client's mouth. ___ ___ ___ _____

11. Allowed client to floss. ___ ___ ___ _____

12. Allowed client to rinse mouth thoroughly with tepid water after flossing. ___ ___ ___ _____

13. Repositioned client comfortably after procedure. ___ ___ ___ _____

14. Disposed of equipment and soiled linen properly. ___ ___ ___ _____

15. Washed hands. ___ ___ ___ _____

EVALUATION

1. Assessed client's comfort level. ___ ___ ___ _____

2. Applied gloves and inspected condition of oral cavity. ___ ___ ___ _____

3. Asked client to describe proper hygiene techniques. ___ ___ ___ _____

4. Observed client brushing. ___ ___ ___ _____

5. Identified unexpected outcomes. ___ ___ ___ _____

RECORDING AND REPORTING

1. Recorded procedure on flowsheet. Included condition of oral cavity. ___ ___ ___ _____

2. Reported any unusual findings to nurse in charge or physician. ___ ___ ___ _____

Student _____   Date _____

Instructor _____   Date _____

PERFORMANCE CHECKLIST 6-3 **ORAL CARE PART II—CLEANING DENTURES**

	S	U	NP	Comments

ASSESSMENT

1. Assessed condition of gums, mucosa, and surfaces of dentures.

2. Determined if dentures are loose-fitting.

3. Assessed type of denture cleaner client uses.

4. Assessed home routines for denture care.

NURSING DIAGNOSIS

1. Developed appropriate nursing diagnoses based on assessment data.

PLANNING

1. Identified expected outcomes.

2. Explained procedure to client.

IMPLEMENTATION

1. Washed hands.

2. Arranged supplies on bedside table or near sink.

3. Added tepid water to emesis basin or sink lined with washcloth.

4. Applied disposable gloves.

5. Asked client to remove dentures. If client unable to remove dentures, removed dentures by grasping upper denture at front with thumb and index finger wrapped in gauze and pulling downward; lifted lower denture and rotated one side downward; placed dentures in emesis basin or sink.

6. Thoroughly brushed all denture surfaces with denture or regular toothbrush and dentifrice.

7. Thoroughly rinsed dentures with tepid water.

8. Stored dentures securely in denture cup containing tepid water.

9. Emptied emesis basin and added fresh water; used soft toothbrush to brush client's gums, palate, and tongue.

10. Had client rinse mouth thoroughly.

	S	U	NP	Comments
11. Reinserted dentures according to client's preferences (moistened denture before reinsertion); checked to see if dentures were sealed in place.	___	___	___	_____
12. Disposed of gloves. Cleaned and stored supplies after procedure. Washed hands.	___	___	___	_____

EVALUATION

	S	U	NP	Comments
1. Questioned client about comfort of dentures.	___	___	___	_____
2. Inspected condition of oral cavity.	___	___	___	_____
3. Asked client to explain steps in denture care.	___	___	___	_____
4. Identified unexpected outcomes.	___	___	___	_____

Student _____ Date _____

Instructor _____ Date _____

PERFORMANCE CHECKLIST 6-4 **PERFORMING MOUTH CARE FOR THE UNCONSCIOUS OR DEBILITATED CLIENT**

	S	U	NP	Comments
ASSESSMENT				
1. Washed hands. Applied disposable gloves.	___	___	___	_____
2. Tested client for presence of gag reflex.	___	___	___	_____
3. Conducted physical assessment of oral cavity.	___	___	___	_____
4. Removed gloves. Washed hands.	___	___	___	_____
5. Assessed client's risk for oral hygiene problems.	___	___	___	_____
NURSING DIAGNOSIS				
1. Developed appropriate nursing diagnoses based on assessment data.	___	___	___	_____
PLANNING				
1. Identified expected outcomes.	___	___	___	_____
2. Positioned client on side with head turned toward dependent side and head of bed lowered. Raised side rail.	___	___	___	_____
3. Explained procedure to client.	___	___	___	_____
IMPLEMENTATION				
1. Washed hands and applied disposable gloves.	___	___	___	_____
2. Properly arranged equipment and turned on suction device.	___	___	___	_____
3. Closed curtain or room door for privacy.	___	___	___	_____
4. Raised bed and lowered side rail to have easy access to client; raised side rail when client was unattended.	___	___	___	_____
5. Positioned client on side of bed near you; kept client positioned on side with head turned toward mattress to prevent aspiration.	___	___	___	_____
6. Placed towel under client's face and positioned emesis basin under client's chin.	___	___	___	_____
7. Separated client's upper and lower teeth correctly with tongue blade.	___	___	___	_____

	S	U	NP	Comments
8. Cleaned client's teeth and mucosa using brush or padded tongue blade moistened in water and peroxide; thoroughly swabbed areas of accumulated crusts or secretions; thoroughly rinsed oral cavity.	___	___	___	_____
9. Suctioned secretions as necessary.	___	___	___	_____
10. Applied water-soluble jelly to lips.	___	___	___	_____
11. Informed client that procedure was completed.	___	___	___	_____
12. Raised side rail. Removed gloves and disposed of them in proper receptacle.	___	___	___	_____
13. Repositioned client safely and comfortably after procedure.	___	___	___	_____
14. Disposed of equipment and soiled linen properly.	___	___	___	_____
15. Washed hands.	___	___	___	_____

EVALUATION

1. Applied gloves and inspected client's oral cavity.	___	___	___	_____
2. Assessed client's level of comfort.	___	___	___	_____
3. Assessed client's respirations on an ongoing basis.	___	___	___	_____
4. Identified unexpected outcomes.	___	___	___	_____

RECORDING AND REPORTING

1. Recorded procedure including description of the condition of the oral cavity.	___	___	___	_____
2. Reported any unusual findings to nurse in charge or physician.	___	___	___	_____

Student _____   Date _____

Instructor _____   Date _____

PERFORMANCE CHECKLIST 6-5 **HAIR CARE PART I—SHAMPOOING THE HAIR OF A BEDRIDDEN CLIENT**

	S	U	NP	Comments
ASSESSMENT				
1. Identified any factors that contraindicated shampooing or restricted positioning.	___	___	___	_____
2. Assessed client's hair and scalp.	___	___	___	_____
NURSING DIAGNOSIS				
1. Developed appropriate nursing diagnoses based on assessment data.	___	___	___	_____
PLANNING				
1. Identified expected outcomes.	___	___	___	_____
2. Explained procedure to client.	___	___	___	_____
IMPLEMENTATION				
1. Washed hands.	___	___	___	_____
2. Arranged equipment within easy reach and lowered side rail.	___	___	___	_____
3. Protected bed linen with waterproof pad; properly positioned client supine with shampoo trough under head and washbasin at end of trough.	___	___	___	_____
4. Placed rolled towel under client's neck; draped client's shoulders with towel.	___	___	___	_____
5. Brushed and combed client's hair before shampooing.	___	___	___	_____
6. Checked water temperature.	___	___	___	_____
7. Provided client with towel to cover eyes during shampooing.	___	___	___	_____
8. Rinsed hair thoroughly before shampooing.	___	___	___	_____
9. Lathered hair thoroughly; worked from hairline toward back of neck to sides of head; used fingertips to massage scalp.	___	___	___	_____
10. Rinsed hair thoroughly.	___	___	___	_____
11. Repeated Steps 8-10, if needed.	___	___	___	_____
12. Applied conditioner or cream rinse as client desired.	___	___	___	_____

	S	U	NP	Comments
13. Used bath towel to wrap client's head and dried moisture from around eyes, face, and neck.	___	___	___	_____
14. Dried hair thoroughly.	___	___	___	_____
15. Combed hair gently to remove tangles and completed drying with dryer if desired.	___	___	___	_____
16. Applied oil or conditioner if desired.	___	___	___	_____
17. Brushed and styled hair with client in comfortable position.	___	___	___	_____
18. Returned equipment to its proper place, disposed of soiled linen, and washed hands.	___	___	___	_____

EVALUATION

1. Asked client how hair felt after shampooing.	___	___	___	_____
2. Inspected condition of hair.	___	___	___	_____
3. Identified unexpected outcomes.	___	___	___	_____

RECORDING AND REPORTING

1. Recorded pertinent findings related to condition of hair or scalp.	___	___	___	_____

Student _____   Date _____

Instructor _____   Date _____

PERFORMANCE CHECKLIST 6-5 **HAIR CARE PART II—SHAVING A CLIENT**

	S	U	NP	Comments

ASSESSMENT

1. Determined if client has a bleeding tendency.

2. Assessed client's ability to manipulate razor.

3. Assessed client's preferences for hygiene products to use to shave.

NURSING DIAGNOSIS

1. Developed appropriate nursing diagnoses based on assessment data.

PLANNING

1. Identified expected outcomes.

2. Prepared client by instructing him to indicate if the shave became uncomfortable, and asked if there were special steps to follow while shaving.

IMPLEMENTATION
Disposable Razor

1. Arranged supplies at bedside table and adjusted lighting.

2. Assisted client to sitting or supine position with head of bed elevated.

3. Placed towel over client's chest and around shoulders.

4. Adjusted water temperature to comfortable level or as client preferred.

5. Applied warm, damp cloth to client's face to soften beard.

6. Applied shaving cream or soap to client's face. Applied gloves, if indicated.

7. Shaved one side of face at a time, using nondominant hand to pull skin taut; used short strokes in same direction as hair grows.

8. Removed cream from blade by dipping razor in water.

9. Rinsed client's face with warm, moist washcloth.

10. Dried face and applied aftershave if client desired.

	S	U	NP	Comments
11. Assisted client to comfortable position.	___	___	___	_____
12. Returned supplies to proper place, discarded soiled linen properly, removed gloves (if worn), and washed hands.	___	___	___	_____

Electric Razor

1. Performed Steps 1-3 for Disposable Razor procedure.	___	___	___	_____
2. Applied skin conditioner or preshave lotion.	___	___	___	_____
3. Turned razor on and shaved one side of face at a time, holding skin taut and using gentle downward strokes.	___	___	___	_____
4. Applied aftershave if client requested.	___	___	___	_____
5. Performed Steps 11 and 12 for Disposable Razor procedure.	___	___	___	_____

Mustache and Beard Care

1. Performed Steps 1-3 for Disposable Razor procedure.	___	___	___	_____
2. Gently combed mustache or beard if necessary.	___	___	___	_____
3. Allowed client to use mirror to direct areas to trim with scissors.	___	___	___	_____

EVALUATION

1. Inspected condition of shaved area and skin underneath beard or mustache.	___	___	___	_____
2. Assessed client's level of comfort and satisfaction with degree of participation.	___	___	___	_____
3. Identified unexpected outcomes.	___	___	___	_____

Student _____   Date _____

Instructor _____   Date _____

PERFORMANCE CHECKLIST 6-6 **PERFORMING NAIL AND FOOT CARE**

	S	U	NP	Comments
ASSESSMENT				
1. Inspected all surfaces of hands, feet, and nails.	___	___	___	_____
2. Assessed circulatory status of toes, feet, and fingers.	___	___	___	_____
3. Observed client's gait and determined relationship to local foot or nail problems.	___	___	___	_____
4. Assessed female client's use of nail polish or polish removal.	___	___	___	_____
5. Assessed type of footwear worn by client.	___	___	___	_____
6. Identified client's risk for foot or nail problems.	___	___	___	_____
7. Assessed client's use of home remedies for foot problems.	___	___	___	_____
8. Assessed client's ability to perform foot and nail care.	___	___	___	_____
9. Assessed client's knowledge of foot and nail care practices.	___	___	___	_____
NURSING DIAGNOSIS				
1. Developed appropriate nursing diagnoses based on assessment data.	___	___	___	_____
PLANNING				
1. Identified expected outcomes.	___	___	___	_____
2. Explained procedure to client.	___	___	___	_____
3. Obtained physician's order to cut nails, if required by agency policy.	___	___	___	_____
IMPLEMENTATION				
1. Washed hands and arranged supplies on overbed table.	___	___	___	_____
2. Closed room door or curtain for privacy.	___	___	___	_____
3. Assisted client to chair (when possible); placed bath mat under client's feet.	___	___	___	_____
4. Prepared washbasin with water; tested water temperature.	___	___	___	_____
5. Placed washbasin on bath mat on floor and helped client place feet in basin; put call light within reach.	___	___	___	_____

	S	U	NP	Comments

6. Adjusted overbed table to low position and placed it over client's lap. ___ ___ ___ _____

7. Filled emesis basin with water and tested temperature; placed emesis basin on overbed table. ___ ___ ___ _____

8. Instructed client to position fingertips in basin, with arms in comfortable position. ___ ___ ___ _____

9. Had client soak fingers and feet for approximately 10-20 minutes and rewarmed water as needed during soaking. ___ ___ ___ _____

10. Used orange stick gently to clean debris from under fingernails while fingers were immersed; removed emesis basin and dried fingers thoroughly. ___ ___ ___ _____

11. Clipped fingernails straight across and shaped with file or emery board; avoided cutting nails at nail bed. Filed nails of client with circulatory problems. ___ ___ ___ _____

12. Used orange stick to gently push back cuticles. ___ ___ ___ _____

13. Moved overbed table away from client. ___ ___ ___ _____

14. Applied disposable gloves before giving foot care; scrubbed calluses of feet with washcloth. ___ ___ ___ _____

15. Cleaned under toenails gently with orange stick; dried feet thoroughly. ___ ___ ___ _____

16. Trimmed toenails using procedures in Steps 11 and 12; avoided filing corners of toenails. ___ ___ ___ _____

17. Applied lotion to feet and hands and assisted client back to bed and into comfortable position. ___ ___ ___ _____

18. Properly disposed of gloves and soiled linen, cleaned and returned equipment and supplies to proper place, washed hands. ___ ___ ___ _____

EVALUATION

1. Inspected nails and skin surfaces after soaking. ___ ___ ___ _____

2. Asked client to explain or demonstrate nail care. ___ ___ ___ _____

3. Assessed client's walk after nail care. ___ ___ ___ _____

4. Identified unexpected outcomes. ___ ___ ___ _____

RECORDING AND REPORTING

1. Recorded procedure and observations related to condition of nails and feet. ___ ___ ___ _____

2. Reported presence of foot ulcers or other breaks in skin to nurse in charge or physician. ___ ___ ___ _____

Student _La Shaun Harriot_   Date _9-16-04_

Instructor _____   Date _____

PERFORMANCE CHECKLIST 6-7   CARE OF THE CLIENT'S ENVIRONMENT PART I— UNOCCUPIED BED

	S	U	NP	Comments

ASSESSMENT

1. Verified client's activity orders and assessed client's ability to get out of bed.

2. Assessed potential for client incontinence or excess drainage on linen.

3. Determined if client should assume any position precautions while out of bed.

NURSING DIAGNOSIS

1. Developed appropriate nursing diagnoses.

PLANNING

1. Identified expected outcomes.

2. Determined best time to change linens. Explained procedure to client; assisted client to chair if needed.

IMPLEMENTATION

1. Washed hands and donned gloves, if needed.

2. Assembled all necessary equipment with linen stacked in order of use (top to bottom). Removed furniture and equipment from around bed before making it.

3. Lowered side rails and removed call light from bed; adjusted bed to a comfortable working height position.

4. Loosened all soiled linen from under mattress.

5. Removed bedspread and blanket separately and discarded properly; did not shake or allow linen to come in contact with uniform.

6. When reusing blanket or spread, folded each correctly into square.

7. Removed soiled pillowcases correctly by slipping each pillow out from case.

8. Checked each piece of soiled linen separately before discarding.

9. Repositioned mattress toward head of bed; cleaned any moisture off mattress with appropriate disinfectant.

	S	U	NP	Comments

10. Stood at side of bed where linen is placed, and spread mattress pad over mattress; smoothed out all wrinkles on pad.

11. Applied all bottom linen on one side before moving to opposite side.

12. Made mitered corner in top corner of bottom sheet or smoothed out fitted sheet.

13. Tucked bottom sheet tightly under mattress; applied drawsheet to bed correctly; tucked excess edge of drawsheet under mattress, keeping palms down.

14. Moved to opposite side of bed.

15. Spread fanfolded bottom sheet smoothly over bed.

16. Mitered top corner of bottom sheet.

17. Used good body mechanics by keeping back straight while tucking linen tightly under mattress. Frequently observed client for tolerance to sitting in chair.

18. Smoothed folded drawsheet over bottom sheet and tucked tightly.

19. Applied waterproof pads according to client's need.

20. Moved to side of bed where linen was placed and applied all top linen to one side of bed at a time.

21. Correctly made horizontal toe pleat in top sheet.

22. Tucked in remaining portion of top sheet under foot of mattress (optional).

23. Placed blanket correctly on bed.

24. Placed bedspread over bed according to Step 8.

25. Made cuff out of top edge of sheet, blanket, and bedspread.

26. Correctly tucked bottom linen together under mattress at foot of bed.

27. Made a modified mitered corner at bottom edge of mattress.

28. Moved to opposite side of bed to complete application of top linen.

29. Correctly applied a clean pillowcase over pillow.

	S	U	NP	Comments

30. Placed pillow at center of head of bed; placed call light within client's reach. Returned bed to low comfortable height. ____ ____ ____ _____

31. Folded back top linen to side or fanfolded linen down to bottom third of bed. ____ ____ ____ _____

32. Rearranged furniture around bedside and placed client's personal items within easy reach. ____ ____ ____ _____

33. Discarded dirty linen properly. Removed gloves and washed hands. ____ ____ ____ _____

EVALUATION

1. Assessed client's tolerance to sitting in chair. ____ ____ ____ _____

2. Assessed client's level of comfort and condition of skin upon return to bed. ____ ____ ____ _____

3. Identified unexpected outcomes. ____ ____ ____ _____

Student _____   Date _____

Instructor _____   Date _____

PERFORMANCE CHECKLIST 6-7 **CARE OF THE CLIENT'S ENVIRONMENT PART II—**
OCCUPIED BED

	S	U	NP	Comments

ASSESSMENT
1. Determined need to apply waterproof pads.

2. Assessed restrictions affecting client's positioning and movement during bed making.

NURSING DIAGNOSIS
1. Developed appropriate nursing diagnoses.

PLANNING
1. Identified expected outcomes.

2. Explained procedure to client.

IMPLEMENTATION
1. Washed hands and donned gloves, if needed.

2. Assembled equipment with linen stacked in order of use (top to bottom). Removed unnecessary equipment.

3. Closed curtain or room door for client's privacy.

4. Adjusted bed to comfortable working height; lowered side rail on working side and removed call light.

5. Loosened top linen sheet at foot of bed.

6. Removed bedspread and blanket separately by folding and discarding into linen bag. Did not allow soiled linen to come in contact with uniform.

7. When reusing blanket or spread, folded each correctly into a square.

8. Covered client with bath blanket and removed top sheet without exposing body parts.

9. Repositioned mattress toward head of bed with assistance from another nurse.

10. Assisted client to side-lying position. Elevated side rail.

11. Loosened bottom linen from head to foot of bed.

12. Fanfolded soiled bottom and drawsheet and tucked them under client's shoulders, back, and buttocks.

	S	U	NP	Comments
13. Cleaned soiled mattress with appropriate disinfectant.		__	__	_____
14. Applied clean mattress pad (if used) and bottom linen to one side of bed at a time.	__	__	__	_____
15. Correctly made mitered corner in top corner of bottom sheet.	__	__	__	_____
16. Tucked bottom sheet tightly under mattress.	__	__	__	_____
17. Put drawsheet in place correctly.	__	__	__	_____
18. Placed waterproof pad on bed.	__	__	__	_____
19. Assisted client to roll slowly over linen. Raised side rail on working side and moved to other side of bed.	__	__	__	_____
20. Lowered side rail and loosened edges of soiled linen from underneath mattress.	__	__	__	_____
21. Discarded linen correctly in linen bag. Cleaned mattress, if necessary.	__	__	__	_____
22. Spread clean, fanfolded linen smoothly over edge of mattress from head to foot of bed.	__	__	__	_____
23. Positioned client supine on bottom linen.	__	__	__	_____
24. Mitered top corner of bottom sheet.	__	__	__	_____
25. Tucked all bottom linen under mattress.	__	__	__	_____
26. Smoothed fanfolded drawsheet and tucked under mattress.	__	__	__	_____
27. Placed top sheet over client and unfolded from head to foot.	__	__	__	_____
28. Removed bath blanket and discarded it into linen bag.	__	__	__	_____
29. Placed blanket correctly on bed.	__	__	__	_____
30. Placed bedspread correctly on bed.	__	__	__	_____
31. Made cuff out of top edge of sheet, blanket, and bedspread.	__	__	__	_____
32. Tucked top sheet, blanket, and spread under mattress.	__	__	__	_____
33. Made modified mitered corner with top sheet, blanket, and spread.	__	__	__	_____
34. Raised side rail. Made other side of bed.	__	__	__	_____
35. Removed and discarded soiled pillow case. Correctly applied clean pillow case over pillow.	__	__	__	_____
36. Repositioned pillow under client's head.	__	__	__	_____

	S	U	NP	Comments

37. Placed call light within client's reach and returned bed to comfortable position. ___ ___ ___ _____

38. Opened room curtains. Rearranged furniture around bedside and placed client's personal items within easy reach. Returned bed to a safe, comfortable height. ___ ___ ___ _____

39. Discarded linen bag properly. Removed gloves and washed hands. ___ ___ ___ _____

EVALUATION

1. Assessed client's level of comfort. ___ ___ ___ _____

2. Inspected skin for irritated areas. ___ ___ ___ _____

3. Observed for signs of fatigue, dyspnea, pain, or discomfort. ___ ___ ___ _____

4. Identified unexpected outcomes. ___ ___ ___ _____

Student _____   Date _____

Instructor _____   Date _____

PERFORMANCE CHECKLIST 7-1 **RISK ASSESSMENT AND PREVENTION STRATEGIES**

	S	U	NP	Comments
ASSESSMENT				
1. Identified client's risk for pressure ulcer formation.	—	—	—	_____
2. Selected risk assessment tool.	—	—	—	_____
3. Obtained client's "Risk Score."	—	—	—	_____
4. Assessed condition of client's skin, particularly over potential pressure sites.	—	—	—	_____
5. Assessed client for additional areas of potential pressure.	—	—	—	_____
6. Observed client for preferred positions when in bed or chair.	—	—	—	_____
7. Assessed client's ability to initiate and assist with position changes.	—	—	—	_____
8. Assessed client's and support person's understanding of risks of pressure ulcers.	—	—	—	_____
NURSING DIAGNOSIS				
1. Developed appropriate nursing diagnoses based on assessment data.	—	—	—	_____
PLANNING				
1. Identified expected outcomes.	—	—	—	_____
2. Explained procedure(s) and purpose to client and family.	—	—	—	_____
3. Washed hands and prepared needed equipment and supplies.	—	—	—	_____
IMPLEMENTATION				
1. Implemented the Pressure Ulcer Prevention Points.	—	—	—	_____
2. Provided for client's privacy.	—	—	—	_____
3. Applied disposable gloves.	—	—	—	_____
4. Assisted client to change position.	—	—	—	_____
5. Assessed for redness in area that was under pressure. Palpated areas of discoloration or mottling.	—	—	—	_____

	S	U	NP	Comments
6. Monitored length of time area of redness persisted.	___	___	___	_____
7. Removed gloves and disposed of them properly. Washed hands.	___	___	___	_____

EVALUATION

	S	U	NP	Comments
1. Assessed condition of skin areas at risk for change in color and texture.	___	___	___	_____
2. Assessed client's tolerance of position changes.	___	___	___	_____
3. Compared subsequent risk assessment scores.	___	___	___	_____
4. Identified unexpected outcomes.	___	___	___	_____

RECORDING AND REPORTING

	S	U	NP	Comments
1. Recorded client's "Risk Score."	___	___	___	_____
2. Recorded appearance of skin area under pressure.	___	___	___	_____
3. Recorded positions, turning intervals, and other preventive measures.	___	___	___	_____
4. Reported need for additional consultations for the high-risk client.	___	___	___	_____

Student _____ Date _____

Instructor _____ Date _____

PERFORMANCE CHECKLIST 7-2 **TREATMENT OF PRESSURE ULCERS**

	S	U	NP	Comments
ASSESSMENT				
1. Assessed client's level of comfort and need for pain medication.	—	—	—	_____
2. Determined presence of allergies to topical agents.	—	—	—	_____
3. Reviewed physician's order for topical agent or dressing.	—	—	—	_____
4. Washed hands and applied clean gloves; closed room door or bedside curtains.	—	—	—	_____
5. Positioned client to allow dressing removal.	—	—	—	_____
6. Assessed pressure ulcer and surrounding skin to determine stage and color of pressure ulcer.	—	—	—	_____
7. Removed gloves and disposed of them properly. Washed hands.	—	—	—	_____
8. Completed an entire assessment of client.	—	—	—	_____
9. Assessed client's and support persons' understanding of pressure ulcer characteristics and purpose of treatment.	—	—	—	_____
NURSING DIAGNOSIS				
1. Developed appropriate nursing diagnoses based on assessment data.	—	—	—	_____
PLANNING				
1. Identified expected outcomes.	—	—	—	_____
2. Explained procedure and its purpose to client and family.	—	—	—	_____
3. Prepared necessary equipment and supplies. Selected appropriate dressing.	—	—	—	_____
IMPLEMENTATION				
1. Assembled needed supplies at bedside. Washed hands and donned gloves. Opened sterile packages and topical solution containers.	—	—	—	_____
2. Removed client's bed linen and gown to expose ulcer and surrounding skin; kept remaining body parts draped.	—	—	—	_____
3. Gently washed skin surrounding ulcer with warm water and soap.	—	—	—	_____

	S	U	NP	Comments
4. Rinsed area thoroughly with water.	___	___	___	_____
5. Gently dried skin by patting with towel.	___	___	___	_____
6. Changed gloves.	___	___	___	_____
7. Cleansed ulcer thoroughly with normal saline or prescribed cleansing agent. Used whirlpool treatments for debridement, as indicated.	___	___	___	_____
8. Applied topical agents if prescribed:	___	___	___	_____
a. Applied enzymes if prescribed.	___	___	___	_____
b. Applied hydrogel agents correctly.	___	___	___	_____
c. Applied calcium alginates correctly.	___	___	___	_____
9. Repositioned client comfortably off pressure ulcer.	___	___	___	_____
10. Removed gloves. Disposed of soiled supplies. Washed hands.	___	___	___	_____

EVALUATION

	S	U	NP	Comments
1. Inspected condition of skin surrounding pressure ulcer.	___	___	___	_____
2. Inspected ulcer and dressing. Monitored for signs and symptoms of infection.	___	___	___	_____
3. Compared subsequent ulcer measurements.	___	___	___	_____
4. Used an appropriate scale to measure healing.	___	___	___	_____
5. Identified unexpected outcomes.	___	___	___	_____

RECORDING AND REPORTING

	S	U	NP	Comments
1. Recorded appearance of ulcer.	___	___	___	_____
2. Described type of topical agent and dressing applied, including client's response.	___	___	___	_____
3. Reported worsening of ulcer to nurse in charge or physician.	___	___	___	_____

Student _____ Date _____

Instructor _____ Date _____

PERFORMANCE CHECKLIST 8-1 **TAKING CARE OF CONTACT LENSES**

	S	U	NP	Comments
ASSESSMENT				
1. Placed towel below client's face.	—	—	—	_____
2. Determined if contact lenses were in place.	—	—	—	_____
3. Assessed for eye discomfort and determined length of time client usually wears lenses.	—	—	—	_____
4. Assessed client's ability to manipulate and hold lenses.	—	—	—	_____
5. Assessed for any unusual visual symptoms.	—	—	—	_____
6. Assessed type of medications client receives.	—	—	—	_____
7. Inspected condition of cornea after removal of lenses.	—	—	—	_____
NURSING DIAGNOSIS				
1. Developed appropriate nursing diagnoses based on assessment data.	—	—	—	_____
PLANNING				
1. Identified expected outcomes.	—	—	—	_____
2. Discussed procedure with client.	—	—	—	_____
3. Positioned client in sitting or supine position. (Side-lying position used, if indicated.)	—	—	—	_____
4. Assembled supplies at bedside.	—	—	—	_____
IMPLEMENTATION				
Removing Soft Lenses				
1. Washed hands. Applied disposable gloves if needed.	—	—	—	_____
2. Placed towel just below client's face.	—	—	—	_____
3. Added 2 to 3 saline drops to client's eye.	—	—	—	_____
4. Told client to look straight ahead.	—	—	—	_____
5. Retracted client's lower eyelid.	—	—	—	_____
6. Slid lens off cornea onto white of eye with pad of index finger.	—	—	—	_____
7. Compressed lens correctly between thumb and index finger.	—	—	—	_____
8. Removed lens from eye.	—	—	—	_____

	S	U	NP	Comments

9. Soaked lens in sterile saline to return lens to normal shape, if needed.   ___ ___ ___ _____

10. Placed lens in correct cup of storage case after cleansing and rinsing.   ___ ___ ___ _____

11. Repeated Steps 3-10 for other lens.   ___ ___ ___ _____

12. Assessed condition of eyes after lenses removed.   ___ ___ ___ _____

13. Disposed of towel, removed gloves, and washed hands.   ___ ___ ___ _____

Removing Rigid Lenses

1. Washed hands. Applied gloves, if needed.   ___ ___ ___ _____

2. Placed towel just below client's face.   ___ ___ ___ _____

3. Determined position of lens before removal.   ___ ___ ___ _____

4. Retracted outer corner of eye toward client's ear.   ___ ___ ___ _____

5. Instructed client to blink.   ___ ___ ___ _____

6. Depressed lower eyelid against edge of lens correctly if lens failed to pop out.   ___ ___ ___ _____

7. Removed lens from eye. Held lens in cupped hand. (Lens suction cup used for confused or unconscious clients.)   ___ ___ ___ _____

8. Placed lens in correct cup of storage case after cleansing and rinsing.   ___ ___ ___ _____

9. Repeated Steps 3-8 for other lens. Secured cover over storage case.   ___ ___ ___ _____

10. Disposed of towel, removed gloves, and washed hands.   ___ ___ ___ _____

Cleansing and Disinfecting Contact Lenses

1. Washed hands and applied gloves if needed.   ___ ___ ___ _____

2. Assembled supplies at bedside. Placed towel over work area. Checked expiration date of all solutions.   ___ ___ ___ _____

3. Opened lens storage case carefully.   ___ ___ ___ _____

4. Removed lens from storage case and applied 1 to 2 drops of cleaner to lens in palm of hand.   ___ ___ ___ _____

5. Used fingertips to distribute cleansing solution over lens surfaces for 20 to 30 seconds.   ___ ___ ___ _____

6. Rinsed lens thoroughly in recommended rinsing solution (soft lenses) or cold tap water (rigid lenses).   ___ ___ ___ _____

7. Placed lenses in storage case with recommended solution.   ___ ___ ___ _____

8. Repeated Steps 3-7 for other lens.   ___ ___ ___ _____

	S	U	NP	Comments

Inserting Soft Lenses

1. Washed hands with mild soap, rinsed well, and dried with lint-free or paper towel. Applied gloves if needed. ___ ___ ___ _____

2. Placed towel over client's chest. ___ ___ ___ _____

3. Removed right lens from storage case and rinsed with recommended solution. ___ ___ ___ _____

4. Checked that lens was not inverted or damaged. ___ ___ ___ _____

5. Retracted upper lid using proper technique. ___ ___ ___ _____

6. Pulled down lower lid using proper finger. ___ ___ ___ _____

7. Instructed client to look straight ahead, and gently placed lens on cornea. ___ ___ ___ _____

8. Correctly positioned lens over cornea if it was on sclera. ___ ___ ___ _____

9. Instructed client to blink a few times. ___ ___ ___ _____

10. Determined if lens was centered properly. ___ ___ ___ _____

11. Repositioned lens if client's vision was blurred after insertion. ___ ___ ___ _____

12. Repeated Steps 3-11 for other eye. ___ ___ ___ _____

13. Assisted client to comfortable position. ___ ___ ___ _____

14. Discarded soiled supplies, rinsed storage case and allowed to air dry, and washed hands. ___ ___ ___ _____

Inserting Rigid Lenses

1. Washed hands with mild soap, rinsed well, and dried with lint-free or paper towel. Applied gloves if needed. ___ ___ ___ _____

2. Placed towel over client's chest. ___ ___ ___ _____

3. Removed right lens from storage case. ___ ___ ___ _____

4. Rinsed lens with cold tap water. ___ ___ ___ _____

5. Wet both sides of lens with prescribed wetting solution. ___ ___ ___ _____

6. Placed right lens concave side up on tip of index finger of dominant hand. ___ ___ ___ _____

7. Instructed client to look straight ahead; retracted eyelids and placed lens over center of cornea. ___ ___ ___ _____

8. Instructed client to close eyes. ___ ___ ___ _____

9. Determined if lens was centered. Repositioned lens if vision blurred and lens not centered. ___ ___ ___ _____

10. Repeated Steps 3-9 for left eye. ___ ___ ___ _____

	S	U	NP	Comments
11. Assisted client to comfortable position.	___	___	___	_____
12. Discarded soiled supplies, rinsed storage case and allowed to air dry, and washed hands.	___	___	___	_____

EVALUATION

1. Determined if lens fit correctly.	___	___	___	_____
2. Inspected eye for signs of infection or injury.	___	___	___	_____
3. Assessed client's visual acuity.	___	___	___	_____
4. Evaluated client's understanding and performance of lens care.	___	___	___	_____
5. Identified unexpected outcomes.	___	___	___	_____

RECORDING AND REPORTING

1. Recorded and reported signs or symptoms of visual alterations noted during procedure.	___	___	___	_____
2. Recorded times of lens insertion and removal.	___	___	___	_____

Student _____   Date _____

Instructor _____   Date _____

PERFORMANCE CHECKLIST 8-2 **TAKING CARE OF AN ARTIFICIAL EYE**

	S	U	NP	Comments

ASSESSMENT

1. Determined which eye is artificial.

2. Inspected condition of eyelids and eye socket.

3. Assessed client's routines for prosthesis care.

4. Assessed client's ability to remove, clean, and replace prosthesis.

NURSING DIAGNOSIS

1. Developed appropriate nursing diagnoses based on assessment data.

PLANNING

1. Identified expected outcomes.

2. Discussed procedure with client.

3. Assisted client to supine position with head elevated.

IMPLEMENTATION

1. Washed hands. Applied disposable gloves.

2. Retracted lower eyelid against lower orbital ridge. Exerted slight pressure below eyelid to loosen prosthesis.

3. Used bulb syringe or medicine dropper bulb to apply direct suction to prosthesis.

4. Removed prosthesis and placed in palm of hand.

5. Washed prosthesis with saline or mild soap and water using thumb and index finger; rinsed and dried prosthesis thoroughly.

6. Stored prosthesis in labeled container when not used.

7. Retracted upper and lower eyelids and washed socket with warm water or saline; dried socket thoroughly; washed lid margin by cleansing from inner to outer canthus; dried eyelids.

8. Dampened prosthesis in water before insertion.

9. Retracted upper eyelid.

10. Inserted prosthesis with notched edge toward nose.

	S	U	NP	Comments

11. Slid prosthesis with notched edge toward nose and pushed down lower lid to allow prosthesis to slip into place. ____ ____ ____ _____

12. Wiped prosthesis from outer to inner canthus if necessary. ____ ____ ____ _____

13. Helped client assume comfortable position. ____ ____ ____ _____

14. Disposed of soiled supplies, removed gloves, and washed hands. ____ ____ ____ _____

EVALUATION

1. Asked client feelings regarding prosthesis removal. ____ ____ ____ _____

2. Observed position of prosthesis. ____ ____ ____ _____

3. Asked client if prosthesis fits comfortably. ____ ____ ____ _____

4. Inspected condition of eyelids and socket. ____ ____ ____ _____

5. Asked client to explain or demonstrate procedure. ____ ____ ____ _____

6. Identified unexpected outcomes. ____ ____ ____ _____

RECORDING AND REPORTING

1. Documented removal of prosthesis for client going to surgery. ____ ____ ____ _____

2. Recorded and reported any alterations in integrity of tissues surrounding eye. ____ ____ ____ _____

Student _____ Date _____

Instructor _____ Date _____

PERFORMANCE CHECKLIST 8-3 **TAKING CARE OF AN IN-THE-EAR HEARING AID**

	S	U	NP	Comments
ASSESSMENT				
1. Assessed client's knowledge of and routines for hearing aid care.	___	___	___	_____
2. Assessed client's hearing with aid in place.	___	___	___	_____
3. Assessed function of aid through battery check.	___	___	___	_____
4. Checked that earmold was intact.	___	___	___	_____
5. Inspected for cerumen around earmold and external ear canal.	___	___	___	_____
NURSING DIAGNOSIS				
1. Developed appropriate nursing diagnoses based on assessment data.	___	___	___	_____
PLANNING				
1. Identified expected outcomes.	___	___	___	_____
2. Asked client for additional suggestions on techniques and explained procedure to be performed.	___	___	___	_____
IMPLEMENTATION				
Cleaning Hearing Aid				
1. Washed hands. Applied disposable gloves if needed.	___	___	___	_____
2. Assembled supplies at bedside table or sink area.	___	___	___	_____
3. Removed cerumen from holes in the aid.	___	___	___	_____
4. Washed, rinsed, and dried ear canal.	___	___	___	_____
5. Placed aid in storage case, if indicated. Kept device dry.	___	___	___	_____
6. Opened battery door to air dry.	___	___	___	_____
7. Labeled client's storage case.	___	___	___	_____
Inserting Hearing Aid				
1. Checked battery function before insertion of hearing aid.	___	___	___	_____
2. Turned aid off and volume control down.	___	___	___	_____
3. Held aid correctly to prepare for insertion in ear.	___	___	___	_____
4. Inserted aid into ear canal correctly.	___	___	___	_____

	S	U	NP	Comments
5. Adjusted volume to comfortable level.	___	___	___	_____
6. Disposed of soiled equipment properly and washed hands.	___	___	___	_____

EVALUATION

1. Determined client's ability to hear with aid in place.	___	___	___	_____
2. Asked client to explain or perform insertion and cleaning.	___	___	___	_____
3. Observed client's response to environmental sounds.	___	___	___	_____
4. Determined client's level of comfort.	___	___	___	_____
5. Identified unexpected outcomes.	___	___	___	_____

RECORDING AND REPORTING

1. Documented removal and storage of aid when client went to surgery or for special procedure.	___	___	___	_____
2. Reported client's communication problems to nursing staff.	___	___	___	_____

Student _____   Date _____

Instructor _____   Date _____

PERFORMANCE CHECKLIST 9-1 **MEASURING BODY TEMPERATURE**

	S	U	NP	Comments

ASSESSMENT

1. Determined need to measure client's temperature.   ___ ___ ___ _____

2. Assessed for factors that normally influence temperature.   ___ ___ ___ _____

3. Assessed site for most appropriate temperature measurement.   ___ ___ ___ _____

4. Determined client's baseline temperature from client's record.   ___ ___ ___ _____

NURSING DIAGNOSIS

1. Developed appropriate nursing diagnoses based on assessment.   ___ ___ ___ _____

PLANNING

1. Identified expected outcomes.   ___ ___ ___ _____

2. Explained procedure to client.   ___ ___ ___ _____

3. Waited 30 minutes before measuring oral temperature if client smoked or ingested hot or cold liquids or foods.   ___ ___ ___ _____

IMPLEMENTATION
Oral Temperature—Glass Thermometer

1. Washed hands.   ___ ___ ___ _____

2. Positioned client comfortably.   ___ ___ ___ _____

3. Applied disposable gloves.   ___ ___ ___ _____

4. Held color-coded end of glass thermometer with fingertips.   ___ ___ ___ _____

5. Read mercury level while gently rotating thermometer at eye level.   ___ ___ ___ _____

6. Shook thermometer down briskly to proper level (below 35.5° C, 96° F).   ___ ___ ___ _____

7. Inserted thermometer into plastic sleeve cover.   ___ ___ ___ _____

8. Placed thermometer under tongue in posterior sublingual pocket.   ___ ___ ___ _____

9. Asked client to hold thermometer with closed lips; cautioned client against biting down on thermometer.   ___ ___ ___ _____

	S	U	NP	Comments

10. Left thermometer in place for 3 minutes or according to agency policy. ___ ___ ___ _____

11. Removed thermometer and disposed of plastic sleeve cover. ___ ___ ___ _____

12. Removed secretions from thermometer by wiping from fingers toward bulb in rotating fashion. Discarded tissue properly. ___ ___ ___ _____

13. Correctly read thermometer at eye level. ___ ___ ___ _____

14. Informed client of temperature reading. ___ ___ ___ _____

15. Cleaned thermometer in lukewarm soapy water, rinsed, dried, and returned to container. ___ ___ ___ _____

16. Removed and disposed of gloves and washed hands. ___ ___ ___ _____

Oral Temperature—Electronic Thermometer

1. Washed hands and applied disposable gloves. ___ ___ ___ _____

2. Positioned client comfortably. ___ ___ ___ _____

3. Correctly attached oral probe to unit. ___ ___ ___ _____

4. Placed disposable plastic cover over probe. ___ ___ ___ _____

5. Inserted thermometer under tongue in posterior sublingual pocket. ___ ___ ___ _____

6. Asked client to hold thermometer with closed lips. ___ ___ ___ _____

7. Left probe in place until audible signal occurred, read temperature on digital display, and informed client of temperature reading. ___ ___ ___ _____

8. Correctly discarded plastic probe cover. ___ ___ ___ _____

9. Returned probe to storage well. ___ ___ ___ _____

10. Removed and disposed of gloves and washed hands. ___ ___ ___ _____

11. Returned thermometer to charger. ___ ___ ___ _____

Rectal Temperature—Glass Thermometer

1. Washed hands and applied disposable gloves. ___ ___ ___ _____

2. Provided for client's privacy and positioned client correctly. ___ ___ ___ _____

3. Prepared thermometer following Steps 4-7 of Oral Temperature Measurement with Glass Thermometer. ___ ___ ___ _____

4. Applied lubricant to thermometer bulb. ___ ___ ___ _____

S   U   NP   Comments

5. Correctly exposed client's anus and instructed client to breathe slowly and relax.

6. Gently inserted thermometer correct distance into anus.

7. Withdrew thermometer if resistance was felt.

8. Held thermometer in place for 2 minutes or according to agency policy.

9. Carefully removed thermometer, disposed of plastic sleeve cover, and wiped off secretions with tissue. Wiped in rotating fashion from fingers toward bulb. Discarded tissue.

10. Read thermometer while gently rotating thermometer at eye level.

11. Wiped client's anal area, disposed of tissue, and helped client return to comfortable position.

12. Informed client of temperature reading.

13. Washed thermometer in lukewarm soapy water, rinsed, dried, and replaced in storage container.

14. Removed and disposed of gloves and washed hands.

Rectal Temperature—Electronic Thermometer

1. Washed hands and applied disposable gloves.

2. Provided for client's privacy.

3. Positioned client correctly.

4. Correctly attached rectal probe to unit.

5. Placed disposable plastic cover over probe. Applied lubricant.

6. Correctly exposed client's anus and asked client to breathe slowly and relax.

7. Gently inserted thermometer correct distance into anus. Withdrew if resistance felt.

8. Held probe in place until audible signal occurred, and read temperature on digital display.

9. Carefully removed probe from rectum and informed client of temperature reading.

10. Correctly discarded plastic probe cover and returned probe to storage well.

11. Wiped client's anal area and removed and disposed of gloves.

12. Helped client return to comfortable position.

	S	U	NP	Comments
13. Washed hands.	——	——	——	_____
14. Returned thermometer to charger.	——	——	——	_____

Axillary Temperature—Glass Thermometer

1. Washed hands.	——	——	——	_____
2. Provided for client's privacy.	——	——	——	_____
3. Positioned client correctly.	——	——	——	_____
4. Moved clothing or gown away from client's shoulder and arm.	——	——	——	_____
5. Prepared glass thermometer following Steps 4-7 of Oral Temperature Measurement with Glass Thermometer.	——	——	——	_____
6. Inserted thermometer in center of axilla, lowered client's arm over thermometer, and placed arm across client's chest.	——	——	——	_____
7. Held thermometer in place for 3 minutes or according to agency policy.	——	——	——	_____
8. Removed thermometer, disposed of plastic sleeve cover, and wiped off secretions with tissue. Wiped in rotating fashion from fingers toward bulb. Discarded tissue.	——	——	——	_____
9. Read temperature while gently rotating thermometer at eye level.	——	——	——	_____
10. Informed client of temperature reading.	——	——	——	_____
11. Washed thermometer in lukewarm soapy water, rinsed, dried, and replaced in storage container.	——	——	——	_____
12. Assisted client in replacing clothing or gown.	——	——	——	_____
13. Washed hands.	——	——	——	_____

Axillary Temperature—Electronic Thermometer

1. Washed hands.	——	——	——	_____
2. Provided for client's privacy.	——	——	——	_____
3. Positioned client correctly.	——	——	——	_____
4. Moved clothing or gown away from client's shoulder and arm.	——	——	——	_____
5. Prepared thermometer following Steps 3 and 4 for Oral Temperature Measurement with Electronic Thermometer.	——	——	——	_____
6. Inserted probe in center of axilla, lowered client's arm over thermometer, and placed arm across client's chest.	——	——	——	_____

	S	U	NP	Comments

7. Held electronic probe in place until audible signal occurred, and read temperature on digital display.   ___ ___ ___ _____

8. Removed probe from axilla and informed client of temperature reading.   ___ ___ ___ _____

9. Correctly discarded plastic probe cover and returned probe to storage well.   ___ ___ ___ _____

10. Assisted client in replacing clothing or gown.   ___ ___ ___ _____

11. Washed hands.   ___ ___ ___ _____

12. Returned thermometer to charger.   ___ ___ ___ _____

Tympanic Membrane Temperature—Electronic Thermometer

1. Washed hands.   ___ ___ ___ _____

2. Assisted client to comfortable position with head turned to side, away from nurse.   ___ ___ ___ _____

3. Noted presence of cerumen in the ear canal.   ___ ___ ___ _____

4. Removed thermometer from charging base without applying pressure to ejection button.   ___ ___ ___ _____

5. Slid disposable speculum cover over tip until locked in place.   ___ ___ ___ _____

6. Inserted speculum into ear canal per manufacturer's instructions and client's age.   ___ ___ ___ _____

7. Depressed scan button on unit. Left thermometer in place until audible signal heard and temperature read.   ___ ___ ___ _____

8. Removed speculum from ear canal, and informed client of temperature reading.   ___ ___ ___ _____

9. Correctly discarded plastic probe cover.   ___ ___ ___ _____

10. Returned unit to charging base.   ___ ___ ___ _____

11. Assisted client to comfortable position.   ___ ___ ___ _____

12. Washed hands.   ___ ___ ___ _____

EVALUATION

1. Established client's temperature as a baseline if within normal range.   ___ ___ ___ _____

2. Compared client's temperature with client's baseline and normal temperature range.   ___ ___ ___ _____

3. Took temperature 30 minutes after antipyretics and every 4 hours for client with fever.   ___ ___ ___ _____

4. Identified unexpected outcomes.   ___ ___ ___ _____

	S	U	NP	Comments

REPORTING AND RECORDING

1. Recorded and reported temperature correctly. ___ ___ ___ _____

2. Reported abnormal findings to nurse in charge or physician. ___ ___ ___ _____

Student _____   Date _____

Instructor _____   Date _____

PERFORMANCE CHECKLIST 9-2 **ASSESSING RADIAL PULSE**

	S	U	NP	Comments

ASSESSMENT

1. Determined need to assess client's pulse: noted conditions or alterations increasing client's risk for pulse alterations and assessed for signs and symptoms of cardiovascular alterations.

2. Identified factors that normally may influence client's pulse.

3. Identified client's baseline heart rate from client's records.

NURSING DIAGNOSIS

1. Developed appropriate nursing diagnoses based on assessment data.

PLANNING

1. Identified expected outcomes.

2. Explained assessment procedure to client and the need to wait 5-10 minutes to assess pulse after client has been active.

IMPLEMENTATION
Radial Pulse

1. Washed hands. Provided privacy, if necessary.

2. Assisted client to a supine or sitting position.

3. If client is supine, placed client's forearm across lower chest with wrist extended and palm down. If client is sitting, bent client's elbow 90 degrees and supported lower arm on chair or on nurse's arm. Slightly extended client's wrist with palm down.

4. Placed fingertips of first two or middle three fingers over radial pulse.

5. Palpated client's radial pulse and determined strength of pulse.

6. Began to count rate when pulse was felt regularly.

7. With regular rate, counted pulse rate for 30 seconds and converted to minute rate.

8. With irregular rate, counted pulse rate for full minute.

	S	U	NP	Comments
9. Assessed regularity frequency of any dysrhythmia. Compared bilateral radial pulses. Assessed for pulse deficit, if indicated.	___	___	___	_____
10. Determined strength and character of pulse.	___	___	___	_____
11. Assisted client in returning to comfortable position.	___	___	___	_____
12. Discussed findings with client.	___	___	___	_____
13. Washed hands.	___	___	___	_____

EVALUATION

1. Established client's baseline pulse.	___	___	___	_____
2. Compared client's pulse rate and character with baseline and/or normal range for age group.	___	___	___	_____
3. Identified unexpected outcomes.	___	___	___	_____

RECORDING AND REPORTING

1. Recorded findings, including site assessed and signs and symptoms of pulse alterations.	___	___	___	_____
2. Reported abnormal findings to nurse in charge or physician.	___	___	___	_____

Student _____   Date _____

Instructor _____   Date _____

PERFORMANCE CHECKLIST 9-3 **ASSESSING APICAL PULSE**

	S	U	NP	Comments

ASSESSMENT

1. Determined need to assess client's pulse: noted conditions or alterations increasing client's risk for pulse alterations and assessed for signs and symptoms of cardiovascular alterations.

2. Identified factors that normally may influence client's pulse.

3. Identified client's baseline heart rate from client's records.

NURSING DIAGNOSIS

1. Developed appropriate nursing diagnoses based on assessment data.

PLANNING

1. Identified expected outcomes.

2. Explained assessment procedure to client and the need to wait 5 to 10 minutes to assess pulse after client has been active.

IMPLEMENTATION
Apical Pulse

1. Washed hands.

2. Provided privacy.

3. Assisted client to supine or sitting position.

4. Exposed client's sternum and left side of chest for auscultation.

5. Used palpation correctly. Located apex of heart at point of maximal impulse.

6. Warmed diaphragm of stethoscope between hands.

7. Placed diaphragm over point of maximal impulse (PMI) and auscultated for S_1 and S_2 heart sounds.

8. Determined rate of S_1 and S_2 sounds accurately.

9. With regular heart rate, counted for 30 seconds and correctly converted to minute rate.

10. With irregular heart rate, counted for 1 minute.

11. Assessed regularity of any existing dysrhythmia.

	S	U	NP	Comments

12. Replaced client's gown. Assisted client in returning to comfortable position.   ___ ___ ___ _____

13. Discussed findings with client.   ___ ___ ___ _____

14. Washed hands.   ___ ___ ___ _____

15. Cleaned stethoscope earpieces and diaphragm with alcohol swab.   ___ ___ ___ _____

EVALUATION

1. Established client's baseline pulse.   ___ ___ ___ _____

2. Compared client's pulse rate and character with baseline and/or normal range for age-group.   ___ ___ ___ _____

3. If pulse character was abnormal, asked another nurse to assess pulse.   ___ ___ ___ _____

4. Identified unexpected outcomes.   ___ ___ ___ _____

RECORDING AND REPORTING

1. Recorded vital signs appropriately.   ___ ___ ___ _____

2. Reported abnormal findings to nurse in charge or physician.   ___ ___ ___ _____

Student _____   Date _____

Instructor _____   Date _____

PERFORMANCE CHECKLIST 9-4 **ASSESSING RESPIRATIONS**

	S	U	NP	Comments
ASSESSMENT				
1. Determined need to assess client's respirations: described conditions that increase client's risk for respiratory alterations and identified common signs and symptoms of respiratory alterations.	___	___	___	_____
2. Assessed factors that normally influence respirations.	___	___	___	_____
3. Assessed results of pertinent laboratory values.	___	___	___	_____
4. Determined client's baseline respiratory rate from client's record.	___	___	___	_____
NURSING DIAGNOSIS				
1. Developed appropriate nursing diagnoses based on assessment data.	___	___	___	_____
PLANNING				
1. Identified expected outcomes.	___	___	___	_____
2. Waited 5 to 10 minutes before assessing respirations if client had been active.	___	___	___	_____
3. Assessed respirations after pulse measurement in adult.	___	___	___	_____
4. Assisted client in assuming comfortable position.	___	___	___	_____
IMPLEMENTATION				
1. Washed hands. Provided privacy.	___	___	___	_____
2. Positioned client and self properly to ensure view of chest wall movement.	___	___	___	_____
3. Was able to observe complete respiratory cycle.	___	___	___	_____
4. Correctly began count of respiration rate.	___	___	___	_____
5. Correctly counted respirations for 30 seconds in normal adult and multiplied by 2; counted rate for full minute in child. If respirations were irregular, counted rate for full minute.	___	___	___	_____
6. Assessed respiratory depth.	___	___	___	_____
7. Assessed respiratory rhythm.	___	___	___	_____
8. Replaced client's gown and covered client with bed linen.	___	___	___	_____

	S	U	NP	Comments
9. Washed hands.	___	___	___	_____
10. Discussed findings with client.	___	___	___	_____

EVALUATION

1. Determined client's baseline respirations.	___	___	___	_____
2. Compared characteristics of client's respirations with previous baseline data and/or normal range for client's age.	___	___	___	_____
3. Correlated respirations with data from other available measurements.	___	___	___	_____
4. Identified unexpected outcomes.	___	___	___	_____

RECORDING AND REPORTING

1. Recorded respiratory rate, rhythm, and depth.	___	___	___	_____
2. Indicated use of oxygen therapy.	___	___	___	_____
3. Reported abnormal findings to nurse in charge or physician.	___	___	___	_____

Student _____   Date _____

Instructor _____   Date _____

PERFORMANCE CHECKLIST 9-5 **ASSESSING ARTERIAL BLOOD PRESSURE**

	S	U	NP	Comments

ASSESSMENT

1. Determined need to assess client's blood pressure: identified conditions or alterations increasing client's risk for blood pressure alterations, identified common signs and symptoms of blood pressure alterations, and determined client's age.   ___ ___ ___ _____

2. Assessed for factors that normally influence blood pressure.   ___ ___ ___ _____

3. Determined best site for blood pressure assessment.   ___ ___ ___ _____

4. Determined client's previous baseline blood pressure from client's record.   ___ ___ ___ _____

5. Selected appropriate cuff size.   ___ ___ ___ _____

NURSING DIAGNOSIS

1. Developed appropriate nursing diagnoses based on assessment data.   ___ ___ ___ _____

PLANNING

1. Identified expected outcomes.   ___ ___ ___ _____

2. Explained procedure to client and had client rest at least 5 minutes before procedure.   ___ ___ ___ _____

3. Postponed assessment for 30 minutes if client had recently exercised, smoked, or ingested caffeine.   ___ ___ ___ _____

4. Assisted client in assuming proper sitting or lying position.   ___ ___ ___ _____

5. Selected appropriate cuff size.   ___ ___ ___ _____

IMPLEMENTATION
Auscultation Method—Upper Extremities

1. Washed hands.   ___ ___ ___ _____

2. Positioned client's forearm at heart level with palm of hand turned up.   ___ ___ ___ _____

3. Removed constricting clothing from around upper arm.   ___ ___ ___ _____

4. Palpated brachial artery, positioned cuff properly above brachial artery, and wrapped deflated cuff evenly and snugly around upper arm.   ___ ___ ___ _____

5. Positioned manometer correctly for viewing.   ___ ___ ___ _____

	S	U	NP	Comments

6. Measured blood pressure.   ___ ___ ___ _____

  a. Two-step method   ___ ___ ___ _____

    1. Identified approximate systolic pressure by palpating brachial or radial pulse during cuff inflation.   ___ ___ ___ _____

    2. Waited 30 seconds after deflating cuff before auscultation.   ___ ___ ___ _____

    3. Checked stethoscope amplification of sound.   ___ ___ ___ _____

    4. Applied stethoscope correctly over brachial artery.   ___ ___ ___ _____

    5. Tightened valve of pressure bulb.   ___ ___ ___ _____

    6. Correctly inflated cuff to 30 mm Hg above that of palpated systolic pressure.   ___ ___ ___ _____

    7. Allowed mercury to fall evenly at rate of 2 to 3 mm Hg/sec during auscultation.   ___ ___ ___ _____

    8. Noted point on manometer when first clear sound was heard.   ___ ___ ___ _____

    9. Continued to deflate cuff gradually, noting point at which sound disappeared in adults.   ___ ___ ___ _____

    10. Deflated cuff completely and removed from client's arm.   ___ ___ ___ _____

  b. One-step method   ___ ___ ___ _____

    1. Placed stethoscope pieces in ears and determined sounds were clear.   ___ ___ ___ _____

    2. Relocated brachial artery and placed diaphragm of stethoscope over it.   ___ ___ ___ _____

    3. Closed valve of pressure bulb.   ___ ___ ___ _____

    4. Quickly inflated cuff to 30 mm Hg above client's usual systolic blood pressure.   ___ ___ ___ _____

    5. Slowly released pressure bulb valve and allowed mercury or needle of aneroid manometer to fall at a rate of 2 to 3 mm Hg/sec.   ___ ___ ___ _____

    6. Noted point on manometer when first clear sound heard.   ___ ___ ___ _____

    7. Continued to deflate cuff gradually, noting point at which sound disappeared in adults.   ___ ___ ___ _____

    8. Repeated procedure on other arm, if first assessment.   ___ ___ ___ _____

S   U   NP   Comments

9. Assisted client in returning to comfortable position.

10. Informed client of blood pressure reading.

11. Washed hands.

12. Cleaned earpieces and diaphragm of stethoscope with alcohol swab.

Auscultation Method—Lower Extremities

1. Washed hands.

2. Assisted client in assuming prone position (supine optional).

3. Removed constricting clothing from around client's leg.

4. Palpated popliteal artery.

5. Applied leg cuff to posterior aspect of middle thigh.

6. Followed Step 6-b of Auscultation Method—Upper Extremities using the popliteal artery.

7. Repeated procedure on other leg if first assessment.

8. Assisted client in returning to comfortable position.

9. Informed client of blood pressure reading.

10. Washed hands.

11. Cleaned earpieces and diaphragm of stethoscope with alcohol swab (optional).

Palpation Method

1. Began palpation by following Steps 1-5 of Auscultation Method.

2. Identified approximate systolic pressure by palpating brachial or radial pulse during cuff inflation.

3. Allowed mercury to fall evenly at rate of 2 to 3 mm Hg/sec.

4. Noted manometer reading when pulse was again palpable.

5. Rapidly deflated cuff completely and removed from client's arm.

6. Assisted client in returning to comfortable position.

	S	U	NP	Comments
7. Informed client of reading.	___	___	___	_____
8. Washed hands.	___	___	___	_____

EVALUATION

1. Established blood pressure as baseline, if assessed for first time and found within normal range.	___	___	___	_____
2. Compared client's blood pressure reading with previous baseline and/or normal average blood pressure for client's age.	___	___	___	_____
3. Identified unexpected outcomes.	___	___	___	_____

RECORDING AND REPORTING

1. Recorded blood pressure appropriately.	___	___	___	_____
2. Reported abnormal findings to nurse in charge or physician.	___	___	___	_____

Student _____ Date _____

Instructor _____ Date _____

PERFORMANCE CHECKLIST 9-6 **MEASURING OXYGEN SATURATION (PULSE OXIMETRY)**

	S	U	NP	Comments
ASSESSMENT				
1. Determined need to measure client's oxygen saturation.	—	—	—	_____
2. Assessed for factors that influence oxygen saturation measurement.	—	—	—	_____
3. Reviewed agency policy or client's medical record for physician's order.	—	—	—	_____
4. Determined previous baseline SaO_2, if available.	—	—	—	_____
5. Assessed site for sensor probe placement.	—	—	—	_____
NURSING DIAGNOSIS				
1. Developed appropriate nursing diagnoses based on assessment data.	—	—	—	_____
PLANNING				
1. Identified expected outcomes.	—	—	—	_____
2. Obtained equipment and placed at bedside.	—	—	—	_____
3. Explained purpose of procedure to client and family.	—	—	—	_____
IMPLEMENTATION				
1. Washed hands.	—	—	—	_____
2. Positioned client comfortably.	—	—	—	_____
3. Instructed client to breathe normally.	—	—	—	_____
4. Removed fingernail polish if using finger site.	—	—	—	_____
5. Attached sensor probe to selected site.	—	—	—	_____
6. Watched pulse bar for pulse sensing.	—	—	—	_____
7. Correlated oximeter with radial pulse rate.	—	—	—	_____
8. Informed client that alarm will sound if probe falls off.	—	—	—	_____
9. Left probe in place until readout reached constant value and full strength. Read oxygen saturation.	—	—	—	_____
10. Discussed findings with client.	—	—	—	_____
11. Set alarms for continuous monitoring; assessed skin integrity and relocated probe regularly.	—	—	—	_____

	S	U	NP	Comments

12. Removed probe and turned oximeter off. ___ ___ ___ _____

13. Assisted client to comfortable position. ___ ___ ___ _____

14. Washed hands. ___ ___ ___ _____

EVALUATION

1. Established SaO$_2$ as baseline, if assessed for first time and within normal limits. ___ ___ ___ _____

2. Compared SaO$_2$ with previous baseline and normals. Noted use of oxygen therapy. ___ ___ ___ _____

3. Assessed skin integrity underneath probe regularly. ___ ___ ___ _____

4. Identified unexpected outcomes. ___ ___ ___ _____

RECORDING AND REPORTING

1. Recorded SaO$_2$; identified use of continuous or intermittent pulse oximetry. ___ ___ ___ _____

2. Reported abnormal findings to nurse in charge or physician. ___ ___ ___ _____

3. Correlated findings with arterial blood gas measurements, if available. ___ ___ ___ _____

4. Reported SaO$_2$ and response to change in therapy to oncoming shift. ___ ___ ___ _____

Student _____   Date _____

Instructor _____   Date _____

PERFORMANCE CHECKLIST 10-1   GENERAL SURVEY

	S	U	NP	Comments
ASSESSMENT				
1. Noted if client is experiencing any acute distress.	___	___	___	_____
2. Checked baseline vital signs and assessed factors that alter readings.	___	___	___	_____
3. Determined client's primary language.	___	___	___	_____
4. Reconfirmed client's primary reason for seeking health care.	___	___	___	_____
5. Identified client's normal height and weight.	___	___	___	_____
6. Reviewed client's past intake and output records.	___	___	___	_____
7. Determined client's perceptions about personal health.	___	___	___	_____
8. Assessed client for latex allergy.	___	___	___	_____
PLANNING				
1. Identified expected outcomes or normal findings.	___	___	___	_____
2. Prepared client for examination.	___	___	___	_____
IMPLEMENTATION				
1. Noted client's verbal and nonverbal behaviors.	___	___	___	_____
2. Obtained vital sign measurements.	___	___	___	_____
3. Observed client's overall appearance.	___	___	___	_____
4. Rephrased questions as necessary.	___	___	___	_____
5. Asked client short, focused questions if responses inappropriate.	___	___	___	_____
6. Offered simple commands or directions if client unable to respond to orientation questions.	___	___	___	_____
7. Assessed client's body posture and mobility.	___	___	___	_____
8. Assessed client's speech pace and clarity.	___	___	___	_____
9. Observed client's hygiene and grooming.	___	___	___	_____
10. Assessed client's eyes:	___	___	___	_____
a. Position, color, and movement	___	___	___	_____
b. Near and far vision	___	___	___	_____
c. Pupil size, shape, and equality	___	___	___	_____
d. Pupillary reflexes	___	___	___	_____

	S	U	NP	Comments
11. Assessed hearing acuity and presence of hearing aid.	___	___	___	_____
12. Inspected client's external nose for shape, skin color, alignment, and abnormalities. Took special care for clients with indwelling tubes.	___	___	___	_____
13. Assessed mouth: oral mucosa, tongue, teeth, and gums. Noted presence and condition of dentures.	___	___	___	_____
14. Asked client about any recent changes in skin integrity.	___	___	___	_____
15. Inspected skin surfaces symetrically; noted variations in color and presence of lesions.	___	___	___	_____
16. Inspected color of face, oral mucosa, lips, conjunctiva, sclera, and nail beds.	___	___	___	_____
17. Palpated skin surfaces to determine skin moisture, texture, and temperature.	___	___	___	_____
18. Applied gloves and inspected character of secretions.	___	___	___	_____
19. Assessed skin turgor.	___	___	___	_____
20. Gently palpated and measured any lesions.	___	___	___	_____
21. Applied clean gloves and palpated IV site.	___	___	___	_____
22. Used the "five rights" to check IV fluids and medications.	___	___	___	_____
23. Assessed client's affect and mood.	___	___	___	_____
24. Observed client's interaction with others.	___	___	___	_____
25. Observed for signs of abuse in the child or adult.	___	___	___	_____

EVALUATION

	S	U	NP	Comments
1. Observed for evidence of physical or emotional distress.	___	___	___	_____
2. Compared assessment findings with previous observations.	___	___	___	_____
3. Asked client if there was information that had not been discussed.	___	___	___	_____
4. Identified unexpected outcomes.	___	___	___	_____

NURSING DIAGNOSIS

	S	U	NP	Comments
1. Developed appropriate nursing diagnoses based on assessment data.	___	___	___	_____

	S	U	NP	Comments

RECORDING AND REPORTING

1. Recorded vital signs.

2. Recorded alterations in client's general appearance.

3. Described client's behaviors and gave a subjective report of signs and symptoms.

4. Reported abnormalities and acute symptoms to nurse in charge or physician.

Student _____   Date _____

Instructor _____   Date _____

PERFORMANCE CHECKLIST 10-2 **ASSESSING THE THORAX AND LUNGS**

	S	U	NP	Comments
ASSESSMENT				
1. Assessed client's smoking history.	___	___	___	_____
2. Assessed for symptoms of respiratory alterations.	___	___	___	_____
3. Determined whether client exposed to environmental pollutants.	___	___	___	_____
4. Reviewed client history for risk factors associated with tuberculosis and infection with human immunodeficiency virus (HIV).	___	___	___	_____
5. Assessed for history of allergies.	___	___	___	_____
6. Reviewed family history for risk factors.	___	___	___	_____
PLANNING				
1. Identified expected outcomes.	___	___	___	_____
IMPLEMENTATION				
1. Assisted client to assume correct positions throughout procedure; exposed chest wall for assessment; explained steps of procedure.	___	___	___	_____
Posterior Thorax				
1. Inspected appearance of thorax.	___	___	___	_____
2. Determined rate and rhythm of breathing.	___	___	___	_____
3. Palpated posterior chest wall and costal and intercostal spaces.	___	___	___	_____
4. Palpated chest excursion.	___	___	___	_____
5. Noted chest symmetry.	___	___	___	_____
6. Percussed intercostal spaces over chest wall.	___	___	___	_____
7. Auscultated breath sounds.	___	___	___	_____
Lateral Thorax				
1. Inspected lateral chest wall with client's arms raised.	___	___	___	_____
2. Extended assessment to lateral sides of chest.	___	___	___	_____
Anterior Thorax				
1. Inspected accessory muscles.	___	___	___	_____
2. Inspected angle of costal margins and tip of sternum.	___	___	___	_____

	S	U	NP	Comments
3. Observed client's respiratory character.	___	___	___	_____
4. Palpated for swelling or tenderness.	___	___	___	_____
5. Palpated anterior chest excursion.	___	___	___	_____
6. Percussed thorax between intercostal spaces.	___	___	___	_____
7. Auscultated breath sounds in anterior thorax.	___	___	___	_____

EVALUATION

1. Compared findings with normal assessment characteristics of thorax and lungs.	___	___	___	_____
2. Had client identify factors leading to lung disease.	___	___	___	_____
3. Identified unexpected outcomes.	___	___	___	_____

NURSING DIAGNOSIS

1. Developed appropriate nursing diagnoses based on assessment data.	___	___	___	_____

RECORDING AND REPORTING

1. Recorded observations and findings.	___	___	___	_____
2. Recorded respiratory rate and character.	___	___	___	_____
3. Reported abnormalities to nurse in charge or physician.	___	___	___	_____

Student _____   Date _____

Instructor _____   Date _____

PERFORMANCE CHECKLIST 10-3 **ASSESSING THE HEART AND NECK VESSELS**

	S	U	NP	Comments
ASSESSMENT				
1. Assessed for risk factors for heart and vascular disease.	___	___	___	_____
2. Determined client's medication history.	___	___	___	_____
3. Assessed for symptoms of heart disease.	___	___	___	_____
4. Determined presence and character of chest pain.	___	___	___	_____
5. Assessed client and family history for heart disease.	___	___	___	_____
6. Assessed client for history of heart problems.	___	___	___	_____
PLANNING				
1. Identified expected outcomes.	___	___	___	_____
IMPLEMENTATION				
1. Assisted client to comfortable position and explained procedure.	___	___	___	_____
2. Made sure room was quiet.	___	___	___	_____
Heart				
1. Located anatomic sites to assess heart function.	___	___	___	_____
2. Used inspection and palpation over anatomic landmarks to detect pulsations.	___	___	___	_____
3. Timed any pulsations in relation to heart sounds.	___	___	___	_____
4. Located PMI by palpation.	___	___	___	_____
5. Turned client to left side when unable to locate PMI.	___	___	___	_____
6. Inspected epigastric area and palpated abdominal aorta.	___	___	___	_____
7. Auscultated heart sounds, repositioning client when indicated.	___	___	___	_____
8. Auscultated heart sounds using diaphragm and bell of stethoscope.	___	___	___	_____
a. Auscultated S_1 sound at various anatomic landmarks.	___	___	___	_____
b. Listened for S_2 sound at each site.	___	___	___	_____
c. Determined apical pulse rate.	___	___	___	_____

	S	U	NP	Comments

d. Assessed heart rhythm.

e. Assessed for a pulse deficit if heart rate irregular.

9. Auscultated for extra heart sounds.

10. Characterized any murmurs present.

Vascular

1. Assessed carotid arteries using inspection, palpation, and auscultation. Palpated each artery separately.

2. Assessed jugular veins separately, measuring from appropriate landmarks.

3. Assessed venous pressure and observed for visible jugular pulsation.

EVALUATION

1. Compared findings with normal assessment characteristics for heart and vascular system.

2. If pulses were not palpable, had another nurse assess for pulses.

3. Asked client to describe behaviors that increase the risk of cardiovascular disease.

4. Identified unexpected outcomes.

NURSING DIAGNOSIS

1. Formulated appropriate nursing diagnoses based on assessment data.

RECORDING AND REPORTING

1. Recorded all findings for heart and vascular assessment.

2. Recorded instructions given to client and client's response.

3. Reported abnormalities to nurse in charge or physician.

Student _____   Date _____

Instructor _____   Date _____

PERFORMANCE CHECKLIST 10-4 **ASSESSING THE ABDOMEN**

	S	U	NP	Comments
ASSESSMENT				
1. Assessed for character of existing abdominal or low back pain.	—	—	—	_____
2. Observed client for signs of pain associated with positioning.	—	—	—	_____
3. Assessed client's bowel habits.	—	—	—	_____
4. Assessed for history of abdominal surgery or trauma.	—	—	—	_____
5. Assessed for weight change or diet intolerance.	—	—	—	_____
6. Assessed for signs and symptoms of abdominal alterations.	—	—	—	_____
7. Asked whether client taking any antiinflammatory medications or antibiotics.	—	—	—	_____
8. Inquired about family history of cancer, kidney disease, alcoholism, hypertension, or heart disease.	—	—	—	_____
9. Determined if female client is pregnant.	—	—	—	_____
10. Reviewed client's history for risk factors of HBV exposure.	—	—	—	_____
PLANNING				
1. Identified expected outcomes.	—	—	—	_____
IMPLEMENTATION				
1. Prepared client by allowing voiding of bladder before assessment, correctly draping and positioning client, and explaining steps of procedure.	—	—	—	_____
2. Described findings in relation to anatomic landmarks.	—	—	—	_____
3. Inspected skin of abdomen. Questioned client if bruising present.	—	—	—	_____
4. Inspected condition of umbilicus.	—	—	—	_____
5. Noted contour and symmetry of abdomen.	—	—	—	_____
6. Had client roll onto side if distention present.	—	—	—	_____
7. Measured abdominal girth if distention suspected.	—	—	—	_____
8. Prepared for auscultation by asking client not to talk or turning nasogastric suction off, if applicable.	—	—	—	_____
9. Auscultated bowel sounds systematically with diaphragm of stethoscope.	—	—	—	_____

	S	U	NP	Comments
10. Used bell of stethoscope to auscultate vascular sounds and notified physician if aortic bruit auscultated.	___	___	___	_____
11. Percussed four abdominal quadrants.	___	___	___	_____
12. Percussed abdomen systematically.	___	___	___	_____
13. Percussed for presence of kidney inflammation.	___	___	___	_____
14. Performed light palpation of abdomen.	___	___	___	_____
15. Palpated bladder area.	___	___	___	_____
16. Noted characteristics of any masses present.	___	___	___	_____
17. Assessed for rebound tenderness if area was tender on palpation.	___	___	___	_____
18. Performed deep palpation.	___	___	___	_____

EVALUATION

	S	U	NP	Comments
1. Compared findings with normal assessment characteristics of the abdomen.	___	___	___	_____
2. Asked client to describe signs and symptoms of colon cancer.	___	___	___	_____
3. Identified unexpected outcomes.	___	___	___	_____

NURSING DIAGNOSIS

	S	U	NP	Comments
1. Formulated appropriate nursing diagnoses based on assessment data.	___	___	___	_____

RECORDING AND REPORTING

	S	U	NP	Comments
1. Recorded results of assessment.	___	___	___	_____
2. Recorded client instruction.	___	___	___	_____
3. Reported abnormalities to nurse in charge or physician.	___	___	___	_____

Student _____   Date _____

Instructor _____   Date _____

PERFORMANCE CHECKLIST 10-5 **ASSESSING THE EXTREMITIES AND PERIPHERAL CIRCULATION**

	S	U	NP	Comments
ASSESSMENT				
1. Reviewed client's history for risk factors.	___	___	___	_____
2. Asked client to describe history of musculoskeletal problems.	___	___	___	_____
3. Assessed characteristics of client's pain.	___	___	___	_____
4. Determined client's ability to perform daily activities.	___	___	___	_____
5. Assessed height decreases of women who are more than 50 years old.	___	___	___	_____
PLANNING				
1. Identified expected outcomes based on communication goals.	___	___	___	_____
IMPLEMENTATION				
1. Prepared client.	___	___	___	_____
2. Integrated musculoskeletal assessment into other aspects of physical assessment.	___	___	___	_____
3. Planned time for rest periods during assessment.	___	___	___	_____
4. Observed client's ability to use arms and hands.	___	___	___	_____
5. Assessed muscle strength of upper extremities.	___	___	___	_____
a. Assessed hand grip strength.	___	___	___	_____
b. Had client move against resistance.	___	___	___	_____
c. Measured muscle size for clients with decreased strength.	___	___	___	_____
6. Observed client's position sitting, supine, prone, or standing.	___	___	___	_____
7. Inspected gait.	___	___	___	_____
8. Observed postural alignment.	___	___	___	_____
9. Observed overall status of extremities.	___	___	___	_____
10. Palpated bones, joints, and surrounding areas gently.	___	___	___	_____
11. Had client put major joints through ROM and observed for equality and abnormality.	___	___	___	_____

	S	U	NP	Comments
12. Assessed muscle tone in major muscle groups.	___	___	___	_____
13. Inspected lower extremities for changes in skin color and condition.	___	___	___	_____
14. Palpated edematous areas and assessed for pitting edema.	___	___	___	_____
15. Checked capillary refill in fingers and toes.	___	___	___	_____
16. Asked if the client experienced discomfort and palpated calf for tenderness, firmness, and swelling.	___	___	___	_____
17. Assessed for Homans' sign.	___	___	___	_____
18. Palpated each peripheral artery symmetrically and assessed pulses: radial, ulnar, brachial, dorsalis pedis, pedal, posterior tibial, popliteal, and femoral. Used ultrasound instrument for pedal pulses, if necessary.	___	___	___	_____
19. Monitored deep tendon reflexes: knee and plantar. Checked for ankle clonus, if indicated.	___	___	___	_____

EVALUATION

	S	U	NP	Comments
1. Compared muscle strength and ROM with previous assessments.	___	___	___	_____
2. Compared pulses and capillary refill bilaterally with previous observations.	___	___	___	_____
3. Compared presence and extent of edema with previous assessments.	___	___	___	_____
4. Evaluated client's level of discomfort after the procedure.	___	___	___	_____
5. Identified unexpected outcomes.	___	___	___	_____

NURSING DIAGNOSIS

	S	U	NP	Comments
1. Developed appropriate nursing diagnoses based on assessment data.	___	___	___	_____

RECORDING AND REPORTING

	S	U	NP	Comments
1. Recorded all assessment findings.	___	___	___	_____
2. Reported acute pain, sudden muscle weakness, or changes in peripheral circulation to nurse in charge or physician.	___	___	___	_____

Student _____ Date _____

Instructor _____ Date _____

PERFORMANCE CHECKLIST 10-6 **ASSESSING INTAKE AND OUTPUT**

	S	U	NP	Comments
ASSESSMENT				
1. Identified conditions that could influence a client's fluid balance status.	—	—	—	_____
2. Identified risk of insufficient fluid intake.	—	—	—	_____
3. Identified medications that could influence a client's fluid balance status.	—	—	—	_____
4. Assessed client for signs of fluid overload or dehydration.	—	—	—	_____
5. Weighed client daily.	—	—	—	_____
6. Monitored laboratory reports.	—	—	—	_____
7. Assess client's and family's knowledge of purpose of procedure.	—	—	—	_____
NURSING DIAGNOSIS				
1. Developed appropriate nursing diagnoses based on assessment data.	—	—	—	_____
PLANNING				
1. Identified expected outcomes.	—	—	—	_____
2. Posted sign indicating I&O was instituted.	—	—	—	_____
3. Placed I&O record in established location.	—	—	—	_____
IMPLEMENTATION				
1. Explained to client and family why I&O measurements are necessary.	—	—	—	_____
2. Measured and recorded all oral and parenteral fluids and all enteral tube feedings.	—	—	—	_____
3. Instructed client not to empty urinal, Foley or wound drainage bag, bedpan, or commode.	—	—	—	_____
4. Observed color and characteristics of urine.	—	—	—	_____
5. Correctly measured and recorded all fluids draining from Foley catheter, nasogastric suction, and wound suction at least every 8 hours.	—	—	—	_____
6. Applied gloves before handling equipment or drainage. Washed hands after measuring and recording output fluids.	—	—	—	_____

	S	U	NP	Comments

EVALUATION

1. Reassessed client's fluid balance correctly. ___ ___ ___ _____

2. Observed characteristics of urinary output and wound drainage. ___ ___ ___ _____

3. Noted I&O balance. ___ ___ ___ _____

4. Identified unexpected outcomes. ___ ___ ___ _____

RECORDING AND REPORTING

1. Calculated and recorded I&O totals at specified time. ___ ___ ___ _____

2. Calculated and recorded 24-hour totals. ___ ___ ___ _____

3. Reported urine output of less than 30 ml/hr or significant changes in weight. ___ ___ ___ _____

Student _____ Date _____

Instructor _____ Date _____

PERFORMANCE CHECKLIST 11-1 **APPLYING A NASAL CANNULA OR OXYGEN MASK**

	S	U	NP	Comments
ASSESSMENT				
1. Observed for signs and symptoms associated with hypoxia.	___	___	___	_____
2. Observed for patent airway and removed airway secretions.	___	___	___	_____
3. Obtained results of client's most recent arterial blood gases (ABGs) study.	___	___	___	_____
4. Reviewed client's medical record for medical order for oxygen therapy; noted method, flow rate, and duration of oxygen therapy.	___	___	___	_____
5. Completed total respiratory system assessment.	___	___	___	_____
NURSING DIAGNOSIS				
1. Developed appropriate nursing diagnoses based on assessment data.	___	___	___	_____
PLANNING				
1. Identified expected outcomes.	___	___	___	_____
2. Explained procedure and its purpose to client and family.	___	___	___	_____
IMPLEMENTATION				
1. Washed hands.	___	___	___	_____
2. Attached nasal cannula or oxygen mask to oxygen tubing and attached oxygen tubing to flow meter.	___	___	___	_____
3. Adjusted oxygen flow rate to prescribed dosage.	___	___	___	_____
4. Applied oxygen delivery device and adjusted to client's comfort. Allowed sufficient slack on oxygen tubing and secured to client's clothing.	___	___	___	_____
5. Observed proper function of oxygen delivery device.	___	___	___	_____
6. Monitored changes in oxygen flow rate with pulse oximetry.	___	___	___	_____
7. Washed hands.	___	___	___	_____
EVALUATION				
1. Reassessed client to determine response to oxygen administration.	___	___	___	_____
2. Observed client's mucous membrane and face for skin breakdown.	___	___	___	_____

	S	U	NP	Comments
3. Monitored ABGs or pulse oximetry.	___	___	___	_____
4. Assessed adequacy of oxygen flow each shift.	___	___	___	_____
5. Identified unexpected outcomes.	___	___	___	_____

RECORDING AND REPORTING

1. Recorded respiratory assessment findings before and during oxygen therapy; method of oxygen delivery, flow rate, patency, and client's response; any adverse reactions or side effects; and any change in physician's orders.   ___ ___ ___ _____

2. Reported unexpected findings to nurse in charge or physician.   ___ ___ ___ _____

Student _____   Date _____

Instructor _____   Date _____

PERFORMANCE CHECKLIST 11-2 **ADMINISTERING OXYGEN THERAPY TO A CLIENT WITH AN ARTIFICIAL AIRWAY**

	S	U	NP	Comments
ASSESSMENT				
1. Observed for signs and symptoms associated with hypoxia.	—	—	—	_____
2. Observed for patent airway and removed airway secretions.	—	—	—	_____
3. Noted client's most recent ABG results or pulse oximetry value.	—	—	—	_____
4. Reviewed client's medical order for oxygen therapy.	—	—	—	_____
5. Completed assessment of respiratory system.	—	—	—	_____
NURSING DIAGNOSIS				
1. Developed appropriate nursing diagnoses based on assessment data.	—	—	—	_____
PLANNING				
1. Identified expected outcomes.	—	—	—	_____
2. Explained purpose of T-tube or tracheostomy collar to client and family.	—	—	—	_____
IMPLEMENTATION				
1. Washed hands. Applied gloves and goggles. Considered need for barrier gown.	—	—	—	_____
2. Attached T-tube or tracheostomy collar to large-bore oxygen tubing and to humidified oxygen source.	—	—	—	_____
3. Adjusted oxygen flow rate at 10 L/min or as ordered and adjusted nebulizer to proper FiO_2 setting. Attached T-tube or tracheostomy collar to endotracheal or tracheostomy tube.	—	—	—	_____
4. Monitored changes in flow rate with pulse oximetry.	—	—	—	_____
5. Monitored ABGs or pulse oximetry after initiating T-tube.	—	—	—	_____
6. Observed for T-tube pulling on endotracheal or tracheostomy tube. Suctioned secretions in T-tube or tracheostomy collar if necessary.	—	—	—	_____
7. Observed oxygen tubing frequently for accumulation of fluid, and drained tubing correctly.	—	—	—	_____

	S	U	NP	Comments
8. Set up suction equipment at client's bedside.	___	___	___	_____
9. Removed gloves and goggles; washed hands.	___	___	___	_____

EVALUATION

	S	U	NP	Comments
1. Assessed client's response to procedure, including respiratory status, LOC, etc.	___	___	___	_____
2. Determined that oxygen delivery device was not pulling on artificial airway.	___	___	___	_____
3. Monitored arterial blood gas levels or pulse oximetry.	___	___	___	_____
4. Identified unexpected outcomes.	___	___	___	_____

RECORDING AND REPORTING

	S	U	NP	Comments
1. Recorded and included in report respiratory assessment findings before and during oxygen therapy and method of oxygen delivery, flow rate, and client's response.	___	___	___	_____
2. Reported unexpected findings to nurse in charge or physician.	___	___	___	_____

Student _____ Date _____

Instructor _____ Date _____

PERFORMANCE CHECKLIST 11-3 **USING INCENTIVE SPIROMETRY**

	S	U	NP	Comments

ASSESSMENT
1. Identified clients who would benefit from incentive spirometry. — — — _____

2. Observed client's respiratory status. — — — _____

3. Reviewed physician's order for incentive spirometry. — — — _____

NURSING DIAGNOSIS
1. Developed appropriate nursing diagnoses based on assessment data. — — — _____

PLANNING
1. Identified expected outcomes. — — — _____

2. Explained to client and family purpose and reason for using incentive spirometry. — — — _____

IMPLEMENTATION
1. Washed hands. — — — _____

2. Instructed client to assume proper upright position. — — — _____

3. Demonstrated how to place mouthpiece. — — — _____

4. Instructed client to inhale slowly and maintain a constant flow through the unit, then hold breath for 2 to 3 seconds and exhale slowly. Instructed client to breathe normally for short period. — — — _____

5. Had client repeat maneuver. — — — _____

6. Washed hands. — — — _____

EVALUATION
1. Reassessed client to determine response and ability to use incentive spirometry. — — NP _____

2. Assessed ability of client to reach target volume or frequency. — — — _____

3. Auscultated chest during respiratory cycle. — — — _____

4. Identified unexpected outcomes. — — — _____

	S	U	NP	Comments

RECORDING AND REPORTING

1. Recorded respiratory assessment before and after incentive spirometry, frequency of use, volumes achieved, and any adverse effects.   ___   ___   ___   _____

2. Reported changes in respiratory status or inability to use equipment.   ___   ___   ___   _____

Student _____   Date _____

Instructor _____   Date _____

PERFORMANCE CHECKLIST 11-4 **ADMINISTERING MECHANICAL VENTILATION**

	S	U	NP	Comments
ASSESSMENT				
1. Observed for signs and symptoms associated with hypoxia.	—	—	—	_____
2. Observed for patent airway and removed airway secretions.	—	—	—	_____
3. Noted client's most recent ABG results or pulse oximetry, if available.	—	—	—	_____
4. Reviewed medical order for mechanical ventilation and ventilation settings.	—	—	—	_____
5. Completed assessment of respiratory system.	—	—	—	_____
NURSING DIAGNOSIS				
1. Developed appropriate nursing diagnoses based on assessment data.	—	—	—	_____
PLANNING				
1. Identified expected outcomes.	—	—	—	_____
2. Explained purpose of mechanical ventilation to client and others.	—	—	—	_____
IMPLEMENTATION				
1. Washed hands and applied gloves and goggles. Considered need for barrier gown.	—	—	—	_____
2. Attached mechanical ventilator to endotracheal or tracheostomy tube. Observed for proper functioning of mechanical ventilator.	—	—	—	_____
3. Verified by auscultation that endotracheal tube is properly posiitoned.	—	—	—	_____
4. Assessed for client anxiety and respiration in synchronization with mechanical ventilation.	—	—	—	_____
5. Monitored vital signs.	—	—	—	_____
6. Secured ventilator tubing to prevent dislodging of artificial airway.	—	—	—	_____
7. Noted level of endotracheal tube at lips or nares.	—	—	—	_____
8. Set up suction equipment.	—	—	—	_____
9. Positioned client to promote best oxygenation.	—	—	—	_____

	S	U	NP	Comments

10. Followed-up with physician frequently about client status and response to therapy.   ___ ___ ___ _____

11. Removed gloves and goggles; washed hands.   ___ ___ ___ _____

EVALUATION

1. Evaluated client's response to mechanical ventilation.   ___ ___ ___ _____

2. Monitored ABG levels and/or pulse oximetry.   ___ ___ ___ _____

3. Assessed integrity of client's ventilator system.   ___ ___ ___ _____

4. Identified unexpected outcomes.   ___ ___ ___ _____

RECORDING AND REPORTING

1. Recorded method of oxygen delivery, flow rate, and client's response.   ___ ___ ___ _____

2. Reported unexpected findings to nurse in charge or physician.   ___ ___ ___ _____

Student _____ Date _____

Instructor _____ Date _____

PERFORMANCE CHECKLIST 11-5 **MEASURING PEAK EXPIRATORY FLOW RATES (PEFR)**

	S	U	NP	Comments
ASSESSMENT				
1. Observed for signs and symptoms of airway obstruction.	—	—	—	_____
2. Observed for patent airway and need for removal of secretions.	—	—	—	_____
3. Completed total respiratory assessment.	—	—	—	_____
4. Reviewed client's medical record for order to measure PEFR and expected rate client is to achieve.	—	—	—	_____
NURSING DIAGNOSES				
1. Formulated appropriate nursing diagnoses based on assessment data.	—	—	—	_____
PLANNING				
1. Identified expected outcomes.	—	—	—	_____
2. Explained procedure to client and family.	—	—	—	_____
IMPLEMENTATION				
1. Placed indicator at the bottom of the numbered scale.	—	—	—	_____
2. Had client stand up and sit on edge of bed or in high-Fowler's position.	—	—	—	_____
3. Had client take deep breath.	—	—	—	_____
4. Had client place meter in mouth and close lips around mouthpiece.	—	—	—	_____
5. Had client blow out as hard and as fast as possible.	—	—	—	_____
6. Had client repeat Steps 1-5 two more times, noting highest number achieved.	—	—	—	_____
EVALUATION				
1. Determined client's PEFR and compared it with the client's personal best.	—	—	—	_____
2. Reassessed client for improvement in symptoms if bronchodilator therapy has been initiated.	—	—	—	_____
3. Observed client performing PEFR.	—	—	—	_____
4. Identified unexpected outcomes.	—	—	—	_____

	S	U	NP	Comments

RECORDING AND REPORTING

1. Recorded and reported PEFR measurement, client's ability to use peak flowmeter, any symptoms client had, and any therapy client may have received as a result of PEFR measurement.

Student _____ Date _____

Instructor _____ Date _____

PERFORMANCE CHECKLIST 12-1 **PERFORMING POSTURAL DRAINAGE**

	S	U	NP	Comments
ASSESSMENT				
1. Assessed for impairment in airway clearance.	—	—	—	_____
2. Identified signs and symptoms that indicated the need to perform postural drainage.	—	—	—	_____
3. Identified, through appropriate measures, which bronchial segments needed to be drained.	—	—	—	_____
4. Determined client's understanding of and ability to perform home postural drainage.	—	—	—	_____
NURSING DIAGNOSIS				
1. Developed appropriate nursing diagnoses based on assessment data.	—	—	—	_____
PLANNING				
1. Identified expected outcomes.	—	—	—	_____
2. Correctly explained purpose, prepared client for procedure, and instructed client to remove any tight or restrictive clothing.	—	—	—	_____
IMPLEMENTATION				
1. Washed hands and applied gloves.	—	—	—	_____
2. Selected areas to be drained.	—	—	—	_____
3. Correctly positioned client to drain congested areas.	—	—	—	_____
4. Had client maintain position for 10 to 15 minutes.	—	—	—	_____
5. Performed percussion, vibration, or rib shaking with hands in correct position.	—	—	—	_____
6. After drainage in first position, had client sit up and cough; saved expectorated secretions.	—	—	—	_____
7. Allowed client to rest.	—	—	—	_____
8. Had client sip water.	—	—	—	_____
9. Repeated Steps 3-8 for all congested areas in accepted time frame.	—	—	—	_____
10. Washed hands.	—	—	—	_____

	S	U	NP	Comments

EVALUATION

1. Evaluated by auscultation changes in chest assessment after drainage.   ___ ___ ___ _____

2. Assessed character of sputum.   ___ ___ ___ _____

3. Reviewed diagnostic reports on client's pulmonary function.   ___ ___ ___ _____

4. Monitored vital signs and pulse oximetry (if used).   ___ ___ ___ _____

5. Evaluated client's understanding of procedure.   ___ ___ ___ _____

6. Identified unexpected outcomes.   ___ ___ ___ _____

RECORDING AND REPORTING

1. Recorded procedure and client's assessment and response.   ___ ___ ___ _____

2. Recorded client education for home care and referrals.   ___ ___ ___ _____

3. Reported unexpected findings to nurse in charge or physician.   ___ ___ ___ _____

Student _____   Date _____

Instructor _____   Date _____

PERFORMANCE CHECKLIST 12-2 **PERFORMING PERCUSSION, VIBRATION, AND RIB SHAKING**

	S	U	NP	Comments
ASSESSMENT				
1. Assessed client's breathing patterns.	——	——	——	_____
2. Identified signs, symptoms, and conditions that indicated the need to perform skills.	——	——	——	_____
3. Assessed client's rib cage and the bronchial segment being drained.	——	——	——	_____
4. Assessed client's understanding and ability to perform procedure at home.	——	——	——	_____
NURSING DIAGNOSIS				
1. Developed appropriate nursing diagnoses based on assessment data.	——	——	——	_____
PLANNING				
1. Identified expected outcomes.	——	——	——	_____
2. Explained purpose and prepared client for procedure.	——	——	——	_____
IMPLEMENTATION				
1. With client in correct position, assessed and identified chest wall area to be percussed and vibrated.	——	——	——	_____
2. Instructed client in relaxation and breathing techniques.	——	——	——	_____
3. Used proper body mechanics.	——	——	——	_____
4. Performed chest wall percussion, properly cupping hands and clapping chest.	——	——	——	_____
5. Performed chest wall vibration, gently resisting and vibrating with flat part of hand.	——	——	——	_____
6. Assessed client's tolerance of vibration.	——	——	——	_____
7. Performed rib shaking as needed, applying appropriate pressure and rocking motion.	——	——	——	_____
8. Completed vibration and rib shaking in each posture.	——	——	——	_____
9. Taught client and family techniques for percussion, vibration, and rib shaking.	——	——	——	_____

	S	U	NP	Comments

EVALUATION

1. Evaluated changes in chest wall after procedure.　＿＿　＿＿　＿＿　＿＿＿＿＿＿＿＿＿＿

2. Assessed character of mucus.　＿＿　＿＿　＿＿　＿＿＿＿＿＿＿＿＿＿

3. Reviewed diagnostic test results for pulmonary function.　＿＿　＿＿　＿＿　＿＿＿＿＿＿＿＿＿＿

4. Observed caregiver performing percussion, vibration, and rib shaking.　＿＿　＿＿　＿＿　＿＿＿＿＿＿＿＿＿＿

5. Identified unexpected outcomes.　＿＿　＿＿　＿＿　＿＿＿＿＿＿＿＿＿＿

RECORDING AND REPORTING

1. Correctly recorded treatment given and client response.　＿＿　＿＿　＿＿　＿＿＿＿＿＿＿＿＿＿

2. Recorded home teaching given to client and family.　＿＿　＿＿　＿＿　＿＿＿＿＿＿＿＿＿＿

3. Reported unexpected findings to nurse in charge or physician.　＿＿　＿＿　＿＿　＿＿＿＿＿＿＿＿＿＿

Student _____ Date _____

Instructor _____ Date _____

PERFORMANCE CHECKLIST 13-1 **PERFORMING ORAL PHARYNGEAL (YANKAUER) SUCTIONING**

	S	U	NP	Comments

ASSESSMENT

1. Observed for signs and symptoms of airway obstruction requiring oral pharyngeal suctioning.

2. Assessed client's knowledge of catheter use.

3. Identified risk factors.

NURSING DIAGNOSIS

1. Developed appropriate nursing diagnoses based on assessment data.

PLANNING

1. Identified expected outcomes.

2. Explained procedure to client.

3. Positioned client correctly; placed towel across client's chest.

IMPLEMENTATION

1. Washed hands and applied gloves. Applied mask or face shield, if indicated.

2. Filled cup or basin with approximately 100 ml of water.

3. Turned suction device to appropriate pressure.

4. Connected tubing properly and checked that apparatus was functioning properly.

5. Removed oxygen mask, if present.

6. Inserted catheter into client's mouth and suctioned correctly. Encouraged client to cough. Replaced oxygen mask.

7. Rinsed catheter. Turned off suction.

8. Assessed client's respiratory status. Repeated procedure, if indicated.

9. Disposed of towel properly and repositioned client.

10. Discarded water and cup, washed and dried basin, and placed catheter in clean, dry area.

	S	U	NP	Comments
11. Removed and disposed of gloves, mask, and face shield. Washed hands.	___	___	___	_____

EVALUATION

	S	U	NP	Comments
1. Compared assessments before and after procedure.	___	___	___	_____
2. Auscultated chest and airways for adventitious sounds.	___	___	___	_____
3. Observed client or caregiver performing procedure.	___	___	___	_____
4. Identified unexpected outcomes.	___	___	___	_____

RECORDING AND REPORTING

	S	U	NP	Comments
1. Recorded procedure, client's respiratory status, and education provided.	___	___	___	_____
2. Reported changes in client's respiratory status.	___	___	___	_____

Student _____   Date _____

Instructor _____   Date _____

PERFORMANCE CHECKLIST 13-2 **AIRWAY MAINTENANCE: SUCTIONING**

	S	U	NP	Comments
ASSESSMENT				
1. Identified signs and symptoms of upper and lower airway obstruction requiring nasal and oral tracheal suctioning.	—	—	—	_____
2. Assessed for risk factors for airway obstruction.	—	—	—	_____
3. Determined factors that normally influence lower airway functioning.	—	—	—	_____
4. Assessed client's understanding of procedure.	—	—	—	_____
NURSING DIAGNOSIS				
1. Developed appropriate nursing diagnoses based on assessment data.	—	—	—	_____
PLANNING				
1. Identified expected outcomes.	—	—	—	_____
2. Explained procedure and importance of coughing to client.	—	—	—	_____
3. Positioned client.	—	—	—	_____
4. Placed towel across client's chest.	—	—	—	_____
IMPLEMENTATION				
Performing Nasal Pharyngeal and Nasal Tracheal Suctioning				
1. Washed hands and applied face shield.	—	—	—	_____
2. Connected tubing to suction machine, turned suction device on, and set vacuum regulator to appropriate pressure.	—	—	—	_____
3. Increased supplemental oxygen as indicated or ordered by physician. Encouraged deep breathing.	—	—	—	_____
4. Prepared suction catheter correctly.	—	—	—	_____
5. Applied sterile gloves properly.	—	—	—	_____
6. Connected catheter to tubing properly.	—	—	—	_____
7. Checked that equipment was functioning correctly.	—	—	—	_____
8. Coated distal end of catheter with water-soluble lubricant.	—	—	—	_____
9. Removed oxygen delivery device, if present. Inserted catheter gently into naris on inhalation.	—	—	—	_____

	S	U	NP	Comments

10. Applied intermittent suction for up to 10 seconds while withdrawing catheter, encouraging client to cough as appropriate. (Performed tracheal suctioning first.) Replaced oxygen device, if applicable.   ___ ___ ___ _____

11. Rinsed catheter and connecting tubing with saline.   ___ ___ ___ _____

12. Reassessed need to repeat suctioning. Allowed time between suction passes for oxygenation. Asked client to breathe deeply and cough.   ___ ___ ___ _____

13. Performed oral pharyngeal suctioning after trachea and pharynx were cleared of secretions.   ___ ___ ___ _____

14. Discarded catheter correctly. Removed and discarded gloves correctly.   ___ ___ ___ _____

15. Discarded towel and repositioned client.   ___ ___ ___ _____

16. Readjusted oxygen to original level, if indicated.   ___ ___ ___ _____

17. Discarded saline and basin (washed and stored reusable basin).   ___ ___ ___ _____

18. Removed and disposed of face shield. Washed hands.   ___ ___ ___ _____

19. Placed unopened suction kit at head of bed.   ___ ___ ___ _____

20. Assisted client with oral hygiene.   ___ ___ ___ _____

IMPLEMENTATION
Performing Artificial Airway Suctioning

1. Washed hands and applied face shield.   ___ ___ ___ _____

2. Connected tubing to suction machine, turned suction device on, and set vacuum regulator to appropriate pressure.   ___ ___ ___ _____

3. Prepared suction catheter correctly.   ___ ___ ___ _____

4. Applied gloves properly.   ___ ___ ___ _____

5. Connected catheter to tubing properly.   ___ ___ ___ _____

6. Checked that equipment was functioning correctly.   ___ ___ ___ _____

7. Coated distal end of catheter with water-soluble lubricant, if indicated.   ___ ___ ___ _____

8. Oxygenated client.   ___ ___ ___ _____

9. Opened swivel adapter or removed oxygen or humidity device with nondominant hand.   ___ ___ ___ _____

10. Inserted catheter gently and pulled catheter back 1 cm when resistance was met.   ___ ___ ___ _____

	S	U	NP	Comments

11. Applied intermittent suction, encouraging client to cough as appropriate. Observed for respiratory distress.

12. Closed swivel adapter or replaced oxygen delivery device. Encouraged client to breathe deeply.

13. Rinsed catheter and connecting tubing with normal saline.

14. Assessed client's cardiopulmonary status. Repeated Steps 1-13, if needed.

15. Performed nasal and oral pharyngeal suctioning when tracheobroncial tree was clear.

16. Disconnected catheter. Discarded gloves and catheter correctly.

17. Discarded towel.

18. Repositioned client.

19. Discarded saline and basin (washed and stored reusable basin).

20. Removed and discarded face shield. Washed hands.

21. Placed unopened suction kit at head of bed.

EVALUATION

1. Compared assessments before and after suctioning.

2. Asked client if breathing is easier.

3. Observed airway secretions.

4. Identified unexpected outcomes.

RECORDING AND REPORTING

1. Recorded procedure and client assessments.

2. Reported changes in client's respiratory status.

Student _____   Date _____

Instructor _____   Date _____

PERFORMANCE CHECKLIST 13-3 **PERFORMING ENDOTRACHEAL OR TRACHEOSTOMY TUBE SUCTIONING USING A CLOSED SYSTEM (IN-LINE) CATHETER**

	S	U	NP	Comments
ASSESSMENT				
1. Observed for signs and symptoms of lower airway obstruction requiring endotracheal or tracheostomy tube suctioning.	___	___	___	_____
2. Determined factors that influence normal airway function.	___	___	___	_____
3. Examined sputum microbiology data.	___	___	___	_____
4. Assessed client's understanding of procedure and feelings about need to be suctioned.	___	___	___	_____
NURSING DIAGNOSIS				
1. Formulated appropriate nursing diagnoses based on assessment data.	___	___	___	_____
PLANNING				
1. Identified expected outcomes.	___	___	___	_____
2. Explained procedure and importance of coughing to client.	___	___	___	_____
3. Positioned client comfortably.	___	___	___	_____
4. Placed towel across client's chest.	___	___	___	_____
IMPLEMENTATION				
1. Washed hands. Applied gloves.	___	___	___	_____
2. Attached suction according to agency policy and prepared suction apparatus correctly.	___	___	___	_____
3. Hyperinflated and/or hyperoxygenated client according to institutional protocol and clinical status.	___	___	___	_____
4. Unlocked suction control mechanism, if required. Opened saline port and attached saline.	___	___	___	_____
5. Picked up enclosed suction catheter with dominant hand. Advanced catheter and administered saline correctly, if indicated.	___	___	___	_____
6. Inserted catheter correctly after saline dispension.	___	___	___	_____
7. Encouraged client to cough, applied suction correctly, and withdrew catheter.	___	___	___	_____

	S	U	NP	Comments
8. Assessed need for repeated suctioning and performed suctioning, if needed. Reassessed cardiopulmonary status.	___	___	___	_____
9. Withdrew catheter completely and rinsed properly.	___	___	___	_____
10. Performed oral or nasal suctioning, if indicated.	___	___	___	_____
11. Repositioned client.	___	___	___	_____
12. Removed and disposed of gloves. Washed hands.	___	___	___	_____
13. Turned off suction device.	___	___	___	_____

EVALUATION

	S	U	NP	Comments
1. Compared client's respiratory assessments before and after suctioning.	___	___	___	_____
2. Observed airway secretions.	___	___	___	_____
3. Asked client if breathing is easier.	___	___	___	_____
4. Identified unexpected outcomes.	___	___	___	_____

RECORDING AND REPORTING

	S	U	NP	Comments
1. Recorded respiratory assessments before and after suctioning; size of suction catheter used; amount of negative suction pressure used; duration of suctioning period; route(s) used to suction; secretions obtained and odor, amount, color, and consistency; frequency of suctioning; and client's tolerance of procedure.	___	___	___	_____
2. Reported changes in respiratory status.	___	___	___	_____

Student _____   Date _____

Instructor _____   Date _____

PERFORMANCE CHECKLIST 13-4 **PERFORMING ENDOTRACHEAL TUBE CARE**

	S	U	NP	Comments
ASSESSMENT				
1. Observed for signs and symptoms of need to perform endotracheal (ET) tube care.	___	___	___	_____
2. Identified factors placing client at greater risk.	___	___	___	_____
3. Assessed client's knowledge of procedure.	___	___	___	_____
NURSING DIAGNOSIS				
1. Developed appropriate nursing diagnoses based on assessment data.	___	___	___	_____
PLANNING				
1. Identified expected outcomes.	___	___	___	_____
2. Asked another nurse to assist with procedure.	___	___	___	_____
3. Explained procedure and client's participation.	___	___	___	_____
4. Positioned client.	___	___	___	_____
5. Placed towel across client's chest.	___	___	___	_____
IMPLEMENTATION				
1. Washed hands. Applied face shield, if indicated.	___	___	___	_____
2. Administered endotracheal nasal and oral pharyngeal suction.	___	___	___	_____
3. Left suction catheter connected to suction source.	___	___	___	_____
4. Prepared adhesive tape correctly.	___	___	___	_____
5. Applied gloves and instructed assistant to apply gloves and hold ET tube firmly.	___	___	___	_____
6. Removed tape carefully from tube and client's face and discarded tape properly.	___	___	___	_____
7. Cleared excess adhesive from client's face.	___	___	___	_____
8. Removed oral airway or bite block and placed on towel.	___	___	___	_____
9. Cleaned mouth, gums, and teeth opposite ET tube.	___	___	___	_____
10. For oral ET tube only, moved ET tube to opposite side of mouth with assistant's help.	___	___	___	_____
11. Repeated oral cleaning as in Step 9 for second side of mouth.	___	___	___	_____

	S	U	NP	Comments
12. Cleaned and dried client's face and neck. Shaved male client as necessary.	___	___	___	_____
13. Applied small amount of skin protectant to face.	___	___	___	_____
14. Positioned tape carefully under head and neck.	___	___	___	_____
15. Secured tape from ear to naris and secured tape across upper lip if oral ET tube or across top of nose if nasal ET tube.	___	___	___	_____
16. Secured tape to remaining side of face and secured tape to tube correctly.	___	___	___	_____
17. Cleaned and rinsed oral airway.	___	___	___	_____
18. Reinserted oral airway. Secured with tape, if indicated.	___	___	___	_____
19. Discarded soiled items.	___	___	___	_____
20. Repositioned client.	___	___	___	_____
21. Nurse and assistant removed gloves and washed hands. Removed face shield.	___	___	___	_____

EVALUATION

	S	U	NP	Comments
1. Compared assessments before and after procedure.	___	___	___	_____
2. Observed depth and position of ET tube.	___	___	___	_____
3. Assessed security of tape.	___	___	___	_____
4. Assessed skin around mouth and oral mucous membranes.	___	___	___	_____
5. Identified unexpected outcomes.	___	___	___	_____

RECORDING AND REPORTING

	S	U	NP	Comments
1. Recorded appropriate depth of ET tube, frequency of care, procedure, and client assessments.	___	___	___	_____
2. Reported unexpected findings.	___	___	___	_____

Student _____   Date _____

Instructor _____   Date _____

PERFORMANCE CHECKLIST 13-5 **PERFORMING TRACHEOSTOMY CARE**

	S	U	NP	Comments
ASSESSMENT				
1. Observed for signs and symptoms of need to perform tracheostomy care.	___	___	___	_____
2. Observed for factors influencing tracheostomy airway function.	___	___	___	_____
3. Assessed client's understanding of and ability to perform own tracheostomy care.	___	___	___	_____
4. Checked when tracheostomy care was last performed.	___	___	___	_____
NURSING DIAGNOSIS				
1. Developed appropriate nursing diagnoses based on assessment data.	___	___	___	_____
PLANNING				
1. Identified expected outcomes.	___	___	___	_____
2. Asked another nurse or family member to assist with procedure.	___	___	___	_____
3. Explained procedure to client.	___	___	___	_____
4. Positioned client comfortably.	___	___	___	_____
5. Placed towel across client's chest.	___	___	___	_____
IMPLEMENTATION				
1. Washed hands and donned gloves. Applied face shield, if indicated.	___	___	___	_____
2. Suctioned tracheostomy.	___	___	___	_____
3. Prepared equipment at bedside table.	___	___	___	_____
4. Applied gloves. Kept dominant hand sterile throughout procedure.	___	___	___	_____
*5. Removed oxygen source and inner cannula. Dropped inner cannula into hydrogen peroxide basin.	___	___	___	_____
6. Placed tracheostomy collar oxygen source over outer cannula. Placed T-tube and ventilator oxygen sources near outer cannula.	___	___	___	_____

*For tracheostomy tube with inner cannula, nurse completed Steps 5-17. For tracheostomy tube with no inner cannula or Kistner button, nurse completed Steps 9-17.

	S	U	NP	Comments

7. Removed secretions inside and outside of inner cannula. ___ ___ ___ _____

8. Rinsed inner cannula correctly. ___ ___ ___ _____

9. Replaced inner cannula and secured locking mechanism. ___ ___ ___ _____

10. Cleaned outer cannula surfaces and stoma under faceplate with hydrogen-peroxide–soaked cotton swabs. ___ ___ ___ _____

11. Rinsed outer cannula and stoma under faceplate. ___ ___ ___ _____

12. Patted skin and outer cannula lightly with gauze. ___ ___ ___ _____

13. Cut new ties properly with assistant's help, as needed. ___ ___ ___ _____

14. Placed and knotted new ties properly. ___ ___ ___ _____

15. Inserted fresh tracheostomy dressing under clean ties and faceplate. ___ ___ ___ _____

16. Positioned client comfortably and assessed respiratory status. ___ ___ ___ _____

17. Removed and discarded gloves, face shield, and soiled ties correctly. ___ ___ ___ _____

18. Stored supplies correctly. ___ ___ ___ _____

19. Washed hands. ___ ___ ___ _____

EVALUATION

1. Compared assessments before and after procedure. ___ ___ ___ _____

2. Assessed comfort of new tracheostomy ties. ___ ___ ___ _____

3. Observed inner and outer cannula for secretions. ___ ___ ___ _____

4. Assessed stoma for signs of infection or skin breakdown. ___ ___ ___ _____

5. Identified unexpected outcomes ___ ___ ___ _____

RECORDING AND REPORTING

1. Recorded type and size of tracheostomy tube, frequency of care, procedure, and client assessment. ___ ___ ___ _____

2. Reported unexpected findings. ___ ___ ___ _____

Student _____   Date _____

Instructor _____   Date _____

PERFORMANCE CHECKLIST 13-6   **INFLATING THE CUFF ON AN ENDOTRACHEAL OR TRACHEOSTOMY TUBE**

	S	U	NP	Comments
ASSESSMENT				
1. Observed for signs and symptoms indicating need to perform cuff care.	___	___	___	_____
2. Determined caregiver's understanding of procedure if client discharged with a cuffed tracheostomy tube.	___	___	___	_____
NURSING DIAGNOSIS				
1. Developed appropriate nursing diagnoses based on assessment data.	___	___	___	_____
PLANNING				
1. Identified expected outcomes.	___	___	___	_____
2. Explained procedure to client.	___	___	___	_____
3. Positioned client comfortably.	___	___	___	_____
IMPLEMENTATION				
1. Washed hands. Applied gloves and face shield, if indicated.	___	___	___	_____
2. Suctioned client.	___	___	___	_____
3. Connected syringe to pilot balloon.	___	___	___	_____
4. Assessed proper cuff inflation with stethoscope.	___	___	___	_____
5. Removed all air from cuff if no air leak heard.	___	___	___	_____
6. Correctly inflated cuff and assessed for minimal leak with stethoscope.	___	___	___	_____
7. Slowly reinflated cuff if excessive air was heard.	___	___	___	_____
8. Cleansed stethoscope with alcohol wipe after removal.	___	___	___	_____
9. Removed syringe and discarded in appropriate receptacle.	___	___	___	_____
10. Repositioned client.	___	___	___	_____
11. Removed and disposed of gloves and face shield. Washed hands.	___	___	___	_____

	S	U	NP	Comments

EVALUATION

1. Compared assessments before and after proce-dure.

2. Observed exhaled tidal volume from mechanical ventilator.

3. Auscultated for audible air leak.

4. Observed for signs of excessive cuff inflation.

5. Identified unexpected outcomes.

RECORDING AND REPORTING

1. Recorded presence of minimal leak at end inspira-tion, volume of air injected into cuff, secretions obtained when suctioning, and frequency of cuff care.

Student _____   Date _____

Instructor _____   Date _____

PERFORMANCE CHECKLIST 14-1 **CARING FOR CLIENTS WITH CHEST TUBES CONNECTED TO DISPOSABLE DRAINAGE SYSTEMS**

	S	U	NP	Comments

ASSESSMENT

1. Obtained vital signs, oxygen saturation, and pulmonary assessment.

2. Observed for changes in vital signs, increased apprehension, and chest pain.

3. Assessed client for known allergies.

4. Reviewed client's medical record for anticoagulant therapy.

NURSING DIAGNOSIS

1. Developed appropriate nursing diagnoses based on assessment data.

PLANNING

1. Identified expected outcomes.

2. Determined if informed consent was obtained, if required.

3. Reviewed physician's roles and responsibilities for chest tube placement.

4. Explained procedure to client.

5. Gathered necessary equipment and supplies.

6. Washed hands.

7. Prepared prescribed drainage system according to manufacturer's guidelines.

8. Correctly taped all connections and checked systems for patency.

9. Turned off suction source and unclamped drainage tubing before connecting client to system.

10. Positioned client correctly in upright position, to tolerance.

IMPLEMENTATION

1. Washed hands and applied gloves.

2. Administered parenteral medications, if ordered.

3. Assisted physician in providing psychologic support.

4. Showed anesthetic to physician.

	S	U	NP	Comments

5. Held anesthetic solution bottle upside down with label facing physician for withdrawal of solution.   ___ ___ ___ _____

6. Assisted physician in connecting drainage system.   ___ ___ ___ _____

7. Taped the tube connection between the chest and drainage tubes.   ___ ___ ___ _____

8. Assessed patency of air vents in system.   ___ ___ ___ _____

9. Coiled and secured excess tubing on mattress next to client.   ___ ___ ___ _____

10. Promoted drainage by correctly adjusting tubing to hang in a straight line from mattress to drainage chamber.   ___ ___ ___ _____

11. Recorded time that drainage began on appropriate place on system. Assessed client at appropriate intervals.   ___ ___ ___ _____

12. Stripped or milked chest tube, if ordered or indicated.   ___ ___ ___ _____

13. Provided hemostats to remain at bedside.   ___ ___ ___ _____

14. Assisted client to comfortable position.   ___ ___ ___ _____

15. Disposed of soiled equipment and removed gloves.   ___ ___ ___ _____

16. Washed hands.   ___ ___ ___ _____

EVALUATION

1. Monitored vital signs, oxygen saturation, pulmonary status, drainage, and insertion site.   ___ ___ ___ _____

2. Assessed client's physical and psychologic status.   ___ ___ ___ _____

3. Assessed client's compliance in activities of daily living related to care of the drainage system.   ___ ___ ___ _____

4. Assessed collection system for proper functioning and for type and amount of fluid drainage.   ___ ___ ___ _____

5. Assessed for improvement in respiratory status and vital signs.   ___ ___ ___ _____

6. Identified unexpected outcomes.   ___ ___ ___ _____

RECORDING AND REPORTING

1. Recorded baseline vital signs and oxygen saturation.   ___ ___ ___ _____

2. Recorded postoperative vital signs at appropriate time intervals.   ___ ___ ___ _____

3. Recorded chest drainage output at appropriate time intervals.   ___ ___ ___ _____

	S	U	NP	Comments

4. Checked chest tube insertion site and dressings at appropriate time intervals.   ___ ___ ___   _____

5. Documented proper functioning of system.   ___ ___ ___   _____

6. Recorded client's physical and psychologic status at appropriate time intervals.   ___ ___ ___   _____

7. Reported changes in client's status and/or problems with system.   ___ ___ ___   _____

Student _____   Date _____

Instructor _____   Date _____

PERFORMANCE CHECKLIST 14-2 **ASSISTING IN THE REMOVAL OF CHEST TUBES**

	S	U	NP	Comments
ASSESSMENT				
1. Identified signs that reveal lung reexpansion.	—	—	—	_____
2. Clamped chest tube 12 to 24 hours before removal or as ordered by physician.	—	—	—	_____
NURSING DIAGNOSIS				
1. Developed appropriate nursing diagnoses based on assessment data.	—	—	—	_____
PLANNING				
1. Identified expected outcomes.	—	—	—	_____
2. Explained procedure to client.	—	—	—	_____
IMPLEMENTATION				
1. Administered prescribed premedication approximately 30 minutes before procedure.	—	—	—	_____
2. Washed hands and applied gloves and face shield, if needed.	—	—	—	_____
3. Assisted client to correct position.	—	—	—	_____
4. Remained with client while physician or APN prepared occlusive dressing.	—	—	—	_____
5. Supported client physically and emotionally while physician or APN removed dressing and clipped sutures.	—	—	—	_____
6. Assisted client as physician or APN asked client to take a deep breath and hold it or exhale completely and hold it.	—	—	—	_____
7. Remained with client while physician or APN pulled out chest tube.	—	—	—	_____
8. Applied prepared occlusive dressing.	—	—	—	_____
9. Assisted client to comfortable position.	—	—	—	_____
10. Removed used equipment from bedside.	—	—	—	_____
11. Removed gloves. Washed hands.	—	—	—	_____

	S	U	NP	Comments

EVALUATION

1. Observed client for subcutaneous emphysema or respiratory distress during first few hours after removal. ___ ___ ___ _____

2. Assessed client's vital signs, oxygen saturation, pulmonary status, and psychologic status. ___ ___ ___ _____

3. Reviewed chest x-ray. ___ ___ ___ _____

4. Asked client about level of pain or comfort. ___ ___ ___ _____

5. Assessed chest dressing for drainage and patency. ___ ___ ___ _____

6. Identified unexpected outcomes. ___ ___ ___ _____

RECORDING AND REPORTING

1. Recorded removal of tube, amount of drainage, wound appearance, and client assessment. ___ ___ ___ _____

2. Reported client's response to chest tube removal. ___ ___ ___ _____

Student _____ Date _____

Instructor _____ Date _____

PERFORMANCE CHECKLIST 14-3 **REINFUSION OF CHEST TUBE DRAINAGE**

	S	U	NP	Comments
ASSESSMENT				
1. Obtained vital signs, oxygen saturation, and pulmonary status.	—	—	—	_____
2. Observed for changes in vital signs, increased apprehension, and chest pain.	—	—	—	_____
3. Assessed client for known allergies.	—	—	—	_____
4. Reviewed client's medical record for anticoagulant therapy.	—	—	—	_____
5. Determined the presence of active bleeding.	—	—	—	_____
NURSING DIAGNOSIS				
1. Formulated appropriate nursing diagnoses based on assessment data.	—	—	—	_____
PLANNING				
1. Identified expected outcomes.	—	—	—	_____
2. Explained procedure to client.	—	—	—	_____
IMPLEMENTATION				
1. Demonstrated correct technique with system set-up, including proper equipment, tight connections, and maintenance of unit sterility.	—	—	—	_____
2. Washed hands and applied gloves.	—	—	—	_____
3. Performed continuous collection correctly.	—	—	—	_____
a. Opened replacement bag properly and relieved excessive negative pressure.	—	—	—	_____
b. Demonstrated proper technique including correct clamp management for removal of initial bag and securing replacement bag.	—	—	—	_____
4. Completed reinfusion process properly.	—	—	—	_____
a. Used new microaggregate filter for each bag.	—	—	—	_____
b. Accessed bag correctly, and, after priming filter, hung bag for reinfusion.	—	—	—	_____
c. Added any ordered anticoagulants.	—	—	—	_____
5. Discontinued autotransfusion correctly.	—	—	—	_____

	S	U	NP	Comments
6. Reconnected chest drainage tube to unit properly when autotransfusion completed.	___	___	___	_____
7. Discarded used supplies and washed hands.	___	___	___	_____

EVALUATION

	S	U	NP	Comments
1. Monitored vital signs, hematocrit, and hemoglobin.	___	___	___	_____
2. Monitored chest drainage system and client's lung sounds.	___	___	___	_____
3. Assessed the IV infusion site for infiltration and phlebitis.	___	___	___	_____
4. Identified unexpected outcomes.	___	___	___	_____

RECORDING AND REPORTING

	S	U	NP	Comments
1. Recorded drainage and reinfusion, with times and amounts of each.	___	___	___	_____
2. Described the condition of the IV infusion site.	___	___	___	_____
3. Reported unusual findings and client's responses to nurse in charge or physician.	___	___	___	_____

Student _____   Date _____

Instructor _____   Date _____

PERFORMANCE CHECKLIST 15-1   **REMOVING A FOREIGN BODY AIRWAY OBSTRUCTION (FBOAM)**

	S	U	NP	Comments

ASSESSMENT

1. Identified physical signs and symptoms indicating need to perform the foreign body obstruction airway maneuver (FBOAM).   ___ ___ ___ _____

2. Identified factors influencing use of the FBOAM.   ___ ___ ___ _____

3. Identified client and family understanding of the FBOAM and anticipated outcomes.   ___ ___ ___ _____

NURSING DIAGNOSIS

1. Developed appropriate nursing diagnoses based on assessment data.   ___ ___ ___ _____

PLANNING

1. Identified expected outcomes.   ___ ___ ___ _____

2. Positioned client appropriately.   ___ ___ ___ _____

3. Removed dentures or other nonpermanent dental work.   ___ ___ ___ _____

4. Activated emergency medical services.   ___ ___ ___ _____

IMPLEMENTATION

Heimlich Maneuver

Conscious Client, Sitting or Standing

1. Stood behind client and wrapped arms around waist.   ___ ___ ___ _____

2. Kept elbows bent.   ___ ___ ___ _____

3. Made a fist with one hand and placed thumb side against client's abdomen at midline, slightly above the naval and below the xiphoid process.   ___ ___ ___ _____

4. Grasped fist with other hand and pressed into client's abdomen with a quick upward thrust.   ___ ___ ___ _____

5. Repeated abdominal thrusts until object was expelled or client became unconscious.   ___ ___ ___ _____

6. Stopped periodically to assess client.   ___ ___ ___ _____

7. Continued thrusts if client still conscious and obstructed.   ___ ___ ___ _____

	S	U	NP	Comments

Unconscious, Supine Client

1. Positioned client face up.

2. Performed finger sweep.

3. Opened airway and attempted ventilation.

4. Straddled client.

5. Placed heel of one hand against client's abdomen at midline, slightly above the navel and below the xiphoid process.

6. Placed second hand directly on top of first, locking fingers if desired.

7. Pressed into client's abdomen with a quick upward thrust.

8. Repeated up to five times, then attempted finger sweep and ventilation again. Continued until object dislodged or emergency personnel arrived.

Chest Thrusts

Sitting or Standing Client

1. Stood behind client and encircled chest with both arms under client's armpits.

2. Placed thumb side of one fist in middle of client's breastbone, avoiding the xiphoid process and rib cage margin.

3. Grabbed fist with other hand and performed backward thrusts.

4. Repeated until foreign body expelled or client became unconscious.

Supine Client

1. Placed client face up and kneeled close to client's side.

2. Placed heel of one hand over lower half of client's sternum.

3. Pressed inward slowly and distinctly 1½ to 2 inches.

4. Repeated sequence until obstruction was removed. Opened client's mouth periodically to perform finger sweep and attempt ventilation. Continued until airway open or emergency personnel arrived.

Back Blows and Chest Thrusts for Infants

1. Held infant prone on forearm with the infant's head lower than the trunk.

2. Delivered up to five forceful back blows with the heel of the hand.

	S	U	NP	Comments

3. Turned the infant over while supporting the head and body.   ___ ___ ___ _____

4. Provided up to five downward thrusts over the lower third of the sternum.   ___ ___ ___ _____

5. Opened airway to check for foreign body. Removed with finger sweep, if possible.   ___ ___ ___ _____

6. Attempted ventilation.   ___ ___ ___ _____

7. Repeated sequence until foreign body expelled.   ___ ___ ___ _____

Finger Sweep

1. Washed hands and applied gloves and face shield, if possible.   ___ ___ ___ _____

2. Opened client's mouth; grasped tongue and lower jaw with thumb and index finger and lifted up.   ___ ___ ___ _____

3. Inserted index finger of other hand; moved finger along cheek to posterior pharynx using a sweeping or hooking motion. Dislodged foreign body and pulled it out of mouth.   ___ ___ ___ _____

4. Assessed airway, respiratory status, and pulse. Began CPR, if necessary.   ___ ___ ___ _____

5. Continued sequence of finger sweep and thrust as long as necessary.   ___ ___ ___ _____

6. Removed and disposed of gloves and face shield. Washed hands.   ___ ___ ___ _____

EVALUATION

1. Observed that foreign body was removed.   ___ ___ ___ _____

2. Compared client's respiratory status before and after FBOAM.   ___ ___ ___ _____

3. If teaching caregivers, evaluated technique.   ___ ___ ___ _____

4. Identified unexpected outcomes.   ___ ___ ___ _____

RECORDING AND REPORTING

1. Recorded and reported client assessment and maneuver performed.   ___ ___ ___ _____

Student _____ Date _____

Instructor _____ Date _____

PERFORMANCE CHECKLIST 15-2 **INSERTING A NASAL AIRWAY**

	S	U	NP	Comments
ASSESSMENT				
1. Identified signs and symptoms indicating need for insertion of nasal airway.	___	___	___	_____
2. Determined size of nasal airway needed.	___	___	___	_____
3. Assessed client's knowledge of procedure.	___	___	___	_____
NURSING DIAGNOSIS				
1. Developed appropriate nursing diagnoses based on assessment data.	___	___	___	_____
PLANNING				
1. Identified expected outcomes.	___	___	___	_____
2. Explained reasons for insertion of airway and client's participation.	___	___	___	_____
3. Positioned client comfortably.	___	___	___	_____
IMPLEMENTATION				
1. Washed hands. Applied gloves and face shield.	___	___	___	_____
2. Prepared nasal airway.	___	___	___	_____
3. Cleaned excess secretions from client's nares. Determined best naris for insertion.	___	___	___	_____
4. Inserted nasal airway using gentle inward and downward pressure. Had client take slow deep breaths.	___	___	___	_____
5. Cleaned excess lubricant from client's face and nares.	___	___	___	_____
6. Secured airway, if necessary.	___	___	___	_____
7. Placed client in comfortable position.	___	___	___	_____
8. Removed gloves and face shield and discarded in appropriate receptacle. Washed hands.	___	___	___	_____
9. Washed nasal airway at least daily with warm soapy water.	___	___	___	_____
10. Assessed pressure points at end of phalange.	___	___	___	_____
11. Auscultated breath sounds.	___	___	___	_____

	S	U	NP	Comments

EVALUATION

1. Observed nares to determine reduction of edema and bleeding.

2. Observed for patency of airway.

3. Assessed respiratory status and secretions.

4. Observed nares for signs of pressure.

5. Identified unexpected outcomes.

RECORDING AND REPORTING

1. Recorded procedure and client assessment.

2. Reported unexpected findings immediately.

Student _____ Date _____

Instructor _____ Date _____

PERFORMANCE CHECKLIST 15-3 INSERTING AN OROPHARYNGEAL AIRWAY

	S	U	NP	Comments
ASSESSMENT				
1. Identified signs and symptoms indicating need for insertion of an oral airway.	___	___	___	_____
2. Determined factors that normally influence upper airway functioning.	___	___	___	_____
3. Assessed for presence of gag reflex.	___	___	___	_____
4. Assessed client's and family's knowledge of procedure.	___	___	___	_____
NURSING DIAGNOSIS				
1. Developed appropriate nursing diagnoses based on assessment data.	___	___	___	_____
PLANNING				
1. Identified unexpected outcomes.	___	___	___	_____
2. Explained reasons for oral airway insertions and techniques used.	___	___	___	_____
3. Positioned client correctly.	___	___	___	_____
IMPLEMENTATION				
1. Washed hands. Applied nonsterile gloves and face shield.	___	___	___	_____
2. Opened client's mouth.	___	___	___	_____
3. Inserted oral airway correctly.	___	___	___	_____
4. Secured oral airway with tape, if necessary.	___	___	___	_____
5. Suctioned secretions, if needed.	___	___	___	_____
6. Reassessed client's respiratory status.	___	___	___	_____
7. Provided client hygiene after procedure.	___	___	___	_____
8. Discarded tissues, washcloth, gloves, and face shield into appropriate receptacle and washed hands.	___	___	___	_____
9. Administered mouth care frequently.	___	___	___	_____

	S	U	NP	Comments

EVALUATION

1. Compared client's respiratory assessments before and after insertion of oral airway.   ___ ___ ___ _____

2. Assessed patency of airway.   ___ ___ ___ _____

3. Identified unexpected outcomes.   ___ ___ ___ _____

RECORDING AND REPORTING

1. Recorded client assessment and procedure.   ___ ___ ___ _____

2. Reported unexpected findings.   ___ ___ ___ _____

Student _____   Date _____

Instructor _____   Date _____

PERFORMANCE CHECKLIST 15-4 **USING AN AMBU-BAG**

	S	U	NP	Comments
ASSESSMENT				
1. Identified signs and symptoms of need for Ambu-bag manual ventilation.	___	___	___	_____
2. Identified factors affecting respiratory drive.	___	___	___	_____
3. Determined alert client's knowledge of procedure or caregiver's knowledge of procedure.	___	___	___	_____
NURSING DIAGNOSIS				
1. Developed appropriate nursing diagnoses based on assessment data.	___	___	___	_____
PLANNING				
1. Identified expected outcomes.	___	___	___	_____
2. Explained procedure and client's participation.	___	___	___	_____
3. Assisted client with positioning.	___	___	___	_____
IMPLEMENTATION				
1. Washed hands. Applied gloves and face shield if not an emergency procedure.	___	___	___	_____
2. Prepared suction apparatus if needed.	___	___	___	_____
3. Provided supplemental oxygen as needed.	___	___	___	_____
4. For intubated client:	___	___	___	_____
a. Removed oxygen delivery device.	___	___	___	_____
b. Instilled saline into airway appropriately.	___	___	___	_____
c. Connected Ambu-bag to artificial airway and administered 1 breath every 3 to 5 seconds to hyperventilate by compressing Ambu-bag with two hands.	___	___	___	_____
d. Suctioned secretions and repeated preceding steps as needed.	___	___	___	_____
5. For nonintubated client:	___	___	___	_____
a. Inserted oropharyngeal airway.	___	___	___	_____
b. Placed Ambu-bag over client's mouth and nose.	___	___	___	_____
c. Hyperextended client's neck unless contraindicated.	___	___	___	_____

	S	U	NP	Comments
d. Administered breaths according to CPR protocol.	___	___	___	_____
e. Suctioned client as necessary.	___	___	___	_____
6. Assessed client throughout procedure. Continued to provide supplemental ventilation and oxygen until assessment indicated this was no longer necessary.	___	___	___	_____
7. Repeated Steps 4-6 as needed. Replaced oxygen delivery device.	___	___	___	_____
8. Discontinued oxygen supply to bag.	___	___	___	_____
9. Repositioned client appropriately.	___	___	___	_____
10. Cleaned equipment.	___	___	___	_____
11. Removed and disposed of gloves and face shield. Washed hands.	___	___	___	_____

EVALUATION

	S	U	NP	Comments
1. Compared assessments before and after Ambu-bag use.	___	___	___	_____
2. Observed for chest expansion with each ventilation.	___	___	___	_____
3. Observed character of suctioned secretions.	___	___	___	_____
4. Provided for return demonstration if instructing caregivers.	___	___	___	_____
5. Identified unexpected outcomes.	___	___	___	_____

RECORDING AND REPORTING

	S	U	NP	Comments
1. Recorded client assessment and procedure.	___	___	___	_____
2. Reported unexpected findings.	___	___	___	_____

Student _____ Date _____

Instructor _____ Date _____

PERFORMANCE CHECKLIST 15-5 **PERFORMING CARDIOPULMONARY RESUSCITATION**

	S	U	NP	Comments
ASSESSMENT				
1. Determined client's level of consciousness.	___	___	___	_____
2. Activated emergency medical services.	___	___	___	_____
3. Determined presence of carotid pulse and respirations.	___	___	___	_____
NURSING DIAGNOSIS				
1. Developed appropriate nursing diagnoses based on assessment data.	___	___	___	_____
PLANNING				
1. Called for assistance.	___	___	___	_____
2. Identified expected outcomes.	___	___	___	_____
IMPLEMENTATION				
1. Placed victim on hard surface.	___	___	___	_____
2. Positioned self in correct position as one- or two-person rescuer.	___	___	___	_____
3. Applied gloves and face shield, if available.	___	___	___	_____
4. Opened airway by using head tilt-chin lift or jaw thrust maneuver.	___	___	___	_____
5. Inserted oral airway, if available.	___	___	___	_____
6. Administered artificial respiration appropriate to victim's age. Used Ambu-bag, if available.	___	___	___	_____
7. Observed for rise and fall of chest.	___	___	___	_____
8. Suctioned secretions, if necessary, or turned victim's head to side.	___	___	___	_____
9. Correctly assessed for presence of pulse after restoring breathing.	___	___	___	_____
10. Began chest compressions if pulse was absent in a manner appropriate to victim's age.	___	___	___	_____
11. Continued ventilation.	___	___	___	_____
12. Palpated for carotid or brachial pulse.	___	___	___	_____
13. Continued CPR in absence of carotid pulse.	___	___	___	_____
14. Removed and discarded gloves, face shield, and pocket mask.	___	___	___	_____

	S	U	NP	Comments

EVALUATION

1. Assessed carotid pulse at 5-minute intervals. ___ ___ ___ _____

2. Observed for spontaneous return of respirations or heart rate. ___ ___ ___ _____

3. Documented that interruption of CPR did not exceed 5 seconds. ___ ___ ___ _____

4. Identified unexpected outcomes. ___ ___ ___ _____

RECORDING AND REPORTING

1. Reported location of respiratory or cardiopulmonary arrest. ___ ___ ___ _____

2. Recorded onset of arrest, assistance given, and victim's response. ___ ___ ___ _____

Student _____ Date _____

Instructor _____ Date _____

PERFORMANCE CHECKLIST 17-1 **ADMINISTERING ORAL MEDICATIONS**

	S	U	NP	Comments
ASSESSMENT				
1. Assessed whether oral medications should be contraindicated for client.	—	—	—	_____
2. Assessed historical data revealing client's need for or potential response to medications.	—	—	—	_____
3. Assessed extent of client's knowledge regarding health status and medications.	—	—	—	_____
4. Asssessed client's fluid preference and any interaction with prescribed medications.	—	—	—	_____
NURSING DIAGNOSIS				
1. Developed appropriate nursing diagnoses based on assessment data.	—	—	—	_____
PLANNING				
1. Identified expected outcomes.	—	—	—	_____
2. Checked medication administration record (MAR) with order and medication label.	—	—	—	_____
3. Recopied forms that were illegible.	—	—	—	_____
4. Identified client and explained procedure.	—	—	—	_____
IMPLEMENTATION				
Preparing Medications				
1. Washed hands.	—	—	—	_____
2. Arranged forms and supplies.	—	—	—	_____
3. Unlocked medicine drawer or cart.	—	—	—	_____
4. Prepared medications for one client at a time.	—	—	—	_____
5. Compared drug label with MAR or form when selecting medication from supply or unit dose drawer.	—	—	—	_____
6. Calculated dosage correctly.	—	—	—	_____
7. Prepared solid tablets or capsules in medicine cup correctly.	—	—	—	_____
8. Prepared unit dose tablets or capsules correctly.	—	—	—	_____
9. Separated medications requiring preadministration assessment from other drugs.	—	—	—	_____
10. Correctly prepared tablets with pill-crushing device if client had difficulty swallowing.	—	—	—	_____

	S	U	NP	Comments
11. Correctly poured liquid medication without contaminating bottle caps or soiling bottle label.	___	___	___	_____
12. Checked expiration date on all medications.	___	___	___	_____
13. Checked narcotic record for count, if administering narcotics.	___	___	___	_____
14. Compared medication and labeled container with MAR or form second time after preparing drug.	___	___	___	_____
15. Compared medication and labeled container with MAR or form third time when returning stock or unused medications to shelf.	___	___	___	_____
16. Arranged medications together with MAR or form on tray or cart.	___	___	___	_____
17. Did not leave drugs unattended.	___	___	___	_____

Administering Medications

	S	U	NP	Comments
1. Administered drugs at correct time.	___	___	___	_____
2. Identified client by checking name on MAR or form with identification bracelet and asking client to state name.	___	___	___	_____
3. Conducted necessary preadministration assessment.	___	___	___	_____
4. Explained purpose of medications to client.	___	___	___	_____
5. Assisted client to sitting or side-lying position.	___	___	___	_____
6. Administered oral medications correctly, depending on form.	___	___	___	_____
7. Assisted client as needed with placing medication in mouth.	___	___	___	_____
8. If tablet fell, discarded it and repeated procedure.	___	___	___	_____
9. Remained with client and confirmed that medication had been taken.	___	___	___	_____
10. Offered snack after administration of medications irritating to gastric lining.	___	___	___	_____
11. Assisted client in returning to comfortable position.	___	___	___	_____
12. Disposed of soiled supplies and washed hands.	___	___	___	_____
13. Recorded medication administration.	___	___	___	_____
14. Returned MAR or forms to medicine room.	___	___	___	_____
15. Replenished supplies and cleaned work area.	___	___	___	_____

	S	U	NP	Comments

EVALUATION

1. Evaluated client's response to medications 30 minutes after administration.

2. Determined client's or family member's level of knowledge gained about the medication.

3. Identified unexpected outcomes.

RECORDING AND REPORTING

1. Accurately recorded medications in medication record.

2. Recorded and reported if drug was withheld.

3. Reported unexpected findings to nurse in charge or physician.

Student _____   Date _____

Instructor _____   Date _____

PERFORMANCE CHECKLIST 17-2   **ADMINISTERING MEDICATIONS BY NASOGASTRIC TUBE**

	S	U	NP	Comments
ASSESSMENT				
1. Assessed for contraindications to client receiving oral medication.	___	___	___	_____
2. Assessed client's medical history, history of allergies, medications, and diet.	___	___	___	_____
3. Reviewed assessment and laboratory data that may influence drug administration.	___	___	___	_____
4. Verified placement of nasogastric tube before administration of medications.	___	___	___	_____
NURSING DIAGNOSIS				
1. Developed appropriate nursing diagnoses based on assessment data.	___	___	___	_____
PLANNING				
1. Identified expected outcomes.	___	___	___	_____
2. Compared MAR with order and medication label.	___	___	___	_____
3. Identified client.	___	___	___	_____
4. Explained procedure.	___	___	___	_____
IMPLEMENTATION				
1. Washed hands.	___	___	___	_____
2. Prepared medications for administration through tube. Prepared 50 to 100 ml of water in graduated container.	___	___	___	_____
3. Assisted client to high Fowler's position.	___	___	___	_____
4. Applied clean gloves.	___	___	___	_____
5. Verified placement of nasogastric tube.	___	___	___	_____
6. Aspirated stomach contents, noted return, and returned aspirate to client.	___	___	___	_____
7. Prepared syringe for medication delivery.	___	___	___	_____
8. Instilled 30 ml of water and then administered medication, followed by another 30 ml of water.	___	___	___	_____
9. Administered multiple medications with a 5 ml rinse with water between doses.	___	___	___	_____
10. Followed last dose of medication with 30 to 60 ml of water.	___	___	___	_____

	S	U	NP	Comments
11. Clamped off and capped end of tube.	___	___	___	_____
12. Removed gloves, disposed of supplies, and rinsed graduated container. Washed hands.	___	___	___	_____

EVALUATION

	S	U	NP	Comments
1. Returned within 30 minutes to determine client's response to medications or reinstitute continuous tube feedings.	___	___	___	_____
2. Identified unexpected outcomes.	___	___	___	_____

RECORDING AND REPORTING

	S	U	NP	Comments
1. Recorded method used to check tube placement, volume of aspirate, and pH of aspirate (if indicated).	___	___	___	_____
2. Recorded actual time of drug administration on MAR or computer printout.	___	___	___	_____
3. Recorded and reported if drug was withheld.	___	___	___	_____
4. Reported unexpected findings.	___	___	___	_____

Student _____ Date _____

Instructor _____ Date _____

PERFORMANCE CHECKLIST 17-3 **ADMINISTERING SKIN APPLICATIONS**

	S	U	NP	Comments
ASSESSMENT				
1. Assessed condition of client's skin.	—	—	—	_____
2. Inspected area where medication is to be applied.	—	—	—	_____
3. Assessed for presence of drug allergy.	—	—	—	_____
4. Determined amount of topical agent required and directions for use.	—	—	—	_____
5. Assessed client's knowledge regarding medication therapy.	—	—	—	_____
6. Assessed client's ability to self-administer medication.	—	—	—	_____
NURSING DIAGNOSIS				
1. Developed appropriate nursing diagnoses based on assessment data.	—	—	—	_____
PLANNING				
1. Identified expected outcomes.	—	—	—	_____
2. Compared MAR with order and topical agent.	—	—	—	_____
3. Identified client correctly.	—	—	—	_____
4. Explained procedure to client.	—	—	—	_____
IMPLEMENTATION				
1. Washed hands. Arranged supplies at bedside and applied gloves.	—	—	—	_____
2. Closed door or curtain for privacy and positioned client comfortably.	—	—	—	_____
3. Used correct procedure when applying any of the following: cream, ointment, or oil-based lotion; antianginal ointment; patch; aerosol spray; suspension-based lotion; or powder.	—	—	—	_____
4. Covered skin area with dressing when ordered.	—	—	—	_____
5. Assisted client in returning to a comfortable position after application.	—	—	—	_____
6. Removed gloves and properly disposed of soiled supplies. Washed hands.	—	—	—	_____

	S	U	NP	Comments

EVALUATION

1. Evaluated client's or caregiver's knowledge of prescribed medication.   ___ ___ ___ _____

2. Had client keep a diary of dosages taken.   ___ ___ ___ _____

3. Observed client administering medication.   ___ ___ ___ _____

4. Evaluated condition of client's skin between applications.   ___ ___ ___ _____

5. Identified unexpected outcomes.   ___ ___ ___ _____

RECORDING AND REPORTING

1. Recorded condition of client's skin before applying topical agent.   ___ ___ ___ _____

2. Recorded application of topical agent.   ___ ___ ___ _____

3. Recorded and reported if drug was withheld.   ___ ___ ___ _____

4. Reported any abnormalities of skin condition to nurse in charge or physician.   ___ ___ ___ _____

Student _____   Date _____

Instructor _____   Date _____

PERFORMANCE CHECKLIST 17-4 **ADMINISTERING EYE MEDICATIONS**

	S	U	NP	Comments
ASSESSMENT				
1. Reviewed prescriber's medication order.	___	___	___	_____
2. Assessed condition of client's eye.	___	___	___	_____
3. Determined client's history of allergies.	___	___	___	_____
4. Assessed client for symptoms of visual alteration.	___	___	___	_____
5. Assessed client's level of consciousness.	___	___	___	_____
6. Assessed client's knowledge regarding drug therapy.	___	___	___	_____
7. Assessed client's ability to self-administer medication.	___	___	___	_____
NURSING DIAGNOSIS				
1. Developed appropriate nursing diagnoses based on assessment data.	___	___	___	_____
PLANNING				
1. Identified expected outcomes.	___	___	___	_____
2. Compared MAR with order and medication label.	___	___	___	_____
3. Identified client correctly.	___	___	___	_____
4. Explained procedure to client.	___	___	___	_____
IMPLEMENTATION				
1. Washed hands, arranged supplies at bedside, and applied gloves.	___	___	___	_____
2. Positioned client supine or in chair with head slightly hyperextended.	___	___	___	_____
3. Washed existing crusts and drainage from eyelids before drug administration.	___	___	___	_____
4. Placed cotton ball or tissue below lower lid margin.	___	___	___	_____
5. Retracted lower lid downward to expose conjunctival sac.	___	___	___	_____
6. Instructed client to look up.	___	___	___	_____
7. Instilled eye drops correctly.	___	___	___	_____
8. Instilled ointment correctly.	___	___	___	_____

	S	U	NP	Comments
9. Applied intraocular disk correctly. Removed if visible.	___	___	___	_____
10. Wiped away excess medication on eyelids.	___	___	___	_____
11. Applied eye patch, when appropriate.	___	___	___	_____
12. Removed gloves and disposed of soiled supplies properly. Washed hands.	___	___	___	_____
13. Supervised client's self-administration.	___	___	___	_____

EVALUATION

	S	U	NP	Comments
1. Evaluated client's response to medication.	___	___	___	_____
2. Evaluated effects of medication by assessing for visual changes or side effects.	___	___	___	_____
3. Determined client's level of understanding of medication.	___	___	___	_____
4. Had client demonstrate self-administration.	___	___	___	_____
5. Identified unexpected outcomes.	___	___	___	_____

RECORDING AND REPORTING

	S	U	NP	Comments
1. Recorded medication on medication record.	___	___	___	_____
2. Recorded appearance of eye.	___	___	___	_____
3. Recorded and reported if drug was withheld.	___	___	___	_____
4. Reported any undesired effects to nurse in charge or physician.	___	___	___	_____

Student _____   Date _____

Instructor _____   Date _____

PERFORMANCE CHECKLIST 17-5 **ADMINISTERING EAR DROPS**

	S	U	NP	Comments
ASSESSMENT				
1. Reviewed prescriber's medication order.	___	___	___	_____
2. Assessed condition of external ear.	___	___	___	_____
3. Assessed client for symptoms of ear discomfort or hearing impairment.	___	___	___	_____
4. Assessed client's level of cooperation.	___	___	___	_____
5. Assessed client's knowledge of drug therapy.	___	___	___	_____
6. Assessed client's ability to self-administer medication.	___	___	___	_____
NURSING DIAGNOSIS				
1. Developed appropriate diagnoses based on assessment data.	___	___	___	_____
PLANNING				
1. Identified expected outcomes.	___	___	___	_____
2. Compared MAR with order and medication label.	___	___	___	_____
3. Identified client correctly.	___	___	___	_____
4. Explained procedure to client.	___	___	___	_____
IMPLEMENTATION				
1. Washed hands and arranged supplies at bedside.	___	___	___	_____
2. Warmed medication.	___	___	___	_____
3. Assisted client to bedside chair or to side-lying position with ear to be treated facing up.	___	___	___	_____
4. Straightened ear canal correctly.	___	___	___	_____
5. Wiped out cerumen and drainage with cotton applicator.	___	U	___	_____
6. Instilled ordered number of drops, holding dropper 1 cm above ear canal.	___	___	___	_____
7. With client in side-lying position, applied gentle pressure to tragus.	___	___	___	_____
8. Placed cotton ball in outer ear canal, as prescribed.	___	___	___	_____
9. Removed cotton ball after 15 minutes, if prescribed.	___	___	___	_____

	S	U	NP	Comments
10. Disposed of soiled supplies properly and washed hands.	___	___	___	_____
11. Assisted client to comfortable position.	___	___	___	_____

EVALUATION

	S	U	NP	Comments
1. Asked client whether there was discomfort during instillation.	___	___	___	_____
2. Evaluated condition of external ear between drug instillations.	___	___	___	_____
3. Evaluated client's hearing acuity.	___	___	___	_____
4. Asked client to explain technique for instilling ear drops.	___	___	___	_____
5. Had client demonstrate self-administration.	___	___	___	_____
6. Identified unexpected outcomes.	___	___	___	_____

RECORDING AND REPORTING

	S	U	NP	Comments
1. Recorded drug administration correctly on medication form.	___	___	___	_____
2. Recorded condition of ear canal.	___	___	___	_____
3. Reported change in client's hearing acuity.	___	___	___	_____
4. Recorded and reported if drug was withheld.	___	___	___	_____
5. Reported unexpected findings to nurse in charge or physician.	___	___	___	_____

Student _____   Date _____

Instructor _____   Date _____

PERFORMANCE CHECKLIST 17-6 **ADMINISTERING EAR IRRIGATIONS**

	S	U	NP	Comments
ASSESSMENT				
1. Reviewed prescriber's medication order.	___	___	___	_____
2. Reviewed medical record for history of ruptured tympanic membrane.	___	___	___	_____
3. Inspected condition of pinna and external auditory meatus.	___	___	___	_____
4. Determined if client was experiencing discomfort.	___	___	___	_____
5. Assessed client's knowledge regarding medication therapy.	___	___	___	_____
NURSING DIAGNOSIS				
1. Developed appropriate nursing diagnoses based on assessment data.	___	___	___	_____
PLANNING				
1. Identified expected outcomes.	___	___	___	_____
2. Compared MAR with order and medication label.	___	___	___	_____
3. Identified client correctly.	___	___	___	_____
4. Instilled mineral oil into ear for 2 to 3 days prior if client had impacted cerumen.	___	___	___	_____
5. Explained procedure to client.	___	___	___	_____
IMPLEMENTATION				
1. Washed hands. Arranged supplies at bedside and applied gloves.	___	___	___	_____
2. Closed curtain or room door for privacy.	___	___	___	_____
3. Positioned client in sitting or lying position with head turned toward affected ear.	___	___	___	_____
4. Poured irrigation solution into sterile basin.	___	___	___	_____
5. Gently cleaned auricle and ear canal with moistened cotton applicator.	___	___	___	_____
6. Filled irrigation syringe with solution.	___	___	___	_____
7. Correctly positioned ear to allow fluid to flow over length of canal.	___	___	___	_____
8. Slowly instilled irrigation solution.	___	___	___	_____
9. Did not occlude canal with syringe tip.	___	___	___	_____

	S	U	NP	Comments

10. Dried outer ear canal with cotton ball and left cotton ball in place for 5 to 10 minutes.   ___ ___ ___ _____

11. Assisted client to sitting position.   ___ ___ ___ _____

12. Removed gloves and properly disposed of supplies. Washed hands.   ___ ___ ___ _____

EVALUATION

1. Determined if client had discomfort during instillation.   ___ ___ ___ _____

2. Inspected condition of meatus and canal.   ___ ___ ___ _____

3. Assessed client's hearing acuity.   ___ ___ ___ _____

4. Determined client's understanding of procedure and techniques for ear care.   ___ ___ ___ _____

5. Identified unexpected outcomes.   ___ ___ ___ _____

RECORDING AND REPORTING

1. Recorded procedure, amount of solution, time, and ear receiving irrigation.   ___ ___ ___ _____

2. Recorded appearance of external ear and client's hearing acuity.   ___ ___ ___ _____

3. Recorded and reported if drug was withheld.   ___ ___ ___ _____

4. Reported and recorded any side effects to nurse in charge or physician.   ___ ___ ___ _____

Student _____   Date _____

Instructor _____   Date _____

PERFORMANCE CHECKLIST 17-7 **ADMINISTERING NASAL INSTILLATIONS**

	S	U	NP	Comments
ASSESSMENT				
1. Determined affected nasal sinus.	___	___	___	_____
2. Assessed client's history to determine contraindication of drug.	___	___	___	_____
3. Assessed condition of nares and sinuses.	___	___	___	_____
4. Assessed client's knowledge regarding use of nasal instillations.	___	___	___	_____
NURSING DIAGNOSIS				
1. Developed appropriate nursing diagnoses based on assessment data.	___	___	___	_____
PLANNING				
1. Identified expected outcomes.	___	___	___	_____
2. Compared MAR with order and medication label.	___	___	___	_____
3. Identified client correctly.	___	___	___	_____
4. Explained procedure to client.	___	___	___	_____
IMPLEMENTATION				
1. Washed hands and arranged supplies and medications at bedside.	___	___	___	_____
2. Instructed client to blow nose gently, unless contraindicated.	___	___	___	_____
3. Administered nasal drops:	___	___	___	_____
a. Assisted client to supine position.	___	___	___	_____
b. Positioned head to access pharynx or sinuses.	___	___	___	_____
c. Supported client's head with nondominant hand.	___	___	___	_____
d. Instructed client to breathe through mouth.	___	___	___	_____
e. Held dropper 1 cm (½ in) above nares and instilled prescribed drops.	___	___	___	_____
f. Had client remain supine for 5 minutes.	___	___	___	_____
g. Offered tissue to blot nose.	___	___	___	_____
4. Assisted client to comfortable position.	___	___	___	_____
5. Disposed of soiled supplies and washed hands.	___	___	___	_____

	S	U	NP	Comments

EVALUATION

1. Observed client for side effects of medication.   ___ ___ ___ _____

2. Evaluated client's ability to breathe through nose.   ___ ___ ___ _____

3. Inspected condition of nasal passages.   ___ ___ ___ _____

4. Asked client to review knowledge regarding use of decongestant and methods of administration.   ___ ___ ___ _____

5. Had client demonstrate self-administration.   ___ ___ ___ _____

6. Identified unexpected outcomes.   ___ ___ ___ _____

RECORDING AND REPORTING

1. Recorded medication administration correctly on medication record.   ___ ___ ___ _____

2. Recorded client's response to medication.   ___ ___ ___ _____

3. Recorded and reported if drug was withheld.   ___ ___ ___ _____

4. Reported any unusual side effects to nurse in charge or physician.   ___ ___ ___ _____

Student _____ Date _____

Instructor _____ Date _____

PERFORMANCE CHECKLIST 17-8 **USING METERED-DOSE INHALERS**

	S	U	NP	Comments

ASSESSMENT

1. Assessed client's respiratory status.

2. Assessed client's readiness to learn.

3. Assessed client's ability to learn.

4. Assessed client's knowledge of disease and drug therapy.

5. Assessed client's ability to handle inhaler.

6. Assessed drug schedule and number of prescribed inhalations.

7. Assessed client's technique in using inhaler (when applicable).

NURSING DIAGNOSIS

1. Developed appropriate nursing diagnoses based on assessment data.

PLANNING

1. Identified expected outcomes.

2. Compared MAR with order and medication label.

3. Identified client correctly.

4. Explained procedure.

5. Provided adequate time for teaching.

IMPLEMENTATION

1. Washed hands and arranged equipment.

2. Provided client opportunity to handle inhaler, canister, and spacer.

3. Explained metered dosage and problems of overuse, including side effects.

4. Explained each step in using inhaler.

 a. Removed mouthpiece cover.

 b. Shook inhaler well.

 c. Had client take deep breath and exhale.

 d. Instructed client about how to position inhaler.

 e. Had client hold inhaler.

	S	U	NP	Comments

f. Instructed client to tilt head back, inhale slowly and deeply through the mouth, and depress medication canister fully. ___ ___ ___ _____

g. Had client hold breath for 10 seconds. ___ ___ ___ _____

h. Instructed client to exhale slowly through nose or pursed lips. ___ ___ ___ _____

5. Explained each step in using an inhaler with a spacer device: ___ ___ ___ _____

a. Removed mouthpiece covers. ___ ___ ___ _____

b. Inserted metered-dose inhaler into end of spacer device. ___ ___ ___ _____

c. Shook inhaler well. ___ ___ ___ _____

d. Had client place spacer device mouthpiece in mouth and close lips. ___ ___ ___ _____

e. Instructed client to breathe normally through space device mouthpiece. ___ ___ ___ _____

f. Had client depress medication canister, spraying one puff into spacer. ___ ___ ___ _____

g. Instructed client to breathe in slowly and fully for 5 seconds. ___ ___ ___ _____

h. Had client hold breath for 5 to 10 seconds. ___ ___ ___ _____

6. Instructed client on the correct interval between inhalations. ___ ___ ___ _____

7. Warned client against increasing the frequency of inhalations. ___ ___ ___ _____

8. Described common sensations after use of inhaler. ___ ___ ___ _____

9. Instructed client in technique for cleansing inhaler. ___ ___ ___ _____

10. Asked if client had questions. ___ ___ ___ _____

EVALUATION

1. Had client demonstrate use of inhaler. ___ ___ ___ _____

2. Asked client to explain drug schedule. ___ ___ ___ _____

3. Asked client to explain medication side effects. ___ ___ ___ _____

4. Assessed respirations and lung sounds after medication instillation. ___ ___ ___ _____

5. Identified unexpected outcomes. ___ ___ ___ _____

	S	U	NP	Comments

RECORDING AND REPORTING

1. Recorded description of teaching session and client's response. ____ ____ ____ _____

2. Recorded times used and amount (puffs). Reported if drug was withheld. ____ ____ ____ _____

3. Recorded client assessment and response to medication. ____ ____ ____ _____

4. Reported any undesirable effects from medication. ____ ____ ____ _____

Student _____   Date _____

Instructor _____   Date _____

PERFORMANCE CHECKLIST 17-9   **USING SMALL-VOLUME NEBULIZERS**

	S	U	NP	Comments
ASSESSMENT				
1. Assessed client's medical history.	___	___	___	_____
2. Assessed client's ability to manipulate nebulizer equipment.	___	___	___	_____
3. Assessed drug ordered.	___	___	___	_____
4. Assessed client's vital signs.	___	___	___	_____
NURSING DIAGNOSIS				
1. Developed appropriate nursing diagnoses based on assessment data.	___	___	___	_____
PLANNING				
1. Identified expected outcomes.	___	___	___	_____
2. Checked MAR with order and medication label.	___	___	___	_____
3. Identified client.	___	___	___	_____
4. Explained procedure.	___	___	___	_____
IMPLEMENTATION				
1. Washed hands and arranged equipment.	___	___	___	_____
2. Explained use of nebulizer and possible side effects.	___	___	___	_____
3. Assembled equipment according to the manufacturer's instructions.	___	___	___	_____
4. Added prescribed medication and diluent to nebulizer.	___	___	___	_____
5. Had client hold mouthpiece between lips with gentle pressure. Used mask or special adapter, if necessary.	___	___	___	_____
6. Had client take a slow, deep breath, pause, and then exhale passively.	___	___	___	_____
7. Turned on the nebulizer machine and ensured that sufficient mist formed.	___	___	___	_____
8. Tapped nebulizer cup periodically.	___	___	___	_____
9. Reminded client to repeat breathing pattern until medication completely nebulized or as ordered.	___	___	___	_____
10. Monitored client's pulse during procedure.	___	___	___	_____

	S	U	NP	Comments

11. Turned off machine and stored tubing according to agency policy.   ___ ___ ___ _____

12. Shook nebulizer bottle to remove remaining solution. Did not rinse with tap water.   ___ ___ ___ _____

13. Encouraged client to rinse mouth if steroids were used.   ___ ___ ___ _____

EVALUATION

1. Assessed client's pulse, respiratory rate, and lung sounds.   ___ ___ ___ _____

2. Had client explain and demonstrate steps.   ___ ___ ___ _____

3. Asked client to explain drug schedule, side effects, and criteria for calling physician.   ___ ___ ___ _____

4. Identified unexpected outcomes.   ___ ___ ___ _____

RECORDING AND REPORTING

1. Recorded medication immediately after administration.   ___ ___ ___ _____

2. Recorded client's response to medication.   ___ ___ ___ _____

3. Documented instruction provided and client's ability to perform treatment.   ___ ___ ___ _____

4. Recorded and reported if drug was withheld.   ___ ___ ___ _____

5. Reported adverse effects to nurse in charge or physician.   ___ ___ ___ _____

Student _____   Date _____

Instructor _____   Date _____

PERFORMANCE CHECKLIST 17-10 **ADMINISTERING VAGINAL INSTILLATIONS**

	S	U	NP	Comments
ASSESSMENT				
1. Reviewed prescriber's medication order.	___	___	___	_____
2. Reviewed pertinent drug information.	___	___	___	_____
3. Had client void.	___	___	___	_____
4. Determined client's ability to self-administer medication.	___	___	___	_____
5. Reviewed client's knowledge of drug therapy.	___	___	___	_____
NURSING DIAGNOSIS				
1. Developed appropriate nursing diagnoses based on assessment data.	___	___	___	_____
PLANNING				
1. Identified expected outcomes.	___	___	___	_____
2. Compared MAR with order and medication label.	___	___	___	_____
3. Identified client correctly.	___	___	___	_____
4. Explained procedure to client.	___	___	___	_____
IMPLEMENTATION				
1. Washed hands and arranged supplies at bedside.	___	___	___	_____
2. Closed room door or curtain.	___	___	___	_____
3. Assisted client to dorsal recumbent position.	___	___	___	_____
4. Kept lower extremities and abdomen draped.	___	___	___	_____
5. Donned disposable gloves.	___	___	___	_____
6. Illuminated vaginal orifice properly.	___	___	___	_____
7. Inspected condition of external genitalia and vaginal canal.	___	___	___	_____
8. For suppository insertion:	___	___	___	_____
a. Removed suppository from wrapper and applied water-soluble lubricant to smooth or rounded end.	___	___	___	_____
b. Lubricated gloved index finger of dominant hand.	___	___	___	_____
c. Separated labia with nondominant gloved hand.	___	___	___	_____

	S	U	NP	Comments

d. Inserted suppository the entire length of finger along posterior wall of vaginial canal.   ___ ___ ___ _____

e. Withdrew finger and wiped away remaining lubricant.   ___ ___ ___ _____

9. For application of cream or foam: ___ ___ ___ _____

   a. Filled applicator according to directions.   ___ ___ ___ _____

   b. Separated labial folds with nondominant gloved hand.   ___ ___ ___ _____

   c. Inserted applicators 5 to 7.5 cm (2 to 3 in) and pushed on plunger to deposit medication.   ___ ___ ___ _____

   d. Withdrew applicator and wiped off residual cream or foam.   ___ ___ ___ _____

10. For irrigation and douche: ___ ___ ___ _____

   a. Placed client on bedpan with absorbent pad underneath.   ___ ___ ___ _____

   b. Made sure fluid was at body temperature, and primed tubing.   ___ ___ ___ _____

   c. Separated labial folds and directed nozzle toward sacrum, along the floor of the vagina.   ___ ___ ___ _____

   d. Raised container to 30 to 50 cm (12 to 20 in) above the vagina.   ___ ___ ___ _____

   e. Inserted nozzle 7 to 10 cm (3 to 4 in) and allowed solution to flow while rotating nozzle.   ___ ___ ___ _____

   f. Withdrew nozzle after all solution administered.   ___ ___ ___ _____

   g. Assisted client to comfortable sitting position.   ___ ___ ___ _____

   h. Allowed client to remain on bedpan and cleansed perineum with soap and water.   ___ ___ ___ _____

   i. Assisted client off bedpan and dried perineum.   ___ ___ ___ _____

11. Instructed client to lie flat for at least 10 minutes after suppository, cream, or foam insertion.   ___ ___ ___ _____

12. If applicator was used, washed it with soap and water, rinsed, and stored.   ___ ___ ___ _____

13. Offered client perineal pad.   ___ ___ ___ _____

14. Disposed of soiled supplies and equipment.   ___ ___ ___ _____

15. Removed gloves properly and discarded them.   ___ ___ ___ _____

	S	U	NP	Comments

EVALUATION

1. Inspected condition of vaginal canal and external genitalia between applications. ___ ___ ___ _____

2. Evaluated client for symptoms of vaginal irritation. ___ ___ ___ _____

3. Evaluated client's understanding of medication therapy. ___ ___ ___ _____

4. Had client demonstrate self-administration. ___ ___ ___ _____

5. Identified unexpected outcomes. ___ ___ ___ _____

RECORDING AND REPORTING

1. Recorded medication correctly on medication record. ___ ___ ___ _____

2. Recorded appearance of vaginal canal and genitalia and reported any unusual findings to nurse in charge or physician. ___ ___ ___ _____

3. Recorded and reported if drug was withheld. ___ ___ ___ _____

Student _____   Date _____

Instructor _____   Date _____

PERFORMANCE CHECKLIST 17-11 **ADMINISTERING RECTAL SUPPOSITORIES**

	S	U	NP	Comments
ASSESSMENT				
1. Reviewed prescriber's medication order.	___	___	___	_____
2. Reviewed pertinent drug information.	___	___	___	_____
3. Determined whether client had history of rectal surgery or bleeding.	___	___	___	_____
4. Assessed for signs and symptoms of gastrointestinal alterations.	___	___	___	_____
5. Assessed client's ability to self-administer suppository.	___	___	___	_____
6. Reviewed client's knowledge of drug therapy.	___	___	___	_____
NURSING DIAGNOSIS				
1. Developed appropriate nursing diagnoses based on assessment data.	___	___	___	_____
PLANNING				
1. Identified expected outcomes.	___	___	___	_____
2. Compared MAR with order and medication label.	___	___	___	_____
3. Identified client correctly.	___	___	___	_____
4. Explained procedure to client.	___	___	___	_____
IMPLEMENTATION				
1. Washed hands. Arranged supplies at bedside and applied gloves.	___	___	___	_____
2. Closed curtain or room door for privacy.	___	___	___	_____
3. Assisted client to side-lying Sims' position with upper leg flexed upward.	___	___	___	_____
4. Kept client properly draped.	___	___	___	_____
5. Examined condition of anus externally and palpated rectal wall as needed; disposed of gloves properly.	___	___	___	_____
6. Applied new disposable gloves.	___	___	___	_____
7. Removed suppository from wrapper and lubricated rounded end.	___	___	___	_____
8. Instructed client to breathe slowly through mouth and relax anal sphincter.	___	___	___	_____

	S	U	NP	Comments

9. Retracted buttocks and inserted suppository gently through anus for proper distance.

10. Cleaned excess lubricant from anal area.

11. Properly disposed of gloves.

12. Asked client to remain flat or on side for 5 minutes.

13. Placed call light within client's reach after drug administration.

14. Washed hands and disposed of supplies and equipment.

EVALUATION

1. Determined whether suppository was prematurely expelled.

2. Determined whether there was any discomfort during insertion.

3. Evaluated effect of medication.

4. Determined client's understanding of purpose of medication.

5. Had client demonstrate self-administration.

6. Identified unexpected outcomes.

RECORDING AND REPORTING

1. Recorded medication correctly on medication record.

2. Recorded and reported client's response to medication and if drug was withheld.

3. Reported unexpected reactions.

Student _____   Date _____

Instructor _____   Date _____

PERFORMANCE CHECKLIST 18-1 **PREPARING INJECTIONS FROM AMPULES AND VIALS**

	S	U	NP	Comments
ASSESSMENT				
1. Assessed client's body build, muscle size, and weight.	___	___	___	_____
2. Considered medication and type of injection.	___	___	___	_____
PLANNING				
1. Identified expected outcomes.	___	___	___	_____
2. Checked MAR or computer printout.	___	___	___	_____
IMPLEMENTATION				
1. Washed hands.	___	___	___	_____
2. Arranged supplies at work area in medicine room.	___	___	___	_____
3. Checked medication card, form, or printout against label on ampule or vial.	___	___	___	_____
Ampule Preparation				
1. Tapped top of ampule to dislodge fluid in neck.	___	___	___	_____
2. Placed gauze pad around ampule neck.	___	___	___	_____
3. Snapped neck of ampule away from hands.	___	___	___	_____
4. Drew up medication quickly; while holding ampule upright or upside down, inserted needle through opening in center of ampule.	___	___	___	_____
5. Aspirated medication.	___	___	___	_____
6. Kept needle tip below fluid level.	___	___	___	_____
7. Did not expel air into ampule.	___	___	___	_____
8. Expelled air from syringe correctly.	___	___	___	_____
9. Correctly expelled excess fluid within syringe into sink.	___	___	___	_____
10. Covered needle with sheath or cap after preparation and changed needle or syringe.	___	___	___	_____
11. Disposed of soiled supplies and placed ampule in special container. Cleaned work area. Washed hands.	___	___	___	_____
Vial Preparation				
1. Removed metal cap from vial to expose rubber seal.	___	___	___	_____

	S	U	NP	Comments

2. Wiped off surface of seal with alcohol swab. ___ ___ ___ _____

3. Drew up air in syringe (with vial adapter or needle) equivalent to volume of medication desired. ___ ___ ___ _____

4. Inserted needle tip, bevel up, through center of rubber seal. ___ ___ ___ _____

5. Injected air into airspace of vial while holding on to plunger. ___ ___ ___ _____

6. With vial inverted, held vial and syringe properly. ___ ___ ___ _____

7. Kept needle tip/adapter below fluid level. ___ ___ ___ _____

8. Allowed air pressure to fill syringe with fluid. ___ ___ ___ _____

9. Correctly dislodged and expelled air that accumulated in syringe barrel. ___ ___ ___ _____

10. Removed needle/adapter from vial. ___ ___ ___ _____

11. Correctly expelled any remaining air in syringe barrel. ___ ___ ___ _____

12. Changed needle and cover on syringe. ___ ___ ___ _____

13. Labeled multidose vial with date of mixing, drug concentration, and nurse's initials. ___ ___ ___ _____

14. Disposed of soiled supplies in proper container. Cleaned work area and washed hands. ___ ___ ___ _____

Reconstituting Medications
1. Removed cap covering vial containing powder and vial containing diluent. ___ ___ ___ _____

2. Wiped surfaces of seals with alcohol. ___ ___ ___ _____

3. Correctly drew up diluent into syringe. ___ ___ ___ _____

4. Correctly injected diluent into vial with powder. Removed needle. ___ ___ ___ _____

5. Mixed medication thoroughly. ___ ___ ___ _____

6. Prepared to draw correct dosage of reconstituted solution into new syringe. ___ ___ ___ _____

EVALUATION
1. Checked dosage level in syringe. ___ ___ ___ _____

2. Identified unexpected outcomes. ___ ___ ___ _____

Student _____   Date _____

Instructor _____   Date _____

PERFORMANCE CHECKLIST 18-2 **MIXING MEDICATIONS FROM TWO VIALS**

	S	U	NP	Comments
ASSESSMENT				
1. Compared MAR with order and medication label.	___	___	___	_____
2. Assessed client's body build, muscle size, and weight.	___	___	___	_____
3. Considered medications to be mixed and type of injection.	___	___	___	_____
4. Checked expiration date of medication.	___	___	___	_____
PLANNING				
1. Identified expected outcomes.	___	___	___	_____
IMPLEMENTATION				
1. Washed hands.	___	___	___	_____
2. Arranged supplies at work area in medicine room.	___	___	___	_____
Mixing Medications from Vials				
1. Took syringe and aspirated volume of air equal to first medication's dosage (vial A).	___	___	___	_____
2. Injected air into vial A without allowing needle to touch solution.	___	___	___	_____
3. Withdrew needle and syringe and aspirated air equal to second medication's dosage (vial B).	___	___	___	_____
4. Inserted needle into vial B, injected air, and filled syringe with proper volume of medication from vial.	___	___	___	_____
5. Withdrew needle and syringe from vial and checked dose.	___	___	___	_____
6. Determined point on scale for correct dosage of combined medications.	___	___	___	_____
7. Inserted needle into vial A and allowed solution to fill syringe to desired level.	___	___	___	_____
8. Withdrew needle and expelled excess air.	___	___	___	_____
9. Changed needle on syringe.	___	___	___	_____
10. Disposed of soiled needle and supplies in proper container.	___	___	___	_____
11. Washed hands.	___	___	___	_____

	S	U	NP	Comments

Mixing Insulin

1. Took insulin syringe and aspirated volume of air equal to dosage to be withdrawn from modified insulin (cloudy vial). ___ ___ ___ _____

2. Injected air into vial of modified insulin without needle touching solution. ___ ___ ___ _____

3. Withdrew needle and syringe from vial and aspirated air equal to dosage to be withdrawn from unmodified regular insulin (clear vial). ___ ___ ___ _____

4. Inserted needle into vial of unmodified regular insulin (clear vial), injected air, and filled syringe with correct dosage. ___ ___ ___ _____

5. Withdrew needle and syringe from vial and checked dose. ___ ___ ___ _____

6. Determined point on syringe scale for correct dosage of combined medications. ___ ___ ___ _____

7. Inserted needle into vial of modified insulin (cloudy vial), and correctly withdrew desired amount of insulin. ___ ___ ___ _____

8. Withdrew needle and checked fluid level in syringe. ___ ___ ___ _____

9. Disposed of soiled supplies in proper container. ___ ___ ___ _____

10. Washed hands. ___ ___ ___ _____

EVALUATION

1. Checked syringe scale for correct dosage of combined medications. ___ ___ ___ _____

2. Identified unexpected outcomes. ___ ___ ___ _____

Student _____   Date _____

Instructor _____   Date _____

PERFORMANCE CHECKLIST 18-3 **ADMINISTERING INTRADERMAL INJECTIONS**

	S	U	NP	Comments
ASSESSMENT				
1. Reviewed medication order.	___	___	___	_____
2. Assessed type of reaction to expect when testing skin.	___	___	___	_____
3. Assessed client's history of allergies.	___	___	___	_____
4. Assessed client's knowledge regarding procedure.	___	___	___	_____
NURSING DIAGNOSIS				
1. Developed appropriate nursing diagnoses based on assessment data.	___	___	___	_____
PLANNING				
1. Identified expected outcomes.	___	___	___	_____
2. Washed hands.	___	___	___	_____
3. Prepared correct dosage from ampule or vial and checked dosage.	___	___	___	_____
4. Correctly identified client.	___	___	___	_____
5. Explained steps of procedure and expected sensations.	___	___	___	_____
IMPLEMENTATION				
1. Provided for client's privacy.	___	___	___	_____
2. Chose appropriate injection site and inspected skin surface for lesions or discoloration.	___	___	___	_____
3. Positioned client appropriately.	___	___	___	_____
4. Had client flex elbow and support it on flat surface.	___	___	___	_____
5. Washed hands and applied disposable gloves.	___	___	___	_____
6. Cleansed injection site.	___	___	___	_____
7. Held swab correctly.	___	___	___	_____
8. Removed needle cap correctly.	___	___	___	_____
9. Held syringe comfortably with bevel of needle pointing up.	___	___	___	_____
10. Stretched skin over injection site.	___	___	___	_____
11. With needle at 5- to 15-degree angle, injected slowly through epidermis just below skin surface.	___	___	___	_____

	S	U	NP	Comments

12. Injected medication slowly and felt normal resistance.   ___ ___ ___ _____

13. Noticed appearance of small bleb on skin.   ___ ___ ___ _____

14. Withdrew needle slowly with swab supporting site.   ___ ___ ___ _____

15. Did not massage site.   ___ ___ ___ _____

16. Assisted client to comfortable position.   ___ ___ ___ _____

17. Discarded uncapped needles and syringes properly.   ___ ___ ___ _____

18. Removed gloves and washed hands.   ___ ___ ___ _____

EVALUATION

1. Remained with client to observe for allergic reaction.   ___ ___ ___ _____

2. With skin pencil, drew circle around perimeter of injection site and read site within appropriate time.   ___ ___ ___ _____

3. Encouraged client to discuss implications of skin testing.   ___ ___ ___ _____

4. Identified unexpected outcomes.   ___ ___ ___ _____

RECORDING AND REPORTING

1. Recorded test substance data correctly on medication record.   ___ ___ ___ _____

2. Recorded area of injection and appearance of skin.   ___ ___ ___ _____

3. Reported any undesirable effects from medication to nurse in charge or physician.   ___ ___ ___ _____

Student _____   Date _____

Instructor _____   Date _____

PERFORMANCE CHECKLIST 18-4 **ADMINISTERING SUBCUTANEOUS INJECTIONS**

	S	U	NP	Comments
ASSESSMENT				
1. Reviewed medication order.	—	—	—	_____
2. Gathered information pertaining to ordered drug.	—	—	—	_____
3. Assessed contraindications for subcutaneous injections.	—	—	—	_____
4. Assessed indications for subcutaneous injections.	—	—	—	_____
5. Assessed client's medical, medication, and allergy history.	—	—	—	_____
6. Considered adequacy of client's adipose tissue.	—	—	—	_____
7. Assessed client's medication knowledge.	—	—	—	_____
8. Observed client's behavioral reaction to receiving injection.	—	—	—	_____
NURSING DIAGNOSIS				
1. Developed appropriate nursing diagnoses based on assessment data.	—	—	—	_____
PLANNING				
1. Identified expected outcomes.	—	—	—	_____
2. Checked MAR or computer printout.	—	—	—	_____
3. Correctly prepared medication in syringe and checked dosage.	—	—	—	_____
4. Correctly identified client receiving medication.	—	—	—	_____
5. Explained procedure to client.	—	—	—	_____
IMPLEMENTATION				
1. Provided for client's privacy.	—	—	—	_____
2. Washed hands and applied disposable gloves.	—	—	—	_____
3. Kept sheet or gown draped over body parts not requiring exposure.	—	—	—	_____
4. Selected appropriate injection site through inspection and palpation of tissues.	—	—	—	_____
5. If daily administration required, correctly rotated injection site.	—	—	—	_____
6. Accurately determined correct needle size.	—	—	—	_____
7. Assisted client to comfortable position.	—	—	—	_____

	S	U	NP	Comments
8. Relocated site using anatomic landmarks.	___	___	___	_____
9. Cleansed site with antiseptic swab.	___	___	___	_____
10. Held swab between third and fourth fingers of nondominant hand.	___	___	___	_____
11. Removed needle cap correctly.	___	___	___	_____
12. Held syringe comfortably in dominant hand with palm upward.	___	___	___	_____
13. Injected needle quickly at correct angle.	___	___	___	_____
14. Grasped lower end of syringe barrel with non-dominant hand and moved dominant hand to plunger.	___	___	___	_____
15. Withdrew needle quickly while placing swab on skin above injection site.	___	___	___	_____
16. Applied gentle pressure to site. Did not message site.	___	___	___	_____
17. Assisted client to comfortable position.	___	___	___	_____
18. Properly disposed of uncapped needle and syringe.	___	___	___	_____
19. Removed gloves and washed hands.	___	___	___	_____

EVALUATION

1. Evaluated for discomfort at injection site.	___	___	___	_____
2. Evaluated client's response to medication.	___	___	___	_____
3. Evaluated client's understanding of purpose and effects of medication.	___	___	___	_____
4. Identified unexpected outcomes.	___	___	___	_____

RECORDING AND REPORTING

1. Documented administration correctly on medication record.	___	___	___	_____
2. Reported undesirable effects from medication to nurse in charge or physician.	___	___	___	_____
3. Recorded client's response to drugs, if indicated.	___	___	___	_____

Student _____   Date _____

Instructor _____   Date _____

PERFORMANCE CHECKLIST 18-5 **ADMINISTERING INTRAMUSCULAR INJECTIONS**

	S	U	NP	Comments
ASSESSMENT				
1. Reviewed medication order.	___	___	___	_____
2. Assessed pertinent drug information.	___	___	___	_____
3. Assessed contraindications for intramuscular injection.	___	___	___	_____
4. Assessed client's medication, medical, and allergy history.	___	___	___	_____
5. Assessed client's knowledge regarding medications.	___	___	___	_____
6. Observed client's response toward receiving injections.	___	___	___	_____
NURSING DIAGNOSIS				
1. Developed appropriate nursing diagnoses based on assessment data.	___	___	___	_____
PLANNING				
1. Identified expected outcomes.	___	___	___	_____
2. Prepared medication from vial or ampule and checked dosage.	___	___	___	_____
3. Changed needle on syringe. Selected appropriate needle size.	___	___	___	_____
4. Identified client correctly.	___	___	___	_____
5. Explained procedure to client.	___	___	___	_____
IMPLEMENTATION				
1. Provided for client's privacy.	___	___	___	_____
2. Washed hands and applied gloves.	___	___	___	_____
3. Exposed only injection site.	___	___	___	_____
4. Assessed integrity of muscle while selecting injection site.	___	___	___	_____
5. Assisted client to comfortable position according to injection site.	___	___	___	_____
6. Relocated site using anatomic landmarks.	___	___	___	_____
7. Cleansed injection site.	___	___	___	_____
8. Held swab correctly.	___	___	___	_____

	S	U	NP	Comments

9. Removed needle cap correctly.

10. Held syringe comfortably in dominant hand with palm down.

11. With nondominant hand, spread skin tightly and grasped muscle, or used Z-tract method and administered injection at 90-degree angle.

12. Released skin and, with nondominant hand, grasped lower end of syringe barrel (with Z-tract method, continued to spread skin taut), then moved dominant hand to plunger.

13. Aspirated to check for blood return. If blood aspirated, withdrew needle; if not, injected medication slowly.

14. Withdrew needle quickly while placing antiseptic swab on skin above injection site (with Z-tract method, kept needle inserted for 10 seconds, then withdrew and released skin).

15. Applied gentle pressure. Did not massage site.

16. Assisted client to comfortable position. (Encouraged leg exercises after injection to leg muscles.)

17. Discarded uncapped needle and syringe in proper receptacle.

18. Removed gloves and washed hands.

EVALUATION

1. Evaluated client for discomfort at injection site.

2. Inspected injection site.

3. Evaluated client's response to medication.

4. Evaluated client's understanding of purpose and effects of medication.

5. Identified unexpected outcomes.

RECORDING AND REPORTING

1. Documented administration correctly on medication record.

2. Reported undesirable effects from medication to nurse in charge or physician.

3. Recorded client's response to drugs, if indicated.

Student _____   Date _____

Instructor _____   Date _____

PERFORMANCE CHECKLIST 18-6 **ADDING MEDICATIONS TO INTRAVENOUS FLUID CONTAINERS**

	S	U	NP	Comments
ASSESSMENT				
1. Assessed order for IV solution, type of medication, and dosage.	___	___	___	_____
2. Gathered information about drug.	___	___	___	_____
3. Assessed for drug incompatibility if more than one was mixed.	___	___	___	_____
4. Assessed client's fluid balance.	___	___	___	_____
5. Assessed client for drug allergies.	___	___	___	_____
6. Assessed condition of IV insertion site.	___	___	___	_____
7. Assessed client's knowledge regarding medication.	___	___	___	_____
NURSING DIAGNOSIS				
1. Developed appropriate nursing diagnoses based on assessment data.	___	___	___	_____
PLANNING				
1. Identified expected outcomes.	___	___	___	_____
2. Assembled supplies in medication area.	___	___	___	_____
3. Correctly prepared medication from vial or ampule.	___	___	___	_____
4. Identified client.	___	___	___	_____
5. Explained procedure to client.	___	___	___	_____
IMPLEMENTATION				
1. Washed hands.	___	___	___	_____
Adding Medication to New Container				
1. Located injection port on IV bag or removed cap and seal from IV bottle and located injection site.	___	___	___	_____
2. Cleaned injection port or site.	___	___	___	_____
3. Inserted needle/adapter of syringe through injection port or site and injected medication.	___	___	___	_____
4. Withdrew syringe.	___	___	___	_____
5. Mixed medications in IV solution container.	___	___	___	_____

	S	U	NP	Comments

6. Labeled container correctly; applied flow strip (optional).

    ___ ___ ___ _____

7. Spiked IV container and hung container correctly, regulating IV infusion at ordered rate.

    ___ ___ ___ _____

Adding Medication to Existing Container

1. Prepared vented IV bottle or plastic bag by checking volume of solution, closing infusion clamps, and cleaning port; inserted syringe and injected medication, lowered and mixed bag, and regulated infusion.

    ___ ___ ___ _____

2. Completed medication label and affixed to IV container.

    ___ ___ ___ _____

3. Disposed of soiled equipment properly. Did not recap needle.

    ___ ___ ___ _____

4. Washed hands.

    ___ ___ ___ _____

EVALUATION

1. Observed client for drug reaction.

    ___ ___ ___ _____

2. Assessed client for signs and symptoms of fluid volume excess.

    ___ ___ ___ _____

3. Evaluated condition of IV site and rate of infusion.

    ___ ___ ___ _____

4. Assessed for signs and symptoms of IV infiltration or phlebitis.

    ___ ___ ___ _____

5. Evaluated client's understanding of drug therapy.

    ___ ___ ___ _____

6. Identified unexpected outcomes.

    ___ ___ ___ _____

RECORDING AND REPORTING

1. Recorded IV solution and medication on appropriate form.

    ___ ___ ___ _____

2. Reported any drug reactions to nurse in charge or physician.

    ___ ___ ___ _____

Student _____   Date _____

Instructor _____   Date _____

PERFORMANCE CHECKLIST 18-7 **ADMINISTERING INTRAVENOUS MEDICATIONS BY INTERMITTENT INFUSION SETS AND MINIINFUSION PUMPS**

	S	U	NP	Comments
ASSESSMENT				
1. Checked order for IV solution, type of medication, and dosage.	___	___	___	_____
2. Collected pertinent information about drug.	___	___	___	_____
3. Determined compatibility of drug with existing IV solution.	___	___	___	_____
4. Assessed patency and infusion rate of main IV line.	___	___	___	_____
5. Assessed condition of IV insertion site.	___	___	___	_____
6. Assessed client's history of drug allergies.	___	___	___	_____
7. Assessed client's understanding of drug therapy.	___	___	___	_____
NURSING DIAGNOSIS				
1. Developed appropriate nursing diagnoses based on assessment data.	___	___	___	_____
PLANNING				
1. Identified expected outcomes.	___	___	___	_____
2. Assembled supplies.	___	___	___	_____
3. Prepared medications.	___	___	___	_____
IMPLEMENTATION				
1. Washed hands and applied gloves.	___	___	___	_____
2. Correctly identified client.	___	___	___	_____
3. Explained purpose of medication and encouraged client to report signs of discomfort at site.	___	___	___	_____
Piggyback or Tandem Infusion				
1. Connected infusion tubing to medication bag and filled tubing.	___	___	___	_____
2. Hung medication bag at proper level.	___	___	___	_____
3. Connected tubing to appropriate stopcocks or to needleless system.	___	___	___	_____
4. Cleaned injection port of main IV line with antiseptic swab.	___	___	___	_____

	S	U	NP	Comments

5. Inserted needle of secondary line into port of main line if using needles, or attached needleless device. ___ ___ ___ _____

6. Removed cover of stopcock and connected secondary line with main line. ___ ___ ___ _____

7. Regulated secondary line flow rate correctly. ___ ___ ___ _____

8. Checked flow regulator on primary infusion after medication infused. ___ ___ ___ _____

9. Regulated main infusion line to desired rate, if necessary. ___ ___ ___ _____

10. Cared for equipment properly after administration. ___ ___ ___ _____

11. Removed gloves and washed hands. ___ ___ ___ _____

Miniinfusor Administration

1. Connected prefilled syringe to miniinfusion tubing. ___ ___ ___ _____

2. Filled syringe with medication, avoiding air bubbles. ___ ___ ___ _____

3. Placed syringe into miniinfusor pump, securing syringe. ___ ___ ___ _____

4. Correctly connected miniinfusion tubing to main IV line. ___ ___ ___ _____

5. Hung infusion pump with syringe on IV pole and initiated infusion. ___ ___ ___ _____

6. Assessed flow rate and patency of IV line. ___ ___ ___ _____

7. Removed gloves and washed hands. ___ ___ ___ _____

Volume-Control Administration Set

1. Filled Volutrol with proper volume of solution. ___ ___ ___ _____

2. Closed clamp and assessed that clamp in air vent of Volutrol chamber was open. ___ ___ ___ _____

3. Cleaned injection port. ___ ___ ___ _____

4. Injected medication into Volutrol and mixed gently. ___ ___ ___ _____

5. Regulated IV infusion. ___ ___ ___ _____

6. Labeled Volutrol. ___ ___ ___ _____

7. Disposed of uncapped needle and syringe in proper container. ___ ___ ___ _____

8. Removed gloves and washed hands. ___ ___ ___ _____

	S	U	NP	Comments

EVALUATION

1. Evaluated client's response to medication. ___ ___ ___ _____

2. Periodically checked infusion rate and IV site. ___ ___ ___ _____

3. Evaluated client's knowledge of purpose and side effects of medication. ___ ___ ___ _____

4. Identified unexpected outcomes. ___ ___ ___ _____

RECORDING AND REPORTING

1. Recorded medication data correctly on medication form. ___ ___ ___ _____

2. Recorded solution on I&O form. ___ ___ ___ _____

3. Reported any adverse drug reactions to nurse in charge or physician. ___ ___ ___ _____

Student _____   Date _____

Instructor _____   Date _____

PERFORMANCE CHECKLIST 18-8 **ADMINISTERING MEDICATIONS BY INTRAVENOUS BOLUS**

	S	U	NP	Comments
ASSESSMENT				
1. Checked order for drug, dosage, time, and route.	——	——	——	_____
2. Collected information related to drug to be given.	——	——	——	_____
3. Assessed for compatibility with existing infusion.	——	——	——	_____
4. Assessed condition of needle insertion site.	——	——	——	_____
5. Checked client's history of allergies.	——	——	——	_____
6. Assessed client's understanding of purpose of drug therapy.	——	——	——	_____
NURSING DIAGNOSIS				
1. Developed appropriate nursing diagnoses based on assessment data.	——	——	——	_____
PLANNING				
1. Identified expected outcomes.	——	——	——	_____
2. Assembled supplies.	——	——	——	_____
3. Prepared medication from vial or ampule.	——	——	——	_____
IMPLEMENTATION				
1. Washed hands and applied gloves.	——	——	——	_____
2. Checked client's identification.	——	——	——	_____
3. Explained procedure to client and encouraged client to report any discomfort at IV site.	——	——	——	_____
4. IV push (existing line)	——	——	——	_____
a. Selected injection port of IV closest to client.	——	——	——	_____
b. Cleaned injection port with antiseptic swab.	——	——	——	_____
c. Inserted needleless tip or small-gauge needle of syringe correctly through port.	——	——	——	_____
d. Aspirated for blood return while occluding infusion tubing. Released tubing.	——	——	——	_____
e. Injected medication slowly over appropriate time.	——	——	——	_____
f. Released tubing, withdrew syringe, and checked infusion rate.	——	——	——	_____

	S	U	NP	Comments
5. IV push (intravenous lock)	——	——	——	_____
a. Prepared two syringes with 2 to 3 ml of normal saline.	——	——	——	_____
b. Prepared syringe needed when using a heparin flush method.	——	——	——	_____
c. Correctly administered drug over several minutes after cleaning injection port, checking for blood return, flushing with saline syringe, and cleaning the port.	——	——	——	_____
d. Correctly administered syringe with heparin if using heparin flush method.	——	——	——	_____
e. Correctly administered syringe with saline if using saline flush method.	——	——	——	_____
f. Disposed of uncapped needles and syringes in proper container.	——	——	——	_____
g. Removed gloves and washed hands.	——	——	——	_____

EVALUATION

	S	U	NP	Comments
1. Observed client for adverse reactions during and after administration of medication.	——	——	——	_____
2. Observed IV site for swelling during injection.	——	——	——	_____
3. Assessed client's response to medication.	——	——	——	_____
4. Evaluated client's knowledge of drug's purpose and side effects.	——	——	——	_____
5. Identified unexpected outcomes.	——	——	——	_____

RECORDING AND REPORTING

	S	U	NP	Comments
1. Recorded drug data correctly on medication record.	——	——	——	_____
2. Reported any adverse reactions to nurse in charge or physician.	——	——	——	_____

Student _____   Date _____

Instructor _____   Date _____

PERFORMANCE CHECKLIST 18-9   **ADMINISTERING CONTINUOUS SUBCUTANEOUS MEDICATIONS**

	S	U	NP	Comments
ASSESSMENT				
1. Checked prescriber's order.	___	___	___	_____
2. Collected information about medication.	___	___	___	_____
3. Assessed client's medical history.	___	___	___	_____
4. Assessed for factors that contraindicate continuous subcutaneous injection (CSQI).	___	___	___	_____
5. Assessed adequacy of client's adipose tissue to determine site.	___	___	___	_____
6. Assessed client's knowledge regarding medication.	___	___	___	_____
NURSING DIAGNOSIS				
1. Developed appropriate nursing diagnoses based on assessment data.	___	___	___	_____
PLANNING				
1. Identified expected outcomes.	___	___	___	_____
2. Checked MAR with order and medication label.	___	___	___	_____
3. Prepared correct dose from vial or ampule.	___	___	___	_____
4. Obtained and programmed medication pump.	___	___	___	_____
5. Identified client.	___	___	___	_____
6. Explained procedure.	___	___	___	_____
IMPLEMENTATION				
1. Washed hands and arranged equipment.	___	___	___	_____
2. Provided privacy.	___	___	___	_____
3. Initiated CSQI:	___	___	___	_____
a. Selected appropriate site.	___	___	___	_____
b. Assisted client to comfortable position.	___	___	___	_____
c. Cleansed injection site with alcohol and povidone-iodine and allowed to dry.	___	___	___	_____
d. Applied clean gloves.	___	___	___	_____
e. Held needle in dominant hand and removed needle guard.	___	___	___	_____

	S	U	NP	Comments
f. Pinched or lifted up skin with nondominant hand.	——	——	——	_____
g. Inserted needle at 30- to 45-degree angle.	——	——	——	_____
h. Released skin fold and applied tape over wings of needle.	——	——	——	_____
i. Placed occlusive transparent dressing over insertion site.	——	——	——	_____
j. Attached tubing from needle to tubing from infusion pump.	——	——	——	_____
k. Turned infusion pump on.	——	——	——	_____
l. Disposed of sharps in appropriate container.	——	——	——	_____
m. Discarded used supplies, removed gloves, and washed hands.	——	——	——	_____
4. Discontinued CSQI:	——	——	——	_____
a. Verified order for discontinuation.	——	——	——	_____
b. Stopped infusion pump.	——	——	——	_____
c. Applied clean gloves.	——	——	——	_____
d. Removed dressing.	——	——	——	_____
e. Removed tape from wings of needle and pulled needle out along insertion line.	——	——	——	_____
f. Applied pressure at site.	——	——	——	_____
g. Applied 2 × 2 gauze dressing or bandage.	——	——	——	_____
h. Discarded used supplies and washed hands.	——	——	——	_____

EVALUATION

	S	U	NP	Comments
1. Evaluated client's response to medication.	——	——	——	_____
2. Observed site at least every 4 hours.	——	——	——	_____
3. Identified unexpected outcomes.	——	——	——	_____

RECORDING AND REPORTING

	S	U	NP	Comments
1. Recorded medication administration.	——	——	——	_____
2. Recorded client's response to medication and assessment of infusion site.	——	——	——	_____
3. Reported unexpected outcomes to the nurse in charge or physician.	——	——	——	_____

Student _____ Date _____

Instructor _____ Date _____

PERFORMANCE CHECKLIST 19-1   **INITIATING A PERIPHERAL INTRAVENOUS INFUSION**

	S	U	NP	Comments
ASSESSMENT				
1. Checked prescriber's order.	—	—	—	_____
2. Assessed for factors and conditions that are affected by IV fluid administration.	—	—	—	_____
3. Assessed client's previous experience with IV therapy.	—	—	—	_____
4. Collected information about the IV solution, any medications the client is taking, and possible incompatibility.	—	—	—	_____
5. Determined if client is to have surgery or receive blood.	—	—	—	_____
6. Assessed for risk factors associated with IV therapy.	—	—	—	_____
7. Assessed laboratory values and history of allergies.	—	—	—	_____
NURSING DIAGNOSIS				
1. Developed appropriate nursing diagnoses based on assessment data.	—	—	—	_____
PLANNING				
1. Identified expected outcomes.	—	—	—	_____
2. Explained procedure and expected sensations.	—	—	—	_____
3. Assisted client to comfortable position.	—	—	—	_____
4. Washed hands.	—	—	—	_____
5. Assembled equipment.	—	—	—	_____
IMPLEMENTATION				
1. Changed client's gown for easier removal.	—	—	—	_____
2. Opened sterile packages correctly.	—	—	—	_____
3. Prepared IV infusion tubing and solution:	—	—	—	_____
a. Checked "five rights" of drug administration.	—	—	—	_____
b. Opened infusion set.	—	—	—	_____
c. Placed roller clamp about 2 to 5 cm (1-2 inches) below drip chamber.	—	—	—	_____
d. Removed protective sheath over IV tubing port on IV solution bag.	—	—	—	_____
e. Inserted infusion set spike into fluid bag or bottle.	—	—	—	_____

	S	U	NP	Comments

    f. Primed infusion tubing by compressing drip chamber and filling to $\frac{1}{3}$ to $\frac{1}{2}$ full. ___ ___ ___ _____

    g. Removed protector cap on end of tubing (if necessary), released roller clamp, and allowed fluid to fill tubing. ___ ___ ___ _____

    h. Removed air bubbles. ___ ___ ___ _____

    i. Replaced protector cap on end of infusion tubing. ___ ___ ___ _____

4. Prepared heparin or normal saline lock for infusion. ___ ___ ___ _____

5. Applied clean gloves. ___ ___ ___ _____

6. Identified accessible vein. ___ ___ ___ _____

7. Applied flat tourniquet above proposed insertion site. ___ ___ ___ _____

8. Selected appropriate vein for IV insertion. ___ ___ ___ _____

    a. Stroked extremity from distal to proximal below site. ___ ___ ___ _____

    b. Had client open and close fist. ___ ___ ___ _____

    c. Lightly tapped over vein. ___ ___ ___ _____

    d. Applied warmth to area for several minutes. ___ ___ ___ _____

9. Released tourniquet temporarily. ___ ___ ___ _____

10. Placed needle adapter end nearby on sterile surface. ___ ___ ___ _____

11. Replaced tourniquet and checked client's distal pulse. ___ ___ ___ _____

12. Cleansed site with alcohol or povidone-iodine and allowed to dry. ___ ___ ___ _____

13. Performed venipuncture: ___ ___ ___ _____

    a. Anchored vein by placing thumb over vein and stretching skin distal to the selected site. ___ ___ ___ _____

    b. Warned client of sharp, quick stick. ___ ___ ___ _____

    c. Inserted over-the-needle catheter (ONC), IV catheter safety device, or butterfly needle with bevel up at a 20- to 30-degree angle slightly distal to the actual site in the direction of the vein. ___ ___ ___ _____

14. Stabilized catheter/needle with one hand and released tourniquet with the other hand. ___ ___ ___ _____

15. Removed stylet of ONC; did not recap stylet. Glided protective guard over stylet of IV safety device. ___ ___ ___ _____

	S	U	NP	Comments

16. Connected needle adapter of infusion tubing set of heparin/saline lock adapter to hub of ONC or butterfly tubing. ___ ___ ___ _____

17. Intermittent infusion: ___ ___ ___ _____

   a. Held heparin/saline lock firmly with one hand and cleansed with alcohol. ___ ___ ___ _____

   b. Inserted prefilled syringe with flush solution into injection cap. ___ ___ ___ _____

   c. Flushed injection cap slowly with solution. ___ ___ ___ _____

   d. Withdrew syringe while still flushing. ___ ___ ___ _____

18. Continuous infusion: Connected tubing and opened roller clamp to allow solution to infuse. ___ ___ ___ _____

19. Taped or secured catheter/butterfly needle. ___ ___ ___ _____

20. Applied sterile gauze or transparent dressing to site. Avoided taping over insertion site and connections. ___ ___ ___ _____

21. Rechecked flow rates of IV fluid infusions. ___ ___ ___ _____

22. Wrote date and time of IV insertion and catheter/needle size on dressing. ___ ___ ___ _____

23. Disposed of sharps in appropriate container. ___ ___ ___ _____

24. Instructed client how to move around without dislodging the IV. ___ ___ ___ _____

25. Changed peripheral access site per agency policy. ___ ___ ___ _____

26. Replaced IV solution when less than 100 ml remained in bottle or bag. ___ ___ ___ _____

EVALUATION

1. Observed client every 1 to 2 hours to determine condition of IV site and status of infusion. ___ ___ ___ _____

2. Observed client's response to IV therapy. ___ ___ ___ _____

3. Identified unexpected outcomes. ___ ___ ___ _____

RECORDING AND REPORTING

1. Recorded IV insertion and information about infusion and insertion site. ___ ___ ___ _____

2. Recorded client's response to IV infusion and assessment of infusion site. ___ ___ ___ _____

3. Documented use of electronic IV infusion device. ___ ___ ___ _____

4. Reported unexpected outcomes to the nurse in charge or physician. ___ ___ ___ _____

Student _____   Date _____

Instructor _____   Date _____

PERFORMANCE CHECKLIST 19-2 **INSERTING A PERIPHERALLY INSERTED CENTRAL CATHETER**

	S	U	NP	Comments
ASSESSMENT				
1. Reviewed physician's orders.	——	——	——	————————
2. Knew agency's policy regarding peripherally inserted central catheters (PICCs).	——	——	——	————————
3. Reviewed manufacturer's directions.	——	——	——	————————
4. Assessed client's understanding of and readiness for procedure.	——	——	——	————————
5. Assessed client's status and needs.	——	——	——	————————
6. Assessed for drug allergies.	——	——	——	————————
NURSING DIAGNOSIS				
1. Developed appropriate nursing diagnoses based on assessment data.	——	——	——	————————
PLANNING				
1. Identified expected outcomes.	——	——	——	————————
2. Explained procedure to client.	——	——	——	————————
3. Verified that consent form was signed.	——	——	——	————————
4. Measured circumference of client's upper arm.	——	——	——	————————
IMPLEMENTATION				
1. Washed hands.	——	——	——	————————
2. Organized equipment at bedside.	——	——	——	————————
3. Instructed client to wash arms thoroughly. Assisted as necessary.	——	——	——	————————
4. Clipped hair if necessary.	——	——	——	————————
5. Identified an appropriate vein in the antecubital fossa.	——	——	——	————————
6. Positioned client correctly.	——	——	——	————————
7. Measured the distance from insertion site to proposed site for catheter tip.	——	——	——	————————
8. Put on mask, gown, and goggles.	——	——	——	————————
9. Opened sterile supplies or kit correctly.	——	——	——	————————
10. Applied sterile gloves.	——	——	——	————————

	S	U	NP	Comments
11. Prepared lidocaine (optional) and solutions for flushing.	——	——	——	————————
12. Correctly prepared insertion site.	——	——	——	————————
13. Correctly prepared catheter and tubing.	——	——	——	————————
14. Removed gloves. Reapplied tourniquet if non-sterile tourniquet was used.	——	——	——	————————
15. Applied a pair of sterile gloves.	——	——	——	————————
16. Placed sterile 4 × 4 gauze over tourniquet or applied sterile tourniquet.	——	——	——	————————
17. Provided sterile field around venipuncture site.	——	——	——	————————
18. Administered local anesthesia if indicated. Verified placement of introducer.	——	——	——	————————
19. Ensured that vein was securely cannulated.	——	——	——	————————
20. Correctly inserted and advanced catheter through introducer needle.	——	——	——	————————
21. Released tourniquet without contaminating glove.	——	——	——	————————
22. Correctly advanced catheter the required distance.	——	——	——	————————
23. Instructed client to assume correct head position.	——	——	——	————————
24. Continued to advance catheter the required distance.	——	——	——	————————
25. Correctly withdrew introducer without removing catheter.	——	——	——	————————
26. Removed needle from catheter.	——	——	——	————————
27. Removed guidewire.	——	——	——	————————
28. Verified patency of distal lumen.	——	——	——	————————
29. Attached extension tubing and cap to the lumen.	——	——	——	————————
30. Anchored hub of catheter to the skin.	——	——	——	————————
31. Cleansed insertion site with antiseptic if it was oozing blood.	——	——	——	————————
32. Placed 2 × 2 pads over insertion site. Covered with transparent dressing.	——	——	——	————————
33. Coiled extension tubings and secured to arm. Labeled dressing with date and time of insertion and gauge of catheter.	——	——	——	————————
34. Flushed each lumen with heparin solution.	——	——	——	————————
35. Disposed of equipment. Removed gloves and washed hands.	——	——	——	————————

	S	U	NP	Comments

36. Followed agency policy for x-ray examination verification of placement. ___ ___ ___ _____

37. Aspirated regularly for blood return, and flushed catheter. ___ ___ ___ _____

EVALUATION

1. Observed client and inquired about comfort level during insertion. ___ ___ ___ _____

2. Inspected and palpated PICC site after insertion. Noted respiratory status. ___ ___ ___ _____

3. Called for x-ray examination to verify placement. ___ ___ ___ _____

4. Observed the PICC setup to determine status of system according to agency policy. ___ ___ ___ _____

5. Observed client to determine response to fluid and electrolyte therapy. ___ ___ ___ _____

6. Weighed client daily. ___ ___ ___ _____

7. Measured client's body temperature every 4 hours. ___ ___ ___ _____

8. Evaluated client's knowledge of complications and maintenance of catheter. ___ ___ ___ _____

9. Identified unexpected outcomes. ___ ___ ___ _____

RECORDING AND REPORTING

1. Recorded PICC's gauge and length, insertion site, date and time of insertion, radiographic confirmation of location of catheter tip, and presence or absence of signs and symptoms of complications. ___ ___ ___ _____

2. Reported status of PICC, therapy being administered, and development of complications and their treatment. ___ ___ ___ _____

Student _____   Date _____

Instructor _____   Date _____

PERFORMANCE CHECKLIST 19-3 **REGULATING INTRAVENOUS FLOW RATE**

	S	U	NP	Comments

ASSESSMENT

1. Observed patency of the IV line and needle.   ___ ___ ___ _____

2. Checked client's medical record for IV fluid orders.   ___ ___ ___ _____

3. Assessed client's knowledge of how positioning affects flow rate.   ___ ___ ___ _____

4. Verified with client how venipuncture site feels.   ___ ___ ___ _____

NURSING DIAGNOSIS

1. Developed appropriate nursing diagnoses based on assessment data.   ___ ___ ___ _____

PLANNING

1. Identified expected outcomes.   ___ ___ ___ _____

2. Used paper and pencil to calculate flow rate.   ___ ___ ___ _____

3. Stated calibration in drops per milliliter of specific infusion set.   ___ ___ ___ _____

4. Selected formula to calculate flow rate.   ___ ___ ___ _____

IMPLEMENTATION

1. Checked physician's orders and followed "five rights" for correct solution and additives.   ___ ___ ___ _____

2. Calculated hourly rate in milliliters per hour (ml/hr).   ___ ___ ___ _____

3. Placed adhesive tape on IV bottle or bag next to volume markings.   ___ ___ ___ _____

4. Calculated drops per minute (gtt/min).   ___ ___ ___ _____

5. Timed flow rate by watch.   ___ ___ ___ _____

6. Followed correct procedure for using infusion controller or pump.   ___ ___ NP _____

7. Followed correct procedure for using volume control device.   ___ ___ ___ _____

EVALUATION

1. Monitored infusion hourly.   ___ ___ ___ _____

2. Observed client to determine effect of IV therapy.   ___ ___ ___ _____

3. Assessed for signs of infiltration.   ___ ___ ___ _____

4. Identified unexpected outcomes.   ___ ___ ___ _____

	S	U	NP	Comments
RECORDING AND REPORTING				
1. Recorded appropriate infusion rate.	___	___	___	_____
2. Recorded new fluid rates.	___	___	___	_____
3. Documented use of infusion device.	___	___	___	_____
4. Reported appropriate information to nursing personnel.	___	___	___	_____

Student _____   Date _____

Instructor _____   Date _____

PERFORMANCE CHECKLIST 19-4 **CHANGING INTRAVENOUS SOLUTIONS**

	S	U	NP	Comments
ASSESSMENT				
1. Checked physician's orders.	—	—	—	_____
2. Noted date and time when solution was last changed.	—	—	—	_____
3. Determined the compatibility of all IV fluids and additives.	—	—	—	_____
4. Determined client's understanding of need for continued IV therapy.	—	—	—	_____
5. Determined patency of IV site.	—	—	—	_____
NURSING DIAGNOSIS				
1. Developed appropriate nursing diagnoses based on assessment data.	—	—	—	_____
PLANNING				
1. Identified expected outcomes.	—	—	—	_____
2. Checked that next ordered solution was ready at least 1 hour before needed.	—	—	—	_____
3. Checked client's identification.	—	—	—	_____
4. Prepared to change solution when it remained in neck of bottle or bag.	—	—	—	_____
5. Explained procedure to client and family.	—	—	—	_____
6. Maintained drip chamber half full.	—	—	—	_____
IMPLEMENTATION				
1. Washed hands.	—	—	—	_____
2. Prepared solution for changing.	—	—	—	_____
3. Moved roller clamp to reduce flow rate.	—	—	—	_____
4. Removed old solution from IV pole.	—	—	—	_____
5. Removed spike from old solution and correctly inserted spike into new solution.	—	—	—	_____
6. Hung new bag or bottle of solution.	—	—	—	_____
7. Checked for air in IV tubing.	—	—	—	_____
8. Ensured that drip chamber contained solution.	—	—	—	_____
9. Regulated flow rate to prescribed rate.	—	—	—	_____

	S	U	NP	Comments

EVALUATION

1. Reassessed client to determine response to IV fluid therapy.   ___ ___ ___ _____

2. Monitored IV infusion for correct solution and additives.   ___ ___ ___ _____

3. Identified unexpected outcomes.   ___ ___ ___ _____

RECORDING AND REPORTING

1. Recorded amount and type of fluid infused and amount and type of new fluid.   ___ ___ ___ _____

Student _____ Date _____

Instructor _____ Date _____

PERFORMANCE CHECKLIST 19-5 **CHANGING INFUSION TUBING**

	S	U	NP	Comments
ASSESSMENT				
1. Determined when new infusion set was warranted.	—	—	—	_____
2. Determined client's understanding of need for continued IV infusions.	—	—	—	_____
NURSING DIAGNOSIS				
1. Developed appropriate nursing diagnoses based on assessment data.	—	—	—	_____
PLANNING				
1. Identified expected outcomes.	—	—	—	_____
2. Explained procedure to client.	—	—	—	_____
IMPLEMENTATION				
1. Washed hands.	—	—	—	_____
2. Opened new infusion set while protecting sites from contamination.	—	—	—	_____
3. Applied disposable gloves.	—	—	—	_____
4. Removed old dressing, if required.	—	—	—	_____
IV Infusion				
1. Moved roller clamp to "off" position.	—	—	—	_____
2. Regulated drip rate on old tubing to slow rate of infusion.	—	—	—	_____
3. Compressed drip chamber and filled it while old tubing was still in place.	—	—	—	_____
4. Discontinued old tubing from solution and hung drip chamber over IV pole.	—	—	—	_____
5. Placed insertion spike into old IV solution opening and hung solution on IV pole.	—	—	—	_____
6. Compressed and released drip chamber on new tubing.	—	—	—	_____
7. Opened roller clamp, removed protective cap from needle adapter, and flushed tubing with solution.	—	—	—	_____
8. Turned roller clamp on old tubing to "off" position.	—	—	—	_____

	S	U	NP	Comments

Heparin Lock

1. Used sterile technique to connect IV plug to tubing.

2. Removed air from tubing.

3. Removed protective cap from end and placed on sterile surface.

4. Stabilized hub of IV catheter or needle and gently pulled out old IV tubing; maintained stability of hub and inserted needle adapter of new tubing into hub.

5. Opened roller clamp on new tubing.

6. Regulated IV drip rate according to physician's orders and monitored hourly rate.

7. Applied new IV dressing, if necessary.

8. Discarded old tubing properly.

9. Disposed of gloves and washed hands.

EVALUATION

1. Evaluated flow rate and observed connection site for leakage.

2. Identified unexpected outcomes.

RECORDING AND REPORTING

1. Recorded changing of tubing and solution on client's record.

2. Recorded date and time on tape below drip chamber.

Student _____   Date _____

Instructor _____   Date _____

PERFORMANCE CHECKLIST 19-6 **CHANGING A PERIPHERAL INTRAVENOUS DRESSING**

	S	U	NP	Comments
ASSESSMENT				
1. Determined time of last dressing change.	—	—	—	_____
2. Observed present dressing for moisture and intactness.	—	—	—	_____
3. Observed present IV system for proper functioning.	—	—	—	_____
4. Inspected catheter site.	—	—	—	_____
5. Monitored client's temperature.	—	—	—	_____
6. Determined client's understanding of need for continued IV infusion.	—	—	—	_____
NURSING DIAGNOSIS				
1. Developed appropriate nursing diagnoses based on assessment data.	—	—	—	_____
PLANNING				
1. Identified expected outcomes.	—	—	—	_____
2. Explained procedure to client.	—	—	—	_____
IMPLEMENTATION				
1. Washed hands and applied disposable gloves.	—	—	—	_____
2. Removed old dressing. Observed integrity of injection site.	—	—	—	_____
3. Discontinued IV infusion if needed or ordered.	—	—	—	_____
4. Stabilized IV catheter or needle and removed excess adhesive.	—	—	—	_____
5. Applied sterile gloves for PICC line dressing.	—	—	—	_____
6. Cleansed venipuncture site with antiseptic solution or ointment. Allowed to dry.	—	U	NP	_____
7. Secured catheter.	—	—	—	_____
8. Applied new transparent or gauze dressing.	—	—	—	_____
9. Anchored IV tube.	—	—	—	_____
10. Dated new dressing.	—	—	—	_____
11. Discarded equipment, removed gloves, and washed hands.	—	—	—	_____

	S	U	NP	Comments

EVALUATION

1. Assessed functioning and patency of IV system. ___ ___ ___ _____

2. Monitored client's body temperature. ___ ___ ___ _____

3. Identified unexpected outcomes. ___ ___ ___ _____

RECORDING AND REPORTING

1. Documented dressing change in client's record. ___ ___ ___ _____

2. Notified nurse in charge of dressing change and integrity of system. ___ ___ ___ _____

3. Reported complications to physician. ___ ___ ___ _____

Student _____   Date _____

Instructor _____   Date _____

PERFORMANCE CHECKLIST 19-7 **CARING FOR VASCULAR ACCESS DEVICES**

	S	U	NP	Comments

ASSESSMENT

1. Assessed client's diagnosis, state of disease, and therapy plan by reviewing medical record.

2. Reviewed medical order.

3. Identified type of vascular access device (VAD) in place.

4. Assessed need to use VAD for blood sampling.

5. Assessed VAD site for skin integrity and infection.

6. Assessed proper functioning of VAD before therapy.

7. Assessed need for irrigation and dressing change.

8. Assessed client's knowledge of care and maintenance of VAD.

NURSING DIAGNOSIS

1. Developed appropriate nursing diagnoses based on assessment data.

PLANNING

1. Identified expected outcomes.

2. Positioned client in supine position with head slightly elevated.

3. Explained procedure to client.

IMPLEMENTATION
Administration of Infusions or Sampling of Blood from Implanted Infusion Port

1. Washed hands. Masked self and client.

2. Prepared sterile field; opened sterile supplies.

3. Prepared client's skin with alcohol.

4. Prepared client's skin overlying port septum with povidone-iodine.

5. Applied sterile gloves.

6. With assistance from another nurse, filled sterile syringe with saline solution.

7. Properly attached tubing and Huber needle, and filled tubing with saline solution.

	S	U	NP	Comments
8. Applied sterile drape to port site.	___	___	___	_____
9. Palpated port septum with strict aseptic technique.	___	___	___	_____
10. Inserted Huber needle through skin correctly.	___	___	___	_____
11. Checked for correct placement.	___	___	___	_____
12. Flushed port with saline.	___	___	___	_____
13. Observed for swelling.	___	___	___	_____
14. Aspirated and discarded 5 ml of fluid.	___	___	___	_____
15. Withdrew blood for sample using appropriately sized syringe.	___	___	___	_____
16. Flushed with 2 ml heparin.	___	___	___	_____
17. Refilled saline syringe and flushed port with 20 ml saline.	___	___	___	_____
18. Heparinized port by flushing with 5 ml heparin flush solution.	___	___	___	_____
19. Secured needle with sterile gauze or transparent dressing.	___	___	___	_____
20. Connected IV infusion tubing with sterile tubing.	___	___	___	_____
21. Regulated IV infusion.	___	___	___	_____
22. Disposed of all soiled supplies and equipment, sent specimens to laboratory, removed gloves, and washed hands.	___	___	___	_____

Administration of Infusions or Sampling of Blood from Central Venous Catheter

	S	U	NP	Comments
1. Washed hands.	___	___	___	_____
2. Applied gloves, gown, and goggles (per policy).	___	___	___	_____
3. Cleansed injection cap or catheter hub.	___	___	___	_____
4. Prepared two syringes: one with 10 ml normal saline and one with 20 ml normal saline.	___	___	___	_____
5. Clamped catheter if removing cap.	___	___	___	_____
6. With cap in place, inserted needle of syringe containing 10 ml normal saline and flushed catheter; if cap removed, connected syringe to hub, released clamp, flushed and reclamped.	___	___	___	_____
7. Connected syringe for blood sampling, released clamp, aspirated, and reclamped.	___	___	___	_____
8. Attached or inserted syringe to catheter, released clamp, withdrew necessary blood for samples, and reclamped.	___	___	___	_____

	S	U	NP	Comments

9. Flushed with 2 ml heparin. ___ ___ ___ _____

10. Attached or inserted syringe filled with 20 ml normal saline to catheter, clamped, and flushed correctly. ___ ___ ___ _____

11. If no continuous infusion indicated, heparinized catheter. ___ ___ ___ _____

12. Replaced new cap to end of catheter and removed clamp. ___ ___ ___ _____

13. If IV fluids were to be administered, connected IV tubing to end of catheter while maintaining aseptic technique. ___ ___ ___ _____

14. Regulated IV infusion as ordered. ___ ___ ___ _____

15. Taped tubing connections and pinned tubing to client's gown. ___ ___ ___ _____

16. Correctly disposed of soiled equipment and supplies. Washed hands. ___ ___ ___ _____

Dressing Change

1. Washed hands and applied clean gloves. ___ ___ ___ _____

2. Masked self and client, if indicated. ___ ___ ___ _____

3. Removed old dressing correctly. ___ ___ ___ _____

4. Inspected placement or exit site. ___ ___ ___ _____

5. For tunneled catheter, palpated Dacron cuff in subcutaneous tunnel. ___ ___ ___ _____

6. Inspected catheter and hub for intactness. ___ ___ ___ _____

7. Washed hands and applied sterile gloves. ___ ___ ___ _____

8. Cleaned placement or exit site correctly. ___ ___ ___ _____

9. Applied povidone-iodine ointment or solution over exit site. ___ ___ ___ _____

10. Redressed site correctly. ___ ___ ___ _____

11. Secured tubing or needle to client's gown. ___ ___ ___ _____

12. Labeled date, time of dressing, and size of needle in place. ___ ___ ___ _____

13. Disposed of soiled supplies, removed gloves, and washed hands. ___ ___ ___ _____

EVALUATION

1. For continuous infusions, observed and calculated drip rate periodically. ___ ___ ___ _____

2. Routinely assessed vital signs. ___ ___ ___ _____

	S	U	NP	Comments
3. Observed catheter or port exit/placement site when exposed.	___	___	___	_____
4. Observed catheter connection points periodically.	___	___	___	_____
5. Inspected condition of catheter and tubing for malfunctioning.	___	___	___	_____
6. Consulted x-ray reports for catheter placement.	___	___	___	_____
7. Evaluated ability of client or family member to provide care and maintain catheter or infusion port.	___	___	___	_____
8. Identified unexpected outcomes.	___	___	___	_____

RECORDING AND REPORTING

	S	U	NP	Comments
1. Recorded medications, blood products, and parenteral nutrition given or samples obtained.	___	___	___	_____
2. Recorded condition of exit site or port implantation.	___	___	___	_____
3. Recorded dressing change procedure.	___	___	___	_____
4. Recorded patency of catheter, ability to draw blood, and difficulty with infusions.	___	___	___	_____
5. Recorded client and family education measures.	___	___	___	_____
6. Reported complications immediately to nursing or medical personnel.	___	___	___	_____

Student _____   Date _____

Instructor _____   Date _____

PERFORMANCE CHECKLIST 19-8 **DISCONTINUING PERIPHERAL INTRAVENOUS ACCESS**

	S	U	NP	Comments

ASSESSMENT

1. Observed IV site for signs and symptoms of infection, infiltration, and phlebitis.

2. Reviewed physician's order for discontinuation of IV.

3. Determined client's understanding of need for discontinuation of peripheral IV access.

NURSING DIAGNOSIS

1. Developed appropriate nursing diagnoses based on assessment data.

PLANNING

1. Identified expected outcomes.

2. Explained procedure to client.

IMPLEMENTATION

1. Washed hands and applied disposable gloves.

2. Turned IV tubing roller clamp to "off" position.

3. Removed IV site dressing.

4. Cleaned site with alcohol and then with povidone-iodine solution.

5. Placed sterile gauze over venipuncture site and correctly removed catheter or needle. Inspected catheter for intactness.

6. Applied pressure to site for 2 to 3 minutes.

7. Applied folded gauze dressing over site and secured with tape.

8. Discarded used supplies, removed gloves, and washed hands.

EVALUATION

1. Observed site for evidence of bleeding.

2. Observed site for redness, pain, drainage, and swelling.

	S	U	NP	Comments

RECORDING AND REPORTING

1. Recorded time IV discontinued and information obtained during site assessment.   ___ ___ ___ _____

2. Reported to nurse in charge or oncoming shift that IV was discontinued and any pertinent information related to the procedure.   ___ ___ ___ _____

Student _____   Date _____

Instructor _____   Date _____

PERFORMANCE CHECKLIST 20-1 **INITIATING BLOOD THERAPY**

	S	U	NP	Comments
ASSESSMENT				
1. Inspected integrity and intactness of present IV line.	—	—	—	_____
2. Obtained client's transfusion history.	—	—	—	_____
3. Reviewed physician's order.	—	—	—	_____
4. Identified indication for blood product.	—	—	—	_____
5. Obtained vital signs before initiating transfusion.	—	—	—	_____
NURSING DIAGNOSIS				
1. Developed appropriate nursing diagnoses based on assessment data.	—	—	—	_____
PLANNING				
1. Identified expected outcomes.	—	—	—	_____
2. Explained procedure and its purpose to client.	—	—	—	_____
IMPLEMENTATION				
Preadministration				
1. Obtained blood from blood bank following agency protocol.	—	—	—	_____
2. Correctly verified right blood product and right client.	—	—	—	_____
3. Had client void or emptied urine collection container.	—	—	—	_____
4. Collected supplies for venipuncture, if necessary.	—	—	—	_____
Administration				
1. Washed hands and applied disposable gloves.	—	—	—	_____
2. Opened blood administration set.	—	—	—	_____
3. Prepared Y tubing or single tubing administration properly.	—	—	—	_____
4. Initiated infusion of blood product.	—	—	—	_____
5. Remained with client during the first 5 to 15 minutes of transfusion.	—	—	—	_____
6. Monitored client's vital signs appropriately.	—	—	—	_____
7. Regulated infusion according to physician's orders.	—	—	—	_____
8. Cleared infusion tubing with 0.9% normal saline.	—	—	—	_____

	S	U	NP	Comments

9. Disposed of supplies. Removed gloves and washed hands. ___ ___ ___ _____

EVALUATION

1. Monitored IV site and status of infusion. ___ ___ ___ _____

2. Assessed client for chills, flushing, itching, dyspnea, rash, hives, or other signs of transfusion reaction. ___ ___ ___ _____

3. Reassessed client and assessed laboratory values to determine response to administration of blood components. ___ ___ ___ _____

4. Identified unexpected outcomes. ___ ___ ___ _____

RECORDING AND REPORTING

1. Recorded type and amount of blood component administered and client's response to blood therapy on appropriate form. ___ ___ ___ _____

2. Reported signs and symptoms of a transfusion reaction immediately. ___ ___ ___ _____

Student _____   Date _____

Instructor _____   Date _____

PERFORMANCE CHECKLIST 20-2 **AUTOLOGOUS TRANSFUSION**

	S	U	NP	Comments
ASSESSMENT				
1. Determined integrity of existing IV line.	—	—	—	_____
2. Obtained vital signs before transfusion.	—	—	—	_____
3. Identified client's comfort level.	—	—	—	_____
4. Assessed client's understanding of procedure.	—	—	—	_____
NURSING DIAGNOSIS				
1. Developed appropriate nursing diagnoses based on assessment data.	—	—	—	_____
PLANNING				
1. Identified expected outcomes.	—	—	—	_____
2. Explained procedure to client and family. Obtained necessary consents.	—	—	—	_____
IMPLEMENTATION				
1. Washed hands and put on appropriate intraoperative or postoperative attire.	—	—	—	_____
2. Placed collected blood into collection container or cell processing system and followed agency's or manufacturer's procedure.	—	—	—	_____
3. Correctly initiated transfusion procedure.	—	—	—	_____
EVALUATION				
1. Assessed client's status and laboratory values to determine response to administration of transfusion.	—	—	—	_____
2. Monitored IV site and infusion status when vital signs measured.	—	—	—	_____
3. Identified unexpected outcomes.	—	—	—	_____
RECORDING AND REPORTING				
1. Recorded amount of blood received by autologous blood transfusion and client's response to blood therapy.	—	—	—	_____
2. Reported any deterioration in cardiac status to physician or nurse in charge.	—	—	—	_____

Student _____   Date _____

Instructor _____   Date _____

PERFORMANCE CHECKLIST 20-3   **ADVERSE REACTIONS TO TRANSFUSIONS**

	S	U	NP	Comments
ASSESSMENT				
1. Observed for signs of acute hemolytic reaction.	___	___	___	_____
2. Observed for signs of delayed hemolytic reaction.	___	___	___	_____
3. Observed for signs of febrile nonhemolytic reaction.	___	___	___	_____
4. Observed for signs of allergic reaction.	___	___	___	_____
5. Observed for signs of anaphylactic reaction.	___	___	___	_____
6. Observed for signs of graft-versus-host disease.	___	___	___	_____
7. Observed for signs of circulatory overload.	___	___	___	_____
8. Observed for signs of septic shock.	___	___	___	_____
9. Observed for signs of hypothermia and cardiac dysrhythmias.	___	___	___	_____
10. Observed for GI symptoms.	___	___	___	_____
NURSING DIAGNOSIS				
1. Developed appropriate nursing diagnoses based on assessment data.	___	___	___	_____
PLANNING				
1. Identified expected outcomes.	___	___	___	_____
2. Explained treatment of a reaction to client and family.	___	___	___	_____
IMPLEMENTATION				
1. Discontinued transfusion.	___	___	___	_____
2. Removed tubing with blood in it and replaced with new tubing.	___	___	___	_____
3. Notified physician of reaction.	___	___	___	_____
4. Maintained patent IV line using 0.9% NaCl.	___	___	___	_____
5. Notified blood bank.	___	___	___	_____
6. Obtained two blood samples.	___	___	___	_____
7. Returned remaining blood to blood bank.	___	___	___	_____
8. Monitored client's vital signs every 15 minutes.	___	___	___	_____
9. Administered prescribed medications.	___	___	___	_____

	S	U	NP	Comments
10. Initiated CPR if necessary.	___	___	___	_____
11. Obtained first voided urine.	___	___	___	_____

EVALUATION

	S	U	NP	Comments
1. Assessed client to determine improvement or changes in physiologic status.	___	___	___	_____
2. Identified unexpected outcomes.	___	___	___	_____

RECORDING AND REPORTING

	S	U	NP	Comments
1. Recorded pertinent information about transfusion reaction.	___	___	___	_____
2. Reported transfusion reaction immediately to nurse in charge and physician.	___	___	___	_____

Student _____   Date _____

Instructor _____   Date _____

PERFORMANCE CHECKLIST 21-1 **PERFORMING NUTRITIONAL ASSESSMENT**

	S	U	NP	Comments
ASSESSMENT				
1. Determined need to perform nutritional assessment.	___	___	___	_____
2. Obtained baseline knowledge through diet history.	___	___	___	_____
3. Assessed client for usual body weight.	___	___	___	_____
4. Reviewed laboratory results.	___	___	___	_____
5. Determined medications client is taking.	___	___	___	_____
NURSING DIAGNOSIS				
1. Developed appropriate nursing diagnoses based on assessment data.	___	___	___	_____
PLANNING				
1. Identified expected outcomes.	___	___	___	_____
2. Prepared equipment and supplies.	___	___	___	_____
3. Explained procedure to client.	___	___	___	_____
4. Performed assessment in an environment free of distractions.	___	___	___	_____
IMPLEMENTATION				
1. Obtained complete and thorough nursing history.	___	___	___	_____
2. Initiated diet diary or 24-hour recall.	___	___	___	_____
3. Documented findings on nutritional assessment sheet.	___	___	___	_____
4. Assisted client into bed.	___	___	___	_____
5. Performed physical assessment.	___	___	___	_____
6. Assisted client to standing position. Used chair, bed, or sling scale if client unable to stand.	___	___	___	_____
7. Weighed client.	___	___	___	_____
8. Obtained client's height.	___	___	___	_____
9. Calculated ideal body weight.	___	___	___	_____
10. Obtained wrist circumference.	___	___	___	_____
11. Obtained mid-upper–arm circumference.	___	___	___	_____

	S	U	NP	Comments
12. Obtained triceps skinfold measurements.	___	___	___	_____
13. Assisted client to comfortable position.	___	___	___	_____
14. Calculated mid-arm circumference.	___	___	___	_____
15. Washed hands. Told client when nutritional assessment was completed.	___	___	___	_____

EVALUATION

	S	U	NP	Comments
1. Reviewed history and physical examination.	___	___	___	_____
2. Reviewed diet diary and 24-hour recall with client.	___	___	___	_____
3. Compared client's height and weight with normal height and weight for age group.	___	___	___	_____
4. Reviewed anthropometric data.	___	___	___	_____
5. Compared client's laboratory data with normal values.	___	___	___	_____
6. Identified unexpected outcomes.	___	___	___	_____

RECORDING AND REPORTING

	S	U	NP	Comments
1. Documented findings and made recommendations on nutritional assessment form.	___	___	___	_____

Student _____   Date _____

Instructor _____   Date _____

PERFORMANCE CHECKLIST 21-2 **ASSISTING THE ADULT CLIENT WITH ORAL NUTRITION**

	S	U	NP	Comments
ASSESSMENT				
1. Assessed that GI tract is functioning and types of diet client can tolerate.	——	——	——	_____
2. Assessed client's ability to swallow. Assessed gag reflex.	——	——	——	_____
3. Assessed client's ability to feed self.	——	——	——	_____
4. Assessed client's appetite, food likes, and tolerance.	——	——	——	_____
5. Determined food allergies before serving meal.	——	——	——	_____
NURSING DIAGNOSIS				
1. Developed appropriate nursing diagnoses based on assessment data.	——	——	——	_____
PLANNING				
1. Identified expected outcomes.	——	——	——	_____
2. Prepared client's room.	——	——	——	_____
3. Prepared client for meal.	——	——	——	_____
IMPLEMENTATION				
1. Washed hands before preparing client's tray.	——	——	——	_____
2. Assessed tray for completeness and correct diet.	——	——	——	_____
3. Prepared tray for client.	——	——	——	_____
4. Determined how well client was eating independently.	——	——	——	_____
5. Began assisting client who could not eat independently.	——	——	——	_____
6. Assessed appropriate order to feed client, and cut food into bite-sized pieces.	——	——	——	_____
7. Fed client, correctly.	——	——	——	_____
8. Provided fluids as requested.	——	——	——	_____
9. Talked with client.	——	——	——	_____
10. Provided client education as appropriate.	——	——	——	_____
11. Assisted client to wash hands and perform mouth care.	——	——	——	_____

	S	U	NP	Comments
12. Assisted client to resting position.	___	___	___	_____
13. Returned client's tray and washed hands.	___	___	___	_____

EVALUATION

	S	U	NP	Comments
1. Observed client's ability to swallow.	___	___	___	_____
2. Assessed client's tolerance to diet.	___	___	___	_____
3. Assessed client's fluid and food intake.	___	___	___	_____
4. Weighed client daily.	___	___	___	_____
5. Assessed client's ability to assist with feeding.	___	___	___	_____
6. Identified unexpected outcomes.	___	___	___	_____

RECORDING AND REPORTING

	S	U	NP	Comments
1. Documented tolerance of diet, amount eaten, and intake and output.	___	___	___	_____

Student _____   Date _____

Instructor _____   Date _____

PERFORMANCE CHECKLIST 21-3   **ASPIRATION PRECAUTIONS**

	S	U	NP	Comments
ASSESSMENT				
1. Performed nutritional assessment (see Skill 21-1).	___	___	___	_____
2. Assessed clients who are at increased risk of aspiration for dysphagia.	___	___	___	_____
3. Reported signs and symptoms of dysphagia to physician.	___	___	___	_____
4. Noted evidence of dysphagia on client's record.	___	___	___	_____
NURSING DIAGNOSIS				
1. Developed appropriate nursing diagnoses based on assessment data.	___	___	___	_____
PLANNING				
1. Identified expected outcomes.	___	___	___	_____
IMPLEMENTATION				
1. Asked client about difficulties with swallowing or chewing various types of food.	___	___	___	_____
2. Inspected client's mouth for pockets of food using penlight and tongue blade.	___	___	___	_____
3. Positioned client upright in bed or chair.	___	___	___	_____
4. Offered client thicker foods and assessed for difficulty in swallowing.	___	___	___	_____
5. Proceeded to foods with thinner consistency if client able to tolerate thicker foods. Observed client closely for dysphagia.	___	___	___	_____
6. Assisted the client to complete the meal or placed the meal within client's reach for self-feeding if no signs or symptoms of dysphagia are evident.	___	___	___	_____
7. Asked client to remain sitting upright for at least 30 minutes after the meal.	___	___	___	_____
8. Assisted client to wash hands and perform mouth care.	___	___	___	_____
9. Returned client's tray to appropriate place and washed hands.	___	___	___	_____
EVALUATION				
1. Assessed client's ability to ingest foods of various textures and thickness.	___	___	___	_____
2. Assessed client's food and fluid intake.	___	___	___	_____

	S	U	NP	Comments
3. Weighed client weekly.	——	——	——	_____
4. Assessed client's oral cavity after meal to detect pockets of food.	——	——	——	_____
5. Identified unexpected outcomes.	——	——	——	_____

RECORDING AND REPORTING

	S	U	NP	Comments
1. Documented tolerance of various food textures, amount of assistance required, position during meal, absence or presence of dysphagia, and amount eaten.	——	——	——	_____
2. Reported dysphagia to nurse in charge or physician.	——	——	——	_____

Student _____   Date _____

Instructor _____   Date _____

PERFORMANCE CHECKLIST 22-1   **INTUBATING THE CLIENT WITH A SMALL-BORE NASOGASTRIC OR NASOINTESTINAL FEEDING TUBE**

	S	U	NP	Comments
ASSESSMENT				
1. Assessed client's need for tube feedings.	—	—	—	_____
2. Assessed patency of nares.	—	—	—	_____
3. Assessed past medical history.	—	—	—	_____
4. Evaluated gag reflex.	—	—	—	_____
5. Assessed client's mental status.	—	—	—	_____
6. Assessed for bowel sounds.	—	—	—	_____
NURSING DIAGNOSIS				
1. Developed appropriate nursing diagnoses based on assessment data.	—	—	—	_____
PLANNING				
1. Identified expected outcomes.	—	—	—	_____
2. Explained procedure to client.	—	—	—	_____
3. Explained to client how to communicate during procedure.	—	—	—	_____
4. Positioned client.	—	—	—	_____
5. Examined feeding tube for flaws.	—	—	—	_____
6. Determined length of tube to be inserted.	—	—	—	_____
7. Correctly prepared tube for intubation.	—	—	—	_____
8. Cut tape.	—	—	—	_____
IMPLEMENTATION				
1. Applied clean gloves.	—	—	—	_____
2. Inspected nares for irritation or obstruction.	—	—	—	_____
3. Dipped tube with surface lubricant into glass of water.	—	—	—	_____
4. Provided client with glass of water and straw.	—	—	—	_____
5. Inserted tube through nostril to back of throat.	—	—	—	_____
6. Flexed client's head toward chest after tube had passed through nasopharynx.	—	—	—	_____
7. Had client swallow and advanced tube as client swallowed.	—	—	—	_____

	S	U	NP	Comments

8. Emphasized need to mouth-breathe and swallow during procedure. ____ ____ ____ _____

9. Advanced tube each time client swallowed until desired length was passed. ____ ____ ____ _____

10. Did not force tube; checked for position of tube in back of throat. ____ ____ ____ _____

11. Checked placement of tube. ____ ____ ____ _____

12. Applied tube fixation device or applied tincture of benzoin on tip of client's nose and tube. Allowed to dry. ____ ____ ____ _____

13. Removed gloves. Secured tube with tape, if used. ____ ____ ____ _____

14. Fastened tube to gown. ____ ____ ____ _____

15. Positioned client on right side when x-ray confirmed placement. ____ ____ ____ _____

16. Obtained x-ray examination of chest/abdomen. ____ ____ ____ _____

17. Left stylet in place until position confirmed. ____ ____ ____ _____

18. Remained with client. ____ ____ ____ _____

19. Applied gloves and administered oral hygiene. ____ ____ ____ _____

20. Removed gloves, disposed of equipment, and washed hands. ____ ____ ____ _____

EVALUATION

1. Assessed client for reaction to procedure. ____ ____ ____ _____

2. Confirmed x-ray examination results. ____ ____ ____ _____

3. Checked external marking on tube. ____ ____ ____ _____

4. Identified unexpected outcomes. ____ ____ ____ _____

RECORDING AND REPORTING

1. Recorded and reported tube size/length, client's tolerance of procedure, and confirmation of placement by x-ray. ____ ____ ____ _____

Student _____   Date _____

Instructor _____   Date _____

PERFORMANCE CHECKLIST 22-2   **VERIFYING TUBE PLACEMENT FOR A LARGE- OR SMALL-BORE FEEDING TUBE**

	S	U	NP	Comments
ASSESSMENT				
1. Identified signs and symptoms of inadvertent respiratory placement.	——	——	——	_____
2. Identified signs and symptoms that increase risk of tube dislocation.	——	——	——	_____
3. Reviewed client's record for history of prior tube placement.	——	——	——	_____
4. Observed external portion of tube for a change in length.	——	——	——	_____
5. Reviewed medication record for gastric acid inhibitors.	——	——	——	_____
NURSING DIAGNOSIS				
1. Developed appropriate nursing diagnoses based on assessment data.	——	——	——	_____
PLANNING				
1. Identified expected outcomes.	——	——	——	_____
2. Explained procedure to client.	——	——	——	_____
IMPLEMENTATION				
1. Washed hands and applied gloves.	——	——	——	_____
2. Performed measures to verify placement of tube: injected 30 ml of air and aspirated GI contents with a syringe and measured pH of aspirated GI contents.	——	——	——	_____
3. Removed and disposed of gloves; washed hands.	——	——	——	_____
EVALUATION				
1. Observed client for respiratory distress.	——	——	——	_____
2. Observed flow rate of enteral formula.	——	——	——	_____
3. Identified unexpected outcomes.	——	——	——	_____
RECORDING AND REPORTING				
1. Recorded and reported information about tube, results of verification, and client's response.	——	——	——	_____

Student _____   Date _____

Instructor _____   Date _____

PERFORMANCE CHECKLIST 22-3 **IRRIGATING A SMALL-BORE FEEDING TUBE**

	S	U	NP	Comments

ASSESSMENT

1. Checked character of gastric aspirates.

2. Determined ease of infusion through tubing.

3. Monitored volume of tube feeding administered and compared with amount ordered.

4. Referred to agency policy regarding routine irrigations.

NURSING DIAGNOSIS

1. Developed appropriate nursing diagnoses based on assessment data.

PLANNING

1. Identified expected outcomes.

2. Explained procedure to client.

3. Assisted client to high-Fowler's or semi-Fowler's position.

IMPLEMENTATION

1. Washed hands.

2. Prepared equipment at bedside and applied gloves.

3. Checked tube placement.

4. Drew up 30 ml saline or tap water in syringe.

5. Kinked feeding tube while disconnecting from feeding bag or plug and placed end of tubing on towel.

6. Inserted tip of syringe into end of feeding tube.

7. Released kink of tubing and slowly instilled irrigating solution into tube.

8. Repositioned client if unable to instill solution.

9. Removed syringe after fluid instilled and reinstituted tube feeding or replaced plug.

10. Disposed of supplies, removed gloves, and washed hands.

	S	U	NP	Comments

EVALUATION

1. Observed ease of tube feeding infusion.   ___ ___ ___ _____

2. Identified unexpected outcomes.   ___ ___ ___ _____

RECORDING AND REPORTING

1. Recorded time of irrigation, fluid instilled, and results.   ___ ___ ___ _____

2. Recorded on I&O form.   ___ ___ ___ _____

3. Reported unexpected outcomes to the nurse in charge or physician.   ___ ___ ___ _____

Student _____ Date _____

Instructor _____ Date _____

PERFORMANCE CHECKLIST 22-4 **ADMINISTERING ENTERAL FEEDINGS VIA NASOENTERAL TUBE**

	S	U	NP	Comments
ASSESSMENT				
1. Assessed client's nutritional needs.	—	—	—	_____
2. Assessed client for food allergies.	—	—	—	_____
3. Assessed for signs and symptoms of malnutrition.	—	—	—	_____
4. Auscultated for bowel sounds.	—	—	—	_____
5. Obtained baseline weight and laboratory values.	—	—	—	_____
6. Verified physician's order.	—	—	—	_____
NURSING DIAGNOSIS				
1. Developed appropriate nursing diagnoses based on assessment data.	—	—	—	_____
PLANNING				
1. Identified expected outcomes.	—	—	—	_____
2. Washed hands.	—	—	—	_____
3. Prepared bag and tubing or syringe to administer formula.	—	—	—	_____
4. Explained procedure to client.	—	—	—	_____
5. Placed client in proper position.	—	—	—	_____
IMPLEMENTATION				
1. Applied gloves.	—	—	—	_____
2. Checked placement of tube.	—	—	—	_____
3. Checked gastric residual by connecting syringe to tube and aspirating contents.	—	—	—	_____
4. Flushed tubing with 30 ml of water.	—	—	—	_____
5. Initiated syringe or intermittent feeding:	—	—	—	_____
a. Pinched proximal end of feeding tube.	—	—	—	_____
b. Removed plunger from syringe and attached syringe to end of tube.	—	—	—	_____
c. Filled syringe with prescribed amount of formula.	—	—	—	_____
d. Released pinched tube, elevated syringe 45 cm (18 inches) above insertion site, and allowed formula to infuse slowly.	—	—	—	_____

	S	U	NP	Comments
e. Refilled syringe until prescribed amount was administered to client.	—	—	—	_____
f. For feeding bag, attached gavage tubing to end of feeding tube bag. Set rate by adjusting roller clamp on tubing, and allowed bag to empty gradually over 30 to 60 minutes.	—	—	—	_____
6. Initiated continuous drip feeding method:	—	—	—	_____
a. Placed feeding bag and tubing on IV pole.	—	—	—	_____
b. Connected distal end of tubing to proximal end of feeding tube.	—	—	—	_____
c. Connected tubing through infusion pump and set rate.	—	—	—	_____

EVALUATION

	S	U	NP	Comments
1. Measured amount of gastric aspirate every 8 to 12 hours.	—	—	—	_____
2. Monitored blood glucose every 6 hours until maximum administration rate reached.	—	—	—	_____
3. Monitored I&O every 8 hours.	—	—	—	_____
4. Weighed client daily.	—	—	—	_____
5. Observed laboratory values.	—	—	—	_____
6. Observed respiratory status.	—	—	—	_____
7. Observed client's level of comfort.	—	—	—	_____
8. Auscultated bowel sounds.	—	—	—	_____
9. Identified unexpected outcomes.	—	—	—	_____

RECORDING AND REPORTING

	S	U	NP	Comments
1. Recorded amount and type of feeding.	—	—	—	_____
2. Recorded client's response to feeding.	—	—	—	_____
3. Reported unexpected outcomes to nurse in charge or physician.	—	—	—	_____

Student _____ Date _____

Instructor _____ Date _____

PERFORMANCE CHECKLIST 22-5 **ADMINISTERING ENTERAL FEEDINGS VIA GASTROSTOMY/JEJUNOSTOMY TUBE**

	S	U	NP	Comments
ASSESSMENT				
1. Assessed client's need for enteral feedings.	—	—	—	
2. Assessed client for food allergies.	—	—	—	
3. Auscultated for bowel sounds.	—	—	—	
4. Obtained baseline weight and laboratory values.	—	—	—	
5. Verified physician's order.	—	—	—	
6. Assessed gastrostomy/jejunostomy site.	—	—	—	
NURSING DIAGNOSIS				
1. Developed appropriate nursing diagnoses based on assessment data.	—	—	—	
PLANNING				
1. Identified expected outcomes.	—	—	—	
2. Explained procedure to client.	—	—	—	
3. Washed hands.	—	—	—	
4. Prepared bag and tubing or syringe to administer formula.	—	—	—	
5. Placed client in correct position.	—	—	—	
IMPLEMENTATION				
1. Applied gloves.	—	—	—	
2. Verified placement of tube.	—	—	—	
3. Initiated feeding (intermittent or continuous drip method).	—	—	—	
4. Administered water via feeding tube as ordered.	—	—	—	
5. Flushed tube with 30 ml of water every 4 to 6 hours.	—	—	—	
6. Clamped tubing when feeding is not being administered.	—	—	—	
7. Rinsed bag and tubing after feeding.	—	—	—	
8. Advanced tube feeding.	—	—	—	
9. Changed exit site dressing as needed; inspected exit site every shift.	—	—	—	
10. Disposed of supplies and washed hands.	—	—	—	

	S	U	NP	Comments

EVALUATION

1. Evaluated client's tolerance of tube feeding. ___ ___ ___ _____

2. Monitored fingerstick blood glucose every 6 hours. ___ ___ ___ _____

3. Monitored I&O every shift. ___ ___ ___ _____

4. Weighed client daily. ___ ___ ___ _____

5. Observed laboratory values. ___ ___ ___ _____

6. Observed stoma site. ___ ___ ___ _____

7. Identified unexpected outcomes. ___ ___ ___ _____

RECORDING AND REPORTING

1. Recorded amount and type of feeding. ___ ___ ___ _____

2. Recorded client's response to feeding, patency of tube, and any adverse effects. ___ ___ ___ _____

3. Reported appropriate information to oncoming nursing staff. ___ ___ ___ _____

Student _____   Date _____

Instructor _____   Date _____

PERFORMANCE CHECKLIST 23-1 **CARING FOR THE CLIENT RECEIVING CENTRAL VENOUS PLACEMENT FOR CENTRAL PARENTERAL NUTRITION**

	S	U	NP	Comments
ASSESSMENT				
1. Assessed client's need for central parenteral nutrition (CPN).	—	—	—	_____
2. Checked physician's order for parenteral therapy.	—	—	—	_____
3. Assessed client's hydration status.	—	—	—	_____
4. Assessed client for surgical procedures or anatomical irregularities of the upper chest.	—	—	—	_____
5. Considered catheter material to be used.	—	—	—	_____
6. Inspected condition of skin.	—	—	—	_____
7. Assessed for allergy to iodine or lidocaine.	—	—	—	_____
NURSING DIAGNOSIS				
1. Developed appropriate nursing diagnoses based on assessment data.	—	—	—	_____
PLANNING				
1. Identified expected outcomes.	—	—	—	_____
2. Explained procedure to client and need for CPN and follow-up care.	—	—	—	_____
3. Verified that consent form was signed.	—	—	—	_____
IMPLEMENTATION				
1. Nurse and physician washed hands.	—	—	—	_____
2. Physician positioned client with assistance from nurse.	—	—	—	_____
3. Physician donned sterile attire; nurse donned cap, mask, eye wear, and nonsterile gloves.	—	—	—	_____
4. Nurse opened central vein kit and saturated gauze.	—	—	—	_____
5. Physician cleansed skin with povidone-iodine.	—	—	—	_____
6. Discarded gauze.	—	—	—	_____
7. Physician cleansed skin with povidone-iodine scrub.	—	—	—	_____
8. Physician wiped away excess scrub solution.	—	—	—	_____
9. Physician applied sterile gloves.	—	—	—	_____

	S	U	NP	Comments

10. Nurse opened first wrapping of central vein kit and handed to physician.   ___ ___ ___ _____

11. Physician opened second wrapping and prepared sterile field.   ___ ___ ___ _____

12. Physician reviewed kit and put needles on syringes.   ___ ___ ___ _____

13. Nurse set up IV bag and filled tubing.   ___ ___ ___ _____

14. Nurse opened sterile tubing and placed on sterile field.   ___ ___ ___ _____

15. Nurse placed client in Trendelenburg's position and turned client's head away from site of insertion.   ___ ___ ___ _____

16. Nurse wiped off top of 1% lidocaine bottle and turned it upside down.   ___ ___ ___ _____

17. Physician withdrew appropriate amount of lidocaine and injected it into subclavian puncture site.   ___ ___ ___ _____

18. Had client perform Valsalva maneuver.   ___ ___ ___ _____

19. Physician inserted subclavian IV catheter into subclavian vein.   ___ ___ ___ _____

20. Nurse frequently checked client to assess tolerance to procedure.   ___ ___ ___ _____

21. Nurse connected IV tubing to extension tubing and flushed with IV fluid while physician was cannulating central vein.   ___ ___ ___ _____

22. Physician connected IV tubing to client's subclavian catheter after establishing rapid blood return.   ___ ___ ___ _____

23. Nurse opened IV fluids wide.   ___ ___ ___ _____

24. Nurse lowered IV bag below heart level.   ___ ___ ___ _____

25. Nurse raised IV bag and slowed rate to 30 ml/hr until x-ray study obtained.   ___ ___ ___ _____

26. Physician sutured central venous catheter in place.   ___ ___ ___ _____

27. Physician removed sterile clothes and completed procedure.   ___ ___ ___ _____

Applying Occlusive Dressing

1. Applied sterile gloves.   ___ ___ ___ _____

2. With alcohol swab, started at catheter exit site and worked in circular motion outward approximately 2 to 3 inches (performed procedure three times).   ___ ___ ___ _____

	S	U	NP	Comments

3. Repeated above steps with povidone-iodine swabs and allowed area to dry.   — — — _____

4. Applied clear adhesive dressing over site.   — — — _____

5. Looped and secured tubing. Labeled dressing.   — — — _____

6. Assisted with x-ray examination.   — — — _____

7. Connected tubing to infusion pump and set rate.   — — — _____

8. Repositioned client.   — — — _____

9. Disposed of supplies and washed hands.   — — — _____

EVALUATION

1. Inspected site and dressing.   — — — _____

2. Evaluated client for complications associated with parenteral nutrition.   — — — _____

3. Identified unexpected outcomes.   — — — _____

RECORDING AND REPORTING

1. Recorded condition of client before, during, and after the procedure.   — — — _____

2. Documented size, type, and location of catheter; presence or absence of blood return after catheter placement; type of dressing; and type and rate of parenteral nutrition infused.   — — — _____

3. Documented confirmation of central vein catheter placement.   — — — _____

Student _____   Date _____

Instructor _____   Date _____

PERFORMANCE CHECKLIST 23-2 **CARING FOR THE CLIENT RECEIVING CENTRAL PARENTERAL NUTRITION (CPN)**

	S	U	NP	Comments
ASSESSMENT				
1. Assessed client's nutritional status, caloric intake, laboratory values, and weight.	___	___	___	_____
2. Inspected condition of access site.	___	___	___	_____
3. Assessed blood glucose levels.	___	___	___	_____
4. Assessed factors influencing CPN administration.	___	___	___	_____
5. Assessed vital signs and auscultated lung sounds.	___	___	___	_____
6. Verified physician's order for CPN and flow rate.	___	___	___	_____
NURSING DIAGNOSIS				
1. Developed appropriate nursing diagnoses based on assessment data.	___	___	___	_____
PLANNING				
1. Identified expected outcomes.	___	___	___	_____
2. Explained purpose of CPN.	___	___	___	_____
IMPLEMENTATION				
1. Washed hands and applied gloves.	___	___	___	_____
2. Inspected parenteral nutrition solution for solution, additives, particulate matter or separation, and expiration date.	___	___	___	_____
3. Checked client's identification.	___	___	___	_____
4. Placed IV tubing into intravenous infusion pump and regulated prescribed flow rate or connected to appropriate tubing.	___	___	___	_____
5. Discarded used supplies and washed hands.	___	___	___	_____
EVALUATION				
1. Monitored infusion rate.	___	___	___	_____
2. Obtained daily weights.	___	___	___	_____
3. Assessed for fluid retention.	___	___	___	_____
4. Monitored client's glucose and laboratory parameters to determine response to CPN.	___	___	___	_____
5. Inspected central venous access site.	___	___	___	_____
6. Identified unexpected outcomes.	___	___	___	_____

	S	U	NP	Comments

RECORDING AND REPORTING

1. Recorded condition of central venous access device, rate of infusion, I&O, vital signs, and weights.   ___ ___ ___ _____

2. Reported complications to nurse in charge or physician.   ___ ___ ___ _____

Student _____   Date _____

Instructor _____   Date _____

PERFORMANCE CHECKLIST 23-3 **CARING FOR THE CLIENT RECEIVING PERIPHERAL PARENTERAL NUTRITION WITH LIPID (FAT) EMULSION**

	S	U	NP	Comments
ASSESSMENT				
1. Assessed client for potential lipid intolerance.	—	—	—	————————
2. Assessed appropriate IV site for fat emulsion administration.	—	—	—	————————
3. Assessed appropriate time to administer fats.	—	—	—	————————
4. Checked physician's order for volume of fat emulsion.	—	—	—	————————
NURSING DIAGNOSIS				
1. Developed appropriate nursing diagnoses based on assessment data.	—	—	—	————————
PLANNING				
1. Identified expected outcomes.	—	—	—	————————
2. Explained why client was receiving fat emulsions.	—	—	—	————————
3. Placed client in comfortable position.	—	—	—	————————
4. Checked parenteral nutrition solution and expiration date.	—	—	—	————————
5. Warmed solution.	—	—	—	————————
IMPLEMENTATION				
1. Washed hands and applied gloves.	—	—	—	————————
2. Checked client's identification.	—	—	—	————————
3. Connected tubing to solution and ran fat emulsion into IV tubing.	—	—	—	————————
4. Cleaned peripheral line tubing injection port.	—	—	—	————————
5. Inserted fat emulsion infusion into injection port correctly.	—	—	—	————————
6. Set flow rate on infusion pump. Began peripheral parenteral nutrition at ordered rate.	—	—	—	————————
7. Discarded supplies and washed hands.	—	—	—	————————
EVALUATION				
1. Assessed vital signs and general comfort level to determine response to fat emulsion.	—	—	—	————————
2. Monitored temperature every 4 hours and regularly inspected venipuncture site.	—	—	—	————————

	S	U	NP	Comments
3. Monitored laboratory values.	___	___	___	_____
4. Assessed client's response to fluid volume.	___	___	___	_____
5. Identified unexpected outcomes.	___	___	___	_____

RECORDING AND REPORTING

	S	U	NP	Comments
1. Recorded I&O every shift.	___	___	___	_____
2. Recorded temperature every 4 hours.	___	___	___	_____
3. Recorded condition of IV site and status of infusion.	___	___	___	_____
4. Reported complications to nurse in charge or physician.	___	___	___	_____

Student _____   Date _____

Instructor _____   Date _____

PERFORMANCE CHECKLIST 24-1 **ASSISTING A CLIENT TO USE A URINAL**

	S	U	NP	Comments
ASSESSMENT				
1. Assessed client's urinary elimination patterns.	___	___	___	_____
2. Assessed for incontinence.	___	___	___	_____
3. Palpated client for distended bladder.	___	___	___	_____
4. Assessed client's cognitive and physical status.	___	___	___	_____
5. Assessed client's knowledge regarding urinal use.	___	___	___	_____
NURSING DIAGNOSIS				
1. Developed appropriate nursing diagnoses based on assessment data.	___	___	___	_____
PLANNING				
1. Identified expected outcomes.	___	___	___	_____
IMPLEMENTATION				
1. Washed hands and applied gloves.	___	___	___	_____
2. Provided privacy.	___	___	___	_____
3. Assisted client into appropriate position.	___	___	___	_____
4. Placed urinal properly.	___	___	___	_____
5. Assessed output. Emptied, cleaned, and returned urinal.	___	___	___	_____
6. Allowed client to wash hands.	___	___	___	_____
7. Removed and disposed of gloves; washed hands.	___	___	___	_____
EVALUATION				
1. Assessed client's ability to use urinal.	___	___	___	_____
2. Noted characteristics of urine.	___	___	___	_____
3. Identified unexpected outcomes.	___	___	___	_____
RECORDING AND REPORTING				
1. Recorded client's ability to use urinal and characteristics of urinary output.	___	___	___	_____
2. Recorded urinary output.	___	___	___	_____
3. Reported frequency of voiding patterns.	___	___	___	_____

Student _____   Date _____

Instructor _____   Date _____

PERFORMANCE CHECKLIST 24-2   **INSERTING A STRAIGHT OR INDWELLING CATHETER**

	S	U	NP	Comments
ASSESSMENT				
1. Assessed client's general status.	—	—	—	_____
2. Assessed for distended bladder.	—	—	—	_____
3. Inspected perineal area.	—	—	—	_____
4. Determined conditions that may impair passage of catheter.	—	—	—	_____
5. Reviewed client's medical record and physician's order.	—	—	—	_____
6. Assessed client's knowledge of purpose for catheterization.	—	—	—	_____
NURSING DIAGNOSIS				
1. Developed appropriate nursing diagnoses based on assessment data.	—	—	—	_____
PLANNING				
1. Identified expected outcomes.	—	—	—	_____
2. Explained procedure to client.	—	—	—	_____
IMPLEMENTATION				
1. Washed hands.	—	—	—	_____
2. Provided privacy.	—	—	—	_____
3. Raised bed to appropriate height.	—	—	—	_____
4. Positioned self correctly.	—	—	—	_____
5. Raised appropriate side rail.	—	—	—	_____
6. Placed pad under client.	—	—	—	_____
7. Positioned client.	—	—	—	_____
8. Draped client.	—	—	—	_____
9. Using disposable gloves, cleansed perineal area using clean technique.	—	—	—	_____
10. Prepared urinary drainage container.	—	—	—	_____
11. Positioned lamp.	—	—	—	_____
12. Maintained sterile asepsis while opening catheter kit.	—	—	—	_____
13. Applied sterile gloves.	—	—	—	_____

	S	U	NP	Comments
14. Organized supplies on sterile field.		—	—	_____
15. Checked integrity of inflatable balloon of indwelling catheter.		—	—	_____
16. Applied sterile drape over client.		—	—	_____
17. Placed sterile tray in easily accessible place.		—	—	_____
18. Applied lubricant to catheter tip.		—	—	_____
19. Cleansed urethral meatus correctly. Positioned nondominant hand correctly on labia or penis.		—	—	_____
20. Handled catheter properly.		—	—	_____
21. Inserted catheter correctly while asking client to bear down gently.		—	—	_____
22. Advanced catheter to appropriate length if no resistance felt.		—	—	_____
23. Collected urine specimen if needed.		—	—	_____
24. Allowed bladder to empty fully.		—	—	_____
25. If using straight single-use catheter, withdrew it slowly and smoothly.		—	—	_____
26. If using indwelling catheter, inflated balloon correctly.		—	—	_____
27. Attached end of catheter to collecting tube.		—	—	_____
28. Taped catheter or applied Velcro tube holder.		—	—	_____
29. Maintained patent tubing.		—	—	_____
30. Assisted client to comfortable position. Washed and dried perineal area as needed.		—	—	_____
31. Removed gloves and disposed of equipment properly.		—	—	_____
32. Instructed client on proper positions.		—	—	_____
33. Cautioned client against pulling catheter.		—	—	_____
34. Washed hands.		—	—	_____

EVALUATION

	S	U	NP	Comments
1. Palpated client's bladder.		—	—	_____
2. Assessed client's comfort.		—	—	_____
3. Observed character and amount of urine.		—	—	_____
4. Determined that no urine was leaking from catheter or tubing.		—	—	_____
5. Identified unexpected outcomes.		—	—	_____

	S	U	NP	Comments

RECORDING AND REPORTING

1. Reported and recorded pertinent data: catheter description, assessment of urine, and client's response to procedure. ___ ___ ___ _____

2. Initiated I&O records. ___ ___ ___ _____

Replaced urinary tubing and collection bag, if needed.

Maintained proper position of drainage tubing.

Emptied collection bag as necessary.

Catheter removal:

a. Completed Steps 1 through 5.

b. Placed waterproof pad correctly.

c. Obtained sterile urine specimen as required.

d. Removed tape or Velcro tube holder.

e. Aspirated fluid used to inflate catheter balloon.

f. Removed catheter and wrapped in waterproof pad.

g. Unhooked bag and tubing from bed.

h. Positioned client. Provided perineal care, if necessary.

i. Measured contents and emptied collection bag.

Assisted client to comfortable position.

Lowered bed to lowest position.

Disposed of contaminated gloves and supplies; washed hands.

EVALUATION

Inspected urethra and surrounding tissue.

Noted character of urine.

Observed time and amount of first voiding.

RECORDING AND REPORTING

Recorded when care was given and assessment of urethral meatus and urine. Documented removal catheter.

Reported pertinent data to appropriate health care team member(s).

Date _____

Date _____

CATHETERIZED SPECIMENS FOR RESIDUAL

	S	U	NP	Comments
	—	—	—	_____
	—	—	—	_____
	—	—	—	_____
	—	—	—	_____
	—	—	—	_____
	—	—	—	_____
	—	—	—	_____
	—	—	—	_____
	—	—	—	_____
	—	—	—	_____
	—	—	—	_____
	—	—	—	_____
	—	—	—	_____

Student _____   Date _____

Instructor _____   Date _____

PERFORMANCE CHECKLIST 24-5 **PERFORMING CATHETER IRRIGATION**

	S	U	NP	Comments
ASSESSMENT				
1. Reviewed client's medical record.	___	___	___	_____
2. Assessed characteristics of urine, patency of tubing, and status of existing closed system.	___	___	___	_____
3. Reviewed I&O record.	___	___	___	_____
4. Assessed client for presence of bladder spasms and discomfort.	___	___	___	_____
5. Assessed client's knowledge of procedure.	___	___	___	_____
NURSING DIAGNOSIS				
1. Developed appropriate nursing diagnoses based on assessment data.	___	___	___	_____
PLANNING				
1. Identified expected outcomes.	___	___	___	_____
2. Explained procedure to client.	___	___	___	_____
IMPLEMENTATION				
1. Washed hands and applied gloves.	___	___	___	_____
2. Provided privacy.	___	___	___	_____
3. Positioned client correctly and removed tape or Velcro tube holder.	___	___	___	_____
4. Assessed lower abdomen for signs of bladder distention.	___	___	___	_____
5. Performed closed intermittent irrigation:	___	___	___	_____
a. Poured prescribed, room-temperature solution into sterile container.	___	___	___	_____
b. Drew solution into syringe.	___	___	___	_____
c. Clamped indwelling retention catheter below injection port on drainage tubing.	___	___	___	_____
d. Applied gloves.	___	___	___	_____
e. Cleansed injection port with antiseptic.	___	___	___	_____
f. Inserted needle of syringe into injection port at 30-degree angle.	___	___	___	_____
g. Injected fluid into catheter slowly.	___	___	___	_____
h. Withdrew syringe and removed clamp.	___	___	___	_____

6. Performed continuous irrigation: ___ ___ ___ _____

   a. Applied gloves and inserted spike of irrigation tubing into bag of solution. ___ ___ ___ _____

   b. Closed clamp on tubing and placed bag of solution on IV pole. ___ ___ ___ _____

   c. Attached tubing to catheter. ___ ___ ___ _____

   d. Opened clamp and allowed solution to flow. ___ ___ ___ _____

   e. Calculated drip rate and adjusted roller clamp on tubing accordingly. ___ ___ ___ _____

   f. For intermittent flow, clamped tubing on drainage system, allowed prescribed amount to enter bladder, and then closed off irrigation infusion and unclamped catheter drainage system. ___ ___ ___ _____

7. Performed open irrigation: ___ ___ ___ _____

   a. Applied gloves. ___ ___ ___ _____

   b. Opened sterile irrigation tray and set up sterile field. ___ ___ ___ _____

   c. Poured required amount of sterile solution into sterile container. ___ ___ ___ _____

   d. Positioned waterproof pad under catheter. ___ ___ ___ _____

   e. Aspirated 30 ml of solution into syringe. ___ ___ ___ _____

   f. Moved sterile collection basin close to client's thigh. ___ ___ ___ _____

   g. Wiped connection point between catheter and drainage tubing with antiseptic before disconnecting. ___ ___ ___ _____

   h. Disconnected catheter from drainage tubing, thereby allowing urine to flow into sterile collection basin. ___ ___ ___ _____

   i. Covered end of drainage tubing with sterile protective cap, and placed tubing in a secure spot. ___ ___ ___ _____

   j. Inserted tip of syringe into catheter lumen and gently instilled solution. ___ ___ ___ _____

   k. Withdrew syringe, lowered catheter, and allowed solution to drain into basin. ___ ___ ___ _____

   l. Repeated instillation until drainage clear. ___ ___ ___ _____

   m. Had client turn onto side, or aspirated solution if solution did not return. ___ ___ ___ _____

   n. Cleansed and replaced drainage tubing adapter. ___ ___ ___ _____

8. Reanchored catheter to client. ___ ___ ___ _____

	S	U	NP	Comments
9. Assisted client to comfortable position.	—	—	—	_____
10. Lowered bed and side rails, if appropriate.	—	—	—	_____
11. Disposed of contaminated supplies and gloves.	—	—	—	_____
12. Washed hands.	—	—	—	_____

EVALUATION

1. Accurately calculated the difference between the amount of irrigating solution instilled and the amount of drainage returned.	—	—	—	_____
2. Assessed characteristics of output and urine.	—	—	—	_____
3. Observed patency of catheter.	—	—	—	_____
4. Identified unexpected outcomes.	—	—	—	_____

RECORDING AND REPORTING

1. Recorded amount of solution used to irrigate and amount and consistency of drainage returned.	—	—	—	_____
2. Reported occlusion, sudden bleeding, infection, or pain to physician.	—	—	—	_____

Student _____   Date _____

Instructor _____   Date _____

PERFORMANCE CHECKLIST 24-6 **APPLYING A CONDOM CATHETER**

	S	U	NP	Comments
ASSESSMENT				
1. Determined client's elimination pattern.	—	—	—	_____
2. Assessed client's mental status.	—	—	—	_____
3. Assessed condition of penis.	—	—	—	_____
4. Assessed client's knowledge of purpose of condom catheter.	—	—	—	_____
NURSING DIAGNOSIS				
1. Developed appropriate nursing diagnoses based on assessment data.	—	—	—	_____
PLANNING				
1. Identified expected outcomes.	—	—	—	_____
2. Explained procedure.	—	—	—	_____
IMPLEMENTATION				
1. Washed hands.	—	—	—	_____
2. Provided privacy.	—	—	—	_____
3. Raised bed to working height. Lowered appropriate side rail.	—	—	—	_____
4. Positioned client correctly.	—	—	—	_____
5. Prepared urinary drainage collection bag and tubing.	—	—	—	_____
6. Put on disposable gloves and provided perineal care.	—	—	—	_____
7. Clipped hair at base of penis.	—	—	—	_____
8. Applied skin preparation to penis and allowed to dry.	—	—	—	_____
9. Put condom on client's penis.	—	—	—	_____
10. Allowed space between glans and end of condom catheter.	—	—	—	_____
11. Attached Velcro or elastic to condom.	—	—	—	_____
12. Connected tubing to end of condom.	—	—	—	_____
13. Secured excess tubing.	—	—	—	_____
14. Positioned client comfortably.	—	—	—	_____

	S	U	NP	Comments
15. Raised side rail and lowered bed.	___	___	___	_____
16. Disposed of contaminated supplies and gloves. Washed hands.	___	___	___	_____

EVALUATION

1. Observed urinary drainage.	___	___	___	_____
2. Inspected penis within 30 minutes after application of catheter.	___	___	___	_____
3. Routinely assessed skin of penis and color of glans penis while condom was removed.	___	___	___	_____
4. Identified unexpected outcomes.	___	___	___	_____

RECORDING AND REPORTING

1. Recorded and reported pertinent information related to procedure.	___	___	___	_____
2. Monitored I&O as indicated.	___	___	___	_____

Student _____   Date _____

Instructor _____   Date _____

PERFORMANCE CHECKLIST 24-7 **CARE OF A SUPRAPUBIC CATHETER**

	S	U	NP	Comments
ASSESSMENT				
1. Assessed urine in bag for amount and characteristics.	—	—	—	_____
2. Assessed dressing for drainage and intactness.	—	—	—	_____
3. Assessed catheter insertion site for signs of inflammation. Asked client if there is pain at the site.	—	—	—	_____
4. Assessed how catheter is held in place.	—	—	—	_____
5. Assessed tape site for signs of irritation.	—	—	—	_____
6. Assessed for fever.	—	—	—	_____
7. Checked for allergies.	—	—	—	_____
NURSING DIAGNOSIS				
1. Developed appropriate nursing diagnoses based on assessment data.	—	—	—	_____
PLANNING				
1. Identified expected outcomes.	—	—	—	_____
2. Explained procedure to client.	—	—	—	_____
IMPLEMENTATION				
1. Washed hands.	—	—	—	_____
2. Provided privacy.	—	—	—	_____
3. Proceeded with application of a dry sterile dressing.	—	—	—	_____
4. Cleansed site around drain.	—	—	—	_____
5. Applied split gauze around catheter with dominant sterile gloved hand, and applied tape.	—	—	—	_____
6. Secured catheter to abdomen with tape or Velcro tube holder.	—	—	—	_____
7. Checked bag and tubing placement.	—	—	—	_____
EVALUATION				
1. Asked client if there is pain or discomfort from suprapubic catheter.	—	—	—	_____
2. Observed client's urine for sediment, odor, or discoloration.	—	—	—	_____
3. Inspected dressing at least every shift.	—	—	—	_____

	S	U	NP	Comments
4. Monitored for signs of infection.	___	___	___	_____
5. Identified unexpected outcomes.	___	___	___	_____

RECORDING AND REPORTING

	S	U	NP	Comments
1. Reported and recorded dressing replacement, assessment of wound, and client's tolerance of procedure.	___	___	___	_____
2. Reported presence of unexpected outcomes.	___	___	___	_____

Student _____   Date _____

Instructor _____   Date _____

PERFORMANCE CHECKLIST 24-8 **PERITONEAL DIALYSIS AND CONTINUOUS AMBULATORY PERITONEAL DIALYSIS**

	S	U	NP	Comments
ASSESSMENT				
1. Obtained client's weight.	—	—	—	_____
2. Obtained client's vital signs.	—	—	—	_____
3. Assessed respiratory status.	—	—	—	_____
4. Measured abdominal girth.	—	—	—	_____
5. Monitored for fluid and electrolyte balance.	—	—	—	_____
6. Inspected catheter site.	—	—	—	_____
7. Measured body temperature.	—	—	—	_____
8. Reviewed agency's procedure for peritoneal dialysis (PD) or continuous ambulatory peritoneal dialysis (CAPD).	—	—	—	_____
9. Reviewed physician's orders.	—	—	—	_____
10. Verified dialysis solutions and medication.	—	—	—	_____
11. Verified number and duration of exchanges.	—	—	—	_____
12. Obtained laboratory data as ordered.	—	—	—	_____
13. Assessed client's knowledge of procedure.	—	—	—	_____
NURSING DIAGNOSIS				
1. Developed appropriate diagnoses based on assessment data.	—	—	—	_____
PLANNING				
1. Identified expected outcomes.	—	—	—	_____
2. Explained procedure to client.	—	—	—	_____
IMPLEMENTATION				
Initiating Manual Dialysis Exchanges				
1. Washed hands. Donned mask (nurse and client if client performing PD).	—	—	—	_____
2. Positioned client.	—	—	—	_____
3. Added medications as listed in physician's order.	—	—	—	_____
4. Attached two warmed dialysate bags to inflow tubing and attached to IV pole.	—	—	—	_____
5. Applied sterile gloves.	—	—	—	_____

	S	U	NP	Comments

6. Disinfected catheter cap and end of catheter. Removed cap. Disinfected adaptor and connected tubing.

7. Used Y connecter and flushed tubing.

8. Instilled dialysate bag #1 over prescribed time.

9. Clamped inflow tubing for prescribed dwell time.

10. Removed dialysate bag #1 from IV pole and placed warmed bag #3 on pole.

11. Unclamped outflow tubing and allowed to drain.

12. Clamped outflow tubing.

13. Emptied and measured fluid in drainage bag.

14. Repeated Steps 3-11 until all exchanges completed.

15. Monitored client's vital signs every 15 minutes during first exchange.

16. Covered catheter with sterile cap or followed guidelines specific to catheter when exchanges completed.

17. Inspected catheter dressing. Reapplied transparent occlusive dressing, if indicated.

18. Disposed of contaminated supplies properly and washed hands.

EVALUATION

1. Obtained weight.

2. Obtained dialysis fluid balance.

3. Obtained vital signs, including body temperature.

4. Auscultated lungs.

5. Measured abdominal girth.

6. Inspected catheter site.

7. Inspected returned dialysate solution.

8. Observed client performing CAPD.

9. Assessed client's comfort level.

10. Monitored lab work.

11. Identified unexpected outcomes.

	S	U	NP	Comments

RECORDING AND REPORTING

1. Documented client's weight, abdominal girth, and dialysis fluid balance before and after PD.

2. Documented client's vital signs before, during, and after dialysis.

3. Documented temperature and status of catheter site.

4. Recorded presence of pain or discomfort.

5. Recorded color of drainage.

6. Recorded condition of catheter dressing.

7. Reported and noted any unexpected outcomes and actions taken.

Student _____   Date _____

Instructor _____   Date _____

PERFORMANCE CHECKLIST 25-1   **ASSISTING THE CLIENT TO USE A BEDPAN**

	S	U	NP	Comments
ASSESSMENT				
1. Assessed client's normal bowel elimination habits.	——	——	——	——————————
2. Auscultated and palpated abdomen.	——	——	——	——————————
3. Assessed client's mobility status.	——	——	——	——————————
4. Determined appropriate type of bedpan to use.	——	——	——	——————————
5. Assessed for rectal or abdominal pain and irritation of skin surrounding anus.	——	——	——	——————————
6. Determined if stool specimen needed.	——	——	——	——————————
NURSING DIAGNOSIS				
1. Developed appropriate nursing diagnoses based on assessment data.	——	——	——	——————————
PLANNING				
1. Identified expected outcomes.	——	——	——	——————————
2. Explained procedure to client.	——	——	——	——————————
3. Obtained assistance from additional nursing personnel, if indicated.	——	——	——	——————————
IMPLEMENTATION				
1. Washed hands and applied gloves.	——	——	——	——————————
2. Provided privacy.	——	——	——	——————————
3. Warmed bedpan before use.	——	——	——	——————————
4. Put opposite side rail up.	——	——	——	——————————
5. Positioned bed at appropriate working height.	——	——	——	——————————
6. Ensured that client was positioned properly.	——	——	——	——————————
Mobile Client				
a. Raised client's head 30 to 60 degrees.	——	——	——	——————————
b. Removed upper bed linen.	——	——	——	——————————
c. Removed bedpan cover and placed bedpan in accessible location.	——	——	——	——————————
d. Instructed client to flex knees and lift hips.	——	——	——	——————————
e. Correctly assisted client onto bedpan.	——	——	——	——————————

	S	U	NP	Comments

Immobile Client

a. Positioned bed flat or level.

b. Removed upper bed linen.

c. Correctly assisted client to roll onto bedpan.

d. Raised client's head 30 degrees (unless contra-indicated).

7. Ensured client's comfort.

8. Placed call bell and toilet tissue within client's reach.

9. Ensured that bed was in lowest position with side rails up.

10. Removed gloves and washed hands.

11. Allowed client to be alone, but monitored status.

12. Responded to client's call bell immediately.

13. Applied new gloves.

14. Positioned client's bedside chair near working side of bed for placement of bedpan.

15. Collected basin of warm water.

16. Removed upper linens. Covered client with towel.

17. Determined if client was able to wipe perineal area.

18. Removed bedpan.

For Mobile Client

a. Correctly removed bedpan while client lifted up.

b. Offered client opportunity to wash hands.

For Immobile Client

a. Lowered head of bed.

b. Assisted client to roll off bedpan.

c. Wiped client's anal area.

19. Covered bedpan.

20. Returned client to comfortable position.

21. Positioned bed in lowest position and returned client's environment to former status.

22. While wearing gloves, emptied contents of bedpan and rinsed it. Obtained stool specimen, if indicated.

	S	U	NP	Comments
23. Replaced all used equipment.	___	___	___	_____
24. Disposed of soiled linens.	___	___	___	_____
25. Removed gloves and washed hands.	___	___	___	_____

EVALUATION

1. Assessed characteristics of urine and stool.	___	___	___	_____
2. Evaluated client's ability to use bedpan.	___	___	___	_____
3. Inspected condition of client's skin.	___	___	___	_____
4. Evaluated client's overall state of well-being.	___	___	___	_____
5. Identified unexpected outcomes.	___	___	___	_____

RECORDING AND REPORTING

1. Documented character of stool and urinary output if client also voids.	___	___	___	_____
2. Completed laboratory requisition for stool or urine specimen.	___	___	___	_____

Student _____   Date _____

Instructor _____   Date _____

PERFORMANCE CHECKLIST 25-2   **REMOVING FECAL IMPACTION DIGITALLY**

	S	U	NP	Comments
ASSESSMENT				
1. Assessed client's elimination status, vital signs, and abdomen.	——	——	——	_____
2. Checked client's record for physician's order.	——	——	——	_____
NURSING DIAGNOSIS				
1. Developed appropriate nursing diagnoses based on assessment data.	——	——	——	_____
PLANNING				
1. Identified expected outcomes.	——	——	——	_____
2. Explained procedure to client.	——	——	——	_____
IMPLEMENTATION				
1. Washed hands and applied gloves.	——	——	——	_____
2. Obtained assistance to position client, if needed.	——	——	——	_____
3. Provided privacy.	——	——	——	_____
4. Raised bed to working height with opposite rail up.	——	——	——	_____
5. Draped client.	——	——	——	_____
6. Placed waterproof pad under client's buttocks.	——	——	——	_____
7. Placed bedpan next to client.	——	——	——	_____
8. Lubricated index finger of glove.	——	——	——	_____
9. Inserted index finger gradually into client's rectum.	——	——	——	_____
10. Gently loosened fecal mass.	——	——	——	_____
11. Moved mass toward end of rectum.	——	——	——	_____
12. Checked client's heart rate and looked for signs of fatigue.	——	——	——	_____
13. Allowed client to rest at intervals during procedure.	——	——	——	_____
14. Washed anal area after disimpaction.	——	——	——	_____
15. Removed bedpan and inspected and disposed of feces. Removed and disposed of gloves.	——	——	——	_____

	S	U	NP	Comments
16. Assisted client to toilet or to use a clean bedpan.	___	___	___	_____
17. Washed hands.	___	___	___	_____

EVALUATION

1. Performed rectal examination.	___	___	___	_____
2. Reassessed vital signs and compared to baseline values.	___	___	___	_____
3. Assessed bowel sounds.	___	___	___	_____
4. Assessed for soft and nontender abdomen.	___	___	___	_____
5. Identified unexpected outcomes.	___	___	___	_____

RECORDING AND REPORTING

1. Documented and reported client's tolerance, amount and consistency of stool, and any adverse effects.	___	___	___	_____
2. Reported adverse effects to nurse in charge or physician.	___	___	___	_____

Student _____   Date _____

Instructor _____   Date _____

PERFORMANCE CHECKLIST 25-3 **ADMINISTERING AN ENEMA**

	S	U	NP	Comments
ASSESSMENT				
1. Assessed client's status.	___	___	___	_____
2. Inspected abdomen for distention.	___	___	___	_____
3. Determined client's understanding of procedure.	___	___	___	_____
4. Checked client's medical record for contraindications.	___	___	___	_____
5. Reviewed physician's order.	___	___	___	_____
NURSING DIAGNOSIS				
1. Developed appropriate nursing diagnoses based on assessment data.	___	___	___	_____
PLANNING				
1. Identified expected outcomes.	___	___	___	_____
2. Collected equipment and arranged at client's bedside.	___	___	___	_____
3. Explained procedure to client.	___	___	___	_____
IMPLEMENTATION				
1. Washed hands and applied gloves.	___	___	___	_____
2. Provided privacy.	___	___	___	_____
3. Raised bed to working height with opposite side rail up.	___	___	___	_____
4. Positioned client correctly.	___	___	___	_____
5. Placed waterproof pad under client's hips and buttocks.	___	___	___	_____
6. Draped client.	___	___	___	_____
7. Examined perianal region.	___	___	___	_____
8. Placed bedpan within easy reach.	___	___	___	_____
9. Administered enema using prepackaged disposable container.	___	___	___	_____
a. Removed plastic cap from rectal tip and lubricated, if necessary.	___	___	___	_____
b. Separated client's buttocks and located anus.	___	___	___	_____
c. Instructed client to relax by breathing out through the mouth.	___	___	___	_____

	S	U	NP	Comments

d. Expelled air from container. ___ ___ ___ _____

e. Inserted nozzle into anal canal, angling toward the umbilicus. Inserted 7.5 to 10 cm (3-4 inches) for an adult client, 5 to 7.5 cm (2-3 inches) for a child client, and 2.5 to 3.75 cm (1-1½ inches) for an infant client. ___ ___ ___ _____

f. Squeezed bottle until all solution instilled. ___ ___ ___ _____

g. Instructed client to retain solution until urge to defecate occurs. ___ ___ ___ _____

10. Administered enema using enema bag: ___ ___ ___ _____

a. Added warmed solution to enema bag; checked temperature of solution. ___ ___ ___ _____

b. Raised bag, released clamp, and allowed solution to fill tubing. ___ ___ ___ _____

c. Reclamped tubing. ___ ___ ___ _____

d. Lubricated 6 to 8 cm (3-4 inches) of tip of tubing. ___ ___ ___ _____

e. Separated client's buttocks and located anus. ___ ___ ___ _____

f. Instructed client to relax. ___ ___ ___ _____

g. Inserted tip appropriate length. ___ ___ ___ _____

h. Held tubing in client's rectum until end of instillation. ___ ___ ___ _____

i. Opened regulating clamp and allowed solution to enter slowly. ___ ___ ___ _____

j. Raised height of container to appropriate level (7.5-45 cm/3-18 inches). ___ ___ ___ _____

k. Lowered container or slowed infusion if client had cramping. ___ ___ ___ _____

l. Clamped tubing after all fluid instilled. ___ ___ ___ _____

m. Placed toilet tissue around end of tubing and withdrew tubing from client's anus. ___ ___ ___ _____

n. Reassured client that feeling of distention is expected, and instructed client to retain fluid. ___ ___ ___ _____

11. Discarded enema containers and tubing. ___ ___ ___ _____

12. Assisted client to bathroom or commode or onto bedpan. ___ ___ ___ _____

13. Observed character of feces and solution. ___ ___ ___ _____

14. Assisted client with perineal care. ___ ___ ___ _____

15. Removed and discarded gloves. Washed hands. ___ ___ ___ _____

	S	U	NP	Comments

EVALUATION

1. Inspected character of stool and fluid. ___ ___ ___ _____

2. Assessed condition of abdomen. ___ ___ ___ _____

3. Identified unexpected outcomes. ___ ___ ___ _____

RECORDING AND REPORTING

1. Recorded type and volume of enema and results. ___ ___ ___ _____

2. Reported failure of client to defecate. ___ ___ ___ _____

Student _____   Date _____

Instructor _____   Date _____

PERFORMANCE CHECKLIST 25-4   **INSERTING AND MAINTAINING THE NASOGASTRIC TUBE**

	S	U	NP	Comments

ASSESSMENT

1. Inspected condition of client's nasal and oral cavity.

2. Determined history of nasal surgery and noted if deviated nasal septum present.

3. Palpated client's abdomen.

4. Assessed client's level of consciousness and ability to follow instructions.

5. Determined if client had a nasogastric (NG) tube in the past.

6. Checked medical record for order.

NURSING DIAGNOSIS

1. Developed appropriate nursing diagnoses based on assessment data.

PLANNING

1. Identified expected outcomes.

2. Prepared equipment at bedside.

3. Identified client and explained procedure.

IMPLEMENTATION

1. Washed hands and applied gloves.

2. Positioned client in high-Fowler's position with pillows behind head and shoulder.

3. Provided privacy.

4. Stood at correct side of bed.

5. Placed bath towel over client's chest.

6. Determined which nostril to use.

7. Measured distance to insert tube using traditional or Hanson method.

8. Marked length of tube to be inserted from nares to stomach.

9. Prepared a piece of tape to anchor tube.

10. Curved tip of NG tube tightly around index finger and then released.

	S	U	NP	Comments

11. Lubricated 3 to 4 inches of the end of the tube with water-soluble lubricating jelly. ___ ___ ___ _____

12. Instructed client to extend neck, and inserted tube slowly through naris with curved end pointing downward. ___ ___ ___ _____

13. Continued to pass tube along floor of nasal passage. ___ ___ ___ _____

14. If resistance met, rotated tube or withdrew tube, allowed client to rest, relubricated tube, and inserted into other naris. ___ ___ ___ _____

15. Continued tube insertion by gently rotating tube toward opposite naris; stopped tube advancement; allowed client to relax; provided tissues; explained to client that next step requires client to swallow. ___ ___ ___ _____

16. With tube above oropharynx, instructed client to flex head forward and dry swallow or suck in air through a straw; advanced the tube 1 to 2 inches with each swallow. ___ ___ ___ _____

17. If client began to cough, gag, or choke, stopped tube advancement; instructed client to breathe easily and take sips of water. ___ ___ ___ _____

18. If client continued to cough, pulled tube back slightly. ___ ___ ___ _____

19. If client continued to gag, checked back of pharynx. ___ ___ ___ _____

20. After client relaxed, continued to advance tube the desired distance. ___ ___ ___ _____

21. After tube advanced, anchored tube with prepared split tape and marked tube length. ___ ___ ___ _____

Checking Tube Placement

1. Asked client to talk. ___ ___ ___ _____

2. Checked posterior pharynx for coiling of tube. ___ ___ ___ _____

3. Aspirated gently back on syringe to obtain gastric contents. ___ ___ ___ _____

4. Measured pH of aspirate. ___ ___ ___ _____

5. If tube not in stomach, advanced it 1 to 2 inches and repeated Steps 3 and 4 to check tube position. ___ ___ ___ _____

	S	U	NP	Comments

Anchoring Tube

1. After tube was properly inserted, either clamped end or connected to a drainage bag or suction machine. ___ ___ ___ _____

2. Cut 4-inch piece of tape; split one end lengthwise 2 inches; placed tab of tape over bridge of nose; wrapped ½-inch strips around tube as it exited nose; avoided putting pressure on naris. ___ ___ ___ _____

3. Fastened end of NG tube to client's gown with rubber band and safety pin; provided slack for client's movement. ___ ___ ___ _____

4. Kept head of bed elevated 30 degrees. ___ ___ ___ _____

5. Explained that sensation of tube should decrease. ___ ___ ___ _____

6. Removed gloves and washed hands. ___ ___ ___ _____

Tube Irrigation

1. Washed hands and applied gloves. ___ ___ ___ _____

2. Checked tube placement. ___ ___ ___ _____

3. Drew up 30 ml normal saline into Asepto or catheter-tipped syringe. ___ ___ ___ _____

4. Clamped tube proximal to connection site for drainage or suction; disconnected tube and laid end on towel. ___ ___ ___ _____

5. Inserted tip of syringe into end of NG tube; held syringe with tip pointed at the floor and slowly injected solution; did not force. ___ ___ ___ _____

6. If resistance occurred, checked tube for kinks; turned client onto left side. ___ ___ ___ _____

7. After instilling saline, aspirated with syringe to withdraw fluids; measured volume returned. ___ ___ ___ _____

8. Reconnected NG tube to drainage or suction; if solution did not return, repeated irrigation. ___ ___ ___ _____

9. Removed gloves and washed hands. ___ ___ ___ _____

Discontinuation of NG Tube

1. Verified order to discontinue NG tube. ___ ___ ___ _____

2. Explained procedure to client. ___ ___ ___ _____

3. Washed hands and applied disposable gloves. ___ ___ ___ _____

4. Turned off suction; disconnected NG tube from drainage bag or suction; removed tape from nose; unpinned tube from gown. ___ ___ ___ _____

5. Provided client facial tissue and placed towel across client's chest. ___ ___ ___ _____

	S	U	NP	Comments
6. Pulled tube out steadily and smoothly as client held breath.	___	___	___	_____
7. Disposed of tube and drainage unit; measured drainage.	___	___	___	_____
8. Cleaned nares and provided mouth care.	___	___	___	_____
9. Positioned client and explained fluid intake.	___	___	___	_____
10. Cleaned and stored equipment.	___	___	___	_____
11. Removed gloves and washed hands.	___	___	___	_____

EVALUATION

	S	U	NP	Comments
1. Observed amount and character of NG drainage.	___	___	___	_____
2. Palpated client's abdomen and auscultated bowel sounds.	___	___	___	_____
3. Inspected condition of nares and nose.	___	___	___	_____
4. Observed position of tubing.	___	___	___	_____
5. Asked if client felt pharyngeal irritation.	___	___	___	_____
6. Identified unexpected outcomes.	___	___	___	_____

RECORDING AND REPORTING

	S	U	NP	Comments
1. Recorded insertion procedure, client's tolerance, and character of drainage correctly.	___	___	___	_____
2. Recorded tube irrigation and amount and type of aspirate correctly.	___	___	___	_____
3. Recorded balance of fluid instilled and aspirated on I&O sheet.	___	___	___	_____
4. Recorded discontinuation of tube.	___	___	___	_____
5. Reported absence or character of drainage and on-set of abdominal distention.	___	___	___	_____
6. Recorded presence or absence of bowel sounds.	___	___	___	_____

Student _____   Date _____

Instructor _____   Date _____

PERFORMANCE CHECKLIST 26-1   **POUCHING AN ENTEROSTOMY**

	S	U	NP	Comments
ASSESSMENT				
1. Auscultated for bowel sounds.	___	___	___	_____
2. Observed skin barrier and pouch for leakage and length of time in place.	___	___	___	_____
3. Observed stoma for color and condition.	___	___	___	_____
4. Observed abdominal incision for pouch placement.	___	___	___	_____
5. Observed drainage from stoma; kept I&O.	___	___	___	_____
6. Checked for skin irritation.	___	___	___	_____
7. Avoided unnecessary changing of pouch.	___	___	___	_____
8. Assessed client's abdomen, overall condition, and stoma type for best pouching system to use.	___	___	___	_____
9. Assessed skin around stoma after pouch is removed.	___	___	___	_____
10. Determined client's knowledge of ostomy and emotional response.	___	___	___	_____
NURSING DIAGNOSIS				
1. Developed appropriate nursing diagnoses based on assessment data.	___	___	___	_____
PLANNING				
1. Identified expected outcomes.	___	___	___	_____
2. Explained steps of procedure to client.	___	___	___	_____
3. Assembled equipment and provided privacy.	___	___	___	_____
IMPLEMENTATION				
1. Positioned client correctly.	___	___	___	_____
2. Washed hands and applied gloves.	___	___	___	_____
3. Placed towel or barrier under client.	___	___	___	_____
4. Removed used pouch and skin barrier.	___	___	___	_____
5. Cleansed peristomal skin, patted dry, and measured stoma.	___	___	___	_____
6. Selected and prepared pouch by removing backing from barrier and adhesive.	___	___	___	_____
7. Correctly applied skin barrier and pouch.	___	___	___	_____

	S	U	NP	Comments
8. Applied nonallergic tape to skin barrier.	___	___	___	_____
9. Added ostomy deodorant, if desired.	___	___	___	_____
10. Secured clamp to pouch.	___	___	___	_____
11. Properly disposed of old pouch and soiled equipment.	___	___	___	_____
12. Removed gloves and washed hands.	___	___	___	_____
13. Changed pouch every 3 to 7 days unless it was leaking.	___	___	___	_____

EVALUATION

1. Assessed appearance of stoma, skin, and incision. Inspected pouch and skin barrier.	___	___	___	_____
2. Auscultated bowel sounds and observed character of stool.	___	___	___	_____
3. Assessed client's comfort level.	___	___	___	_____
4. Observed client's nonverbal behavior and asked if client had any questions about pouching.	___	___	___	_____
5. Identified unexpected outcomes.	___	___	___	_____

RECORDING AND REPORTING

1. Documented pouching procedure and equipment used.	___	___	___	_____
2. Recorded character of effluent and appearance of stoma and skin.	___	___	___	_____
3. Documented abdominal distention or discomfort.	___	___	___	_____
4. Reported abnormal appearance of stoma or suture line or unusual character of effluent.	___	___	___	_____
5. Reported absence of flatus for 24 to 36 hours or no stool by third day.	___	___	___	_____

Student _____   Date _____

Instructor _____   Date _____

PERFORMANCE CHECKLIST 26-2 **IRRIGATING A COLOSTOMY**

	S	U	NP	Comments

ASSESSMENT

1. Assessed frequency and character of stool, placement of stoma, and nutritional pattern.

2. Assessed time when client normally irrigates colostomy. Conferred with physician about order to irrigate new ostomy.

3. Reviewed procedural orders requiring bowel preparation.

4. Assessed client's understanding and ability to perform irrigation.

NURSING DIAGNOSIS

1. Developed appropriate nursing diagnoses based on assessment data.

PLANNING

1. Identified expected outcomes.

2. Explained procedure to client.

3. Assembled equipment and provided privacy.

IMPLEMENTATION

1. Positioned client correctly.

2. Applied gloves.

3. Filled irrigation bag with proper amount of fluid. Hung on hook at appropriate height.

4. Removed old pouch. Removed gloves and washed hands.

5. Correctly applied irrigation sleeve.

6. Applied gloves, lubricated cone tip, and held against stomal opening. Initiated flow of water.

7. Allowed water to flow in over 5 to 10 minutes. Clamped tubing.

8. After desired amount of water instilled, removed cone after waiting 15 seconds. Discarded gloves and closed top of irrigation sleeve.

	S	U	NP	Comments

9. Allowed 15 to 20 minutes for initial evacuation. Applied gloves. Dried tip of sleeve and clamped bottom. Folded sleeve, discarded gloves, and allowed client to ambulate.   ___ ___ ___ _____

10. Applied gloves; unclamped sleeve and emptied contents; removed sleeve. Rinsed sleeve and hung sleeve to dry.   ___ ___ ___ _____

11. Applied new pouch or stoma covering.   ___ ___ ___ _____

12. Removed gloves and washed hands.   ___ ___ ___ _____

EVALUATION

1. Inspected volume and character of fecal material and fluid.   ___ ___ ___ _____

2. Noted client's response during irrigation.   ___ ___ ___ _____

3. Asked client to describe steps of procedure.   ___ ___ ___ _____

4. Identified unexpected outcomes.   ___ ___ ___ _____

RECORDING AND REPORTING

1. Recorded procedure, volume and type of solution administered, fluid returned, and client's tolerance.   ___ ___ ___ _____

2. Recorded reapplication of pouch.   ___ ___ ___ _____

3. Reported any complications to nurse in charge or physician.   ___ ___ ___ _____

Student _____ Date _____

Instructor _____ Date _____

PERFORMANCE CHECKLIST 26-3 **POUCHING A NONCONTINENT URINARY DIVERSION**

	S	U	NP	Comments
ASSESSMENT				
1. Assessed pouch and condition of skin to determine need to change pouch.	___	___	___	_____
2. Observed output from stoma, stents, or catheters.	___	___	___	_____
3. Assessed abdomen for best type of pouch to use.	___	___	___	_____
4. Assessed bowel sounds.	___	___	___	_____
5. Determined client's knowledge of ostomy, and his or her emotional response.	___	___	___	_____
NURSING DIAGNOSIS				
1. Developed appropriate nursing diagnoses based on assessment data.	___	___	___	_____
PLANNING				
1. Identified expected outcomes.	___	___	___	_____
2. Assembled equipment.	___	___	___	_____
3. Closed door or curtain.	___	___	___	_____
4. Explained steps of procedure to client and encouraged participation.	___	___	___	_____
IMPLEMENTATION				
1. Positioned client correctly.	___	___	___	_____
2. Prepared pouch.	___	___	___	_____
3. Washed hands and applied gloves.	___	___	___	_____
4. Placed towel or barrier under client. Placed wick or gauze pad over stoma.	___	___	___	_____
5. Removed old pouch.	___	___	___	_____
6. Cleansed peristomal skin, patted dry. Used skin barrier or sealant as indicated.	___	___	___	_____
7. Wicked and measured stoma. Applied pouch.	___	___	___	_____
8. Opened drain spout and attached to urinary bag. Placed bag at foot of bed.	___	___	___	_____
9. Properly disposed of used pouch and soiled equipment.	___	___	___	_____
10. Removed gloves and washed hands.	___	___	___	_____

	S	U	NP	Comments
11. Changed pouch every 3 to 7 days unless it was leaking.	___	___	___	_____

EVALUATION

1. Noted condition of stoma, skin, and suture line. Evaluated character and volume of urine.	___	___	___	_____
2. Assessed for discomfort around stoma.	___	___	___	_____
3. Noted client's and/or significant other's willingness to view stoma and ask questions.	___	___	___	_____
4. Identified unexpected outcomes.	___	___	___	_____

RECORDING AND REPORTING

1. Recorded type of pouch, time of change, appearance of stoma and skin, and character of urine.	___	___	___	_____
2. Recorded urinary output on I&O flowsheet.	___	___	___	_____
3. Noted client's or significant other's reaction to procedure.	___	___	___	_____
4. Reported any abnormalities to nurse in charge or physician.	___	___	___	_____

Student _____   Date _____

Instructor _____   Date _____

PERFORMANCE CHECKLIST 26-4 **CATHETERIZING A NONCONTINENT URINARY DIVISION**

	S	U	NP	Comments
ASSESSMENT				
1. Determined need to obtain urine specimen.	___	___	___	_____
2. Obtained physician's order.	___	___	___	_____
3. Assessed client's understanding of procedure.	___	___	___	_____
NURSING DIAGNOSIS				
1. Developed appropriate nursing diagnoses based on assessment data.	___	___	___	_____
PLANNING				
1. Identified expected outcomes.	___	___	___	_____
2. Assembled equipment.	___	___	___	_____
3. Provided for client's privacy.	___	___	___	_____
4. Explained procedure to client and timed procedure in accordance with pouch change.	___	___	___	_____
IMPLEMENTATION				
1. Positioned client correctly.	___	___	___	_____
2. Washed hands and opened barrier. Prepared gauze wicks. Applied nonsterile gloves.	___	___	___	_____
3. Removed old pouch according to Skill 26-3.	___	___	___	_____
4. Removed and discarded gloves. Opened sterile catheterization set or needed equipment. Had client wick stoma while waiting, if possible.	___	___	___	_____
5. Applied sterile gloves. Cleansed "face" of stoma with povidone-iodine swabs.	___	___	___	_____
6. Allowed small amount of urine to flow from stoma.	___	___	___	_____
7. Lubricated catheter.	___	___	___	_____
8. Placed distal end of catheter in specimen container.	___	___	___	_____
9. Using dominant hand, gently inserted catheter into stoma; instructed client to cough or turn slightly.	___	___	___	_____
10. Placed specimen container below level of stoma to collect urinary drainage.	___	___	___	_____

	S	U	NP	Comments
11. Withdrew catheter and placed 4 inch × 4 inch gauze pad over stoma.	___	___	___	_____
12. Secured specimen container and labeled specimen.	___	___	___	_____
13. Reapplied new pouch.	___	___	___	_____
14. Disposed of soiled pouch and equipment.	___	___	___	_____
15. Removed gloves, washed hands, and sent specimen to laboratory.	___	___	___	_____

EVALUATION

	S	U	NP	Comments
1. Compared results of culture and sensitivity with normal expected findings.	___	___	___	_____
2. Observed stoma and peristomal area for breakdown.	___	___	___	_____
3. Checked urinary pouch and skin barrier for leakage.	___	___	___	_____
4. Asked client about signs and symptoms of urinary tract infection.	___	___	___	_____
5. Identified unexpected outcomes.	___	___	___	_____

RECORDING AND REPORTING

	S	U	NP	Comments
1. Recorded specimen collection, client's tolerance of procedure, and appearance of urine, skin, and stoma.	___	___	___	_____
2. Reported results of laboratory test to nurse in charge or physician.	___	___	___	_____

Student _____ Date _____

Instructor _____ Date _____

PERFORMANCE CHECKLIST 26-5 **MAINTAINING A CONTINENT DIVERSION**

	S	U	NP	Comments
ASSESSMENT				
1. Observed all tubes for intactness and patency, nature of drainage, and connection to collection system.	—	—	—	_____
2. Observed condition of stoma, peristomal skin, and suture lines.	—	—	—	_____
3. Assessed bowel and lung sounds. Assessed serum chloride and creatinine values.	—	—	—	_____
4. Palpated lightly around stoma and noted any signs of infection.	—	—	—	_____
5. Determined client's emotional response, knowledge, and understanding of urinary reservoir. Assessed client's family and other support.	—	—	—	_____
NURSING DIAGNOSIS				
1. Formulated appropriate nursing diagnoses based on assessment data.	—	—	—	_____
PLANNING				
1. Identified expected outcomes.	—	—	—	_____
2. Assembled equipment.	—	—	—	_____
3. Provided for client's privacy.	—	—	—	_____
4. Explained procedure to client and encouraged participation.	—	—	—	_____
IMPLEMENTATION				
Postoperative Care to 3 Weeks				
1. Positioned client correctly.	—	—	—	_____
2. Washed hands and opened sterile equipment. Correctly removed lid from sterile specimen cup. Poured 20 to 30 ml sterile saline into cup. Opened syringe and povidone-iodine swabs.	—	—	—	_____
3. Applied sterile gloves and drew 20 to 30 ml saline into syringe. Cleansed connected point of indwelling stomal catheter and drainage tubing with swabs.	—	—	—	_____
4. Disconnected and irrigated stomal catheter.	—	—	—	_____
5. Reconnected drainage system. Recorded I&O. Changed bedside drainage bags according to policy.	—	—	—	_____

	S	U	NP	Comments

6. Used remaining swabs to clean "face" of stoma and to cleanse area around base of stoma. Allowed area to dry and removed iodine with sterile water. ___ ___ ___ _____

7. Discarded soiled equipment; removed gloves. Labeled sterile specimen cup correctly. ___ ___ ___ _____

Postoperative Care at 4 to 6 Weeks

1. Followed Steps 1 and 2 of preceding section. (Omitted setting up sterile cup.) ___ ___ ___ _____

2. Observed aseptic technique while unwrapping supplies. ___ ___ ___ _____

3. Applied sterile gloves and drew 30 to 60 ml of sterile saline into syringe. Cleansed "face" of stoma with povidone-iodine swab. ___ ___ ___ _____

4. Lubricated catheter. Correctly inserted into stoma until urine began to drain. ___ ___ ___ _____

5. Irrigated pouch, if needed. ___ ___ ___ _____

6. Had client cough before removing catheter. ___ ___ ___ _____

7. Cleansed peristomal area and patted dry. ___ ___ ___ _____

8. Covered stoma with stomal covering. ___ ___ ___ _____

9. Discarded soiled equipment; removed gloves. Maintained correctly labeled sterile saline. ___ ___ ___ _____

10. Recorded urinary output and amount used for irrigation. ___ ___ ___ _____

EVALUATION

1. Noted appearance of stoma, peristomal skin, and suture lines. ___ ___ ___ _____

2. Evaluated character and volume of urinary output. ___ ___ ___ _____

3. Palpated for discomfort over pouch site and peristomal skin. ___ ___ ___ _____

4. Observed client's or caregiver's willingness to participate in care. ___ ___ ___ _____

5. Identified unexpected outcomes. ___ ___ ___ _____

RECORDING AND REPORTING

1. Recorded time of irrigation and intubation, size of catheter used, ease of intubation, amount of normal saline used, amount and character of urinary output, and client's tolerance. ___ ___ ___ _____

2. Documented client's, family's, and significant others' responses and their level of participation in care. ___ ___ ___ _____

3. Reported abnormalities of stoma and peristomal skin. ___ ___ ___ _____

Student _____   Date _____

Instructor _____   Date _____

PERFORMANCE CHECKLIST 27-1 **MAINTAINING BODY ALIGNMENT**

	S	U	NP	Comments
ASSESSMENT				
1. Observed alignment of client in standing, sitting, or lying position.	—	—	—	_____
NURSING DIAGNOSIS				
1. Developed appropriate diagnoses based on assessment data.	—	—	—	_____
PLANNING				
1. Identified expected outcomes.	—	—	—	_____
2. Instructed client or family on proper body alignment.	—	—	—	_____
IMPLEMENTATION				
1. Demonstrated to client or family correct body alignment for standing, sitting, or lying.	—	—	—	_____
2. Provided opportunity of return demonstration.	—	—	—	_____
3. Discussed with client or family hazards of prolonged immobility on body alignment and mobility.	—	—	—	_____
4. Provided client or family with community resources.	—	—	—	_____
EVALUATION				
1. Inspected skin surfaces.	—	—	—	_____
2. Had client demonstrate body alignment for standing, sitting, and lying.	—	—	—	_____
3. Asked client to describe benefits of body alignment.	—	—	—	_____
4. Identified unexpected outcomes.	—	—	—	_____
RECORDING AND REPORTING				
1. Recorded information presented to client and client's progress.	—	—	—	_____
2. Reported information taught to client at change-of-shift.	—	—	—	_____
3. Recorded time and position change of client.	—	—	—	_____

Student _____   Date _____

Instructor _____   Date _____

PERFORMANCE CHECKLIST 27-2 USING SAFE AND EFFECTIVE TRANSFER TECHNIQUES

	S	U	NP	Comments
ASSESSMENT				
1. Correctly assessed client's physiologic capacity for transfer.	——	——	——	——————————
2. Correctly assessed client for presence of weakness, dizziness, and postural hypotension.	——	——	——	——————————
3. Correctly assessed client's activity tolerance.	——	——	——	——————————
4. Correctly assessed client's proprioceptive function.	——	——	——	——————————
5. Correctly assessed client's sensory status.	——	——	——	——————————
6. Assessed client for comfort.	——	——	——	——————————
7. Correctly assessed client's cognitive status.	——	——	——	——————————
8. Assessed client's level of motivation.	——	——	——	——————————
9. Assessed previous mode of transfer, if applicable.	——	——	——	——————————
10. Assessed client's risk of injury.	——	——	——	——————————
11. Determined need for special transfer equipment in the home.	——	——	——	——————————
NURSING DIAGNOSIS				
1. Developed appropriate nursing diagnoses based on assessment data.	——	——	——	——————————
PLANNING				
1. Identified expected outcomes.	——	——	——	——————————
2. Explained procedure to client.	——	——	——	——————————
IMPLEMENTATION				
1. Washed hands.	——	——	——	——————————
2. Assisted client to sitting position:	——	——	——	——————————
a. Placed client in supine position.	——	——	——	——————————
b. Removed pillows from bed.	——	——	——	——————————
c. Faced head of bed and removed pillows.	——	——	——	——————————
d. Placed feet apart for broad base of support.	——	——	——	——————————
e. Correctly placed hand under client's shoulders.	——	——	——	——————————

	S	U	NP	Comments

f. Placed other hand on bed surface. ___ ___ ___ _____

g. Correctly raised client to sitting position (weight shifted to rear leg). ___ ___ ___ _____

h. Pushed against bed with hand on bed surface. ___ ___ ___ _____

3. Assisted client to a sitting position on the side of the bed: ___ ___ ___ _____

   a. Placed client in side-lying position. ___ ___ ___ _____

   b. Raised head of bed to 30 degrees. ___ ___ ___ _____

   c. Stood in correct position for transfer and turned diagonally to face client and far corner of bed. ___ ___ ___ _____

   d. Placed feet correctly. ___ ___ ___ _____

   e. Placed arm near bed under client's shoulders. ___ ___ ___ _____

   f. Placed other arm over client's thighs. ___ ___ ___ _____

   g. Moved client's lower legs and feet over side of bed and correctly pivoted leg. ___ ___ ___ _____

   h. Shifted weight to elevate client. ___ ___ ___ _____

   i. Remained in front of client until balance regained. ___ ___ ___ _____

   j. Provided physical support to weak or cognitively impaired client. ___ ___ ___ _____

4. Transferred client from bed to chair: ___ ___ ___ _____

   a. Assisted client to a sitting position on side of bed, with chair placed correctly. ___ ___ ___ _____

   b. Applied transfer belt, if needed. ___ ___ ___ _____

   c. Ensured that client was wearing nonskid shoes; kept weight-bearing leg forward. ___ ___ ___ _____

   d. Stood with feet apart. ___ ___ ___ _____

   e. Flexed knees and hips; aligned knees with client's. ___ ___ ___ _____

   f. Correctly placed arms around client or grasped transfer belt. ___ ___ ___ _____

   g. Rocked client to standing position on count of 3. ___ ___ ___ _____

   h. Used knee to maintain stability of weak (or paralyzed) leg. ___ ___ ___ _____

   i. Pivoted on foot that was farther from chair. ___ ___ ___ _____

   j. Instructed client to use arm rests on chair for support. ___ ___ ___ _____

	S	U	NP	Comments

k. Flexed hips and knees while lowering client into chair. ___ ___ ___ _____

l. Assessed client for proper alignment in sitting position. ___ ___ ___ _____

m. Provided client with support and encouragement. ___ ___ ___ _____

5. Performed three-person carry: ___ ___ ___ _____

   a. Three nurses stood side-by-side, facing side of client's bed. ___ ___ ___ _____

   b. Nurses were correctly positioned at client's head, hips, and thighs. ___ ___ ___ _____

   c. Used correct body mechanics for client transfer. ___ ___ ___ _____

   d. Properly positioned arms with hands securely around client's body. ___ ___ ___ _____

   e. Client correctly log-rolled to nurses' chests. ___ ___ ___ _____

   f. Client correctly lifted, with alignment maintained. ___ ___ ___ _____

   g. Nurses pivoted to stretcher in synchrony. ___ ___ ___ _____

   h. Used correct body alignment when placing client on stretcher. ___ ___ ___ _____

   i. Nurses assessed client's realignment. ___ ___ ___ _____

6. Used mechanical/hydraulic lift: ___ ___ ___ _____

   a. Moved lift to bedside. ___ ___ ___ _____

   b. Placed chair to allow adequate space to maneuver lift. ___ ___ ___ _____

   c. Raised bed to high position. ___ ___ ___ _____

   d. Kept side rail up on side opposite of nurse. ___ ___ ___ _____

   e. Rolled client away from nurse. ___ ___ ___ _____

   f. Placed hammock or a canvas strip under client to form seat. ___ ___ ___ _____

   g. Raised bed rail. ___ ___ ___ _____

   h. Went to opposite side of bed, lowered side rail. ___ ___ ___ _____

   i. Rolled client to opposite side and pulled hammock through. ___ ___ ___ _____

   j. Rolled client supine onto canvas seat. ___ ___ ___ _____

   k. Removed client's glasses, if applicable. ___ ___ ___ _____

	S	U	NP	Comments
l. Placed lift's horseshoe bar under bed.	—	—	—	_____
m. Lowered horizontal bar to sling level; locked valve.	—	—	—	_____
n. Attached strap hooks to holes in sling.	—	—	—	_____
o. Elevated head of bed.	—	—	—	_____
p. Folded client's arms over chest.	—	—	—	_____
q. Pumped handle until client was lifted from the bed.	—	—	—	_____
r. Pulled lift from bed and maneuvered to chair using steering handle.	—	—	—	_____
s. Rolled base around chair.	—	—	—	_____
t. Released check valve slowly; lowered client into chair.	—	—	—	_____
u. Closed check valve.	—	—	—	_____
v. Removed straps and lift.	—	—	—	_____
w. Checked client for proper alignment.	—	—	—	_____
7. Washed hands.	—	—	—	_____

EVALUATION

	S	U	NP	Comments
1. Monitored vital signs. Asked if client felt fatigued.	—	—	—	_____
2. Observed for correct body alignment and presence of pressure points on skin.	—	—	—	_____
3. Observed client's response to transfer.	—	—	—	_____
4. Asked if client had pain during transfer.	—	—	—	_____
5. Identified unexpected outcomes.	—	—	—	_____

RECORDING AND REPORTING

	S	U	NP	Comments
1. Recorded procedure and observations.	—	—	—	_____
2. Reported any unusual occurrence to appropriate personnel.	—	—	—	_____

Student _____   Date _____

Instructor _____   Date _____

PERFORMANCE CHECKLIST 27-3 **MOVING AND POSITIONING CLIENTS IN BED**

	S	U	NP	Comments
ASSESSMENT				
1. Assessed client's body alignment and comfort level.	—	—	—	_____
2. Assessed for risk factors.	—	—	—	_____
3. Assessed client's level of consciousness.	—	—	—	_____
4. Assessed client's ability to assist with positioning.	—	—	—	_____
5. Assessed for presence of tubes, incisions, and equipment.	—	—	—	_____
6. Assessed ability of client and family to participate in care.	—	—	—	_____
NURSING DIAGNOSIS				
1. Developed appropriate nursing diagnoses based on assessment data.	—	—	—	_____
PLANNING				
1. Identified expected outcomes.	—	—	—	_____
2. Raised level of bed to comfortable working height.	—	—	—	_____
3. Removed pillows and other objects.	—	—	—	_____
4. Obtained extra assistance as needed.	—	—	—	_____
5. Explained procedure to client.	—	—	—	_____
IMPLEMENTATION				
1. Washed hands.	—	—	—	_____
2. Provided for client privacy.	—	—	—	_____
3. Put bed in flat position.	—	—	—	_____
4. Moved immobile client up in bed (one nurse):	—	—	—	_____
a. Placed client on back with head of bed flat; stood on one side of bed.	—	—	—	_____
b. Placed pillow at head of bed.	—	—	—	_____
c. Correctly moved client up in bed.	—	—	—	_____
d. Kept arms level with client's hips.	—	—	—	_____
e. Slid client's hip diagonally toward head of bed.	—	—	—	_____
f. Maintained proper body alignment.	—	—	—	_____

	S	U	NP	Comments

g. Supported client's head on nurse's arm nearest the head of bed.

h. Placed other arm under client's chest.

i. Slid client's head, shoulders, and chest toward head of bed.

j. Raised side rail next to client and repositioned self on other side of bed.

k. Repeated procedure until client reached desired height in bed.

l. Correctly centered client in middle of bed.

5. Assisted client to move up in bed (one or two nurses):

a. Placed client on back with head of bed flat.

b. Placed pillow at head of bed.

c. Faced head of bed.

d. Stood in proper position.

e. Asked client to flex knees.

f. Instructed client to flex neck.

g. Instructed client to push feet on bed surface to assist movement.

h. Maintained own body alignment.

i. Instructed client to push heels and elevate trunk.

j. Shifted weight while client elevated trunk.

6. Moved immobile client up in bed using drawsheet or pullsheet (two nurses):

a. Placed drawsheet or pullsheet under client.

b. Placed client on back with bed flat.

c. Positioned one nurse at each side of client.

d. Grasped drawsheet or pullsheet firmly near client.

e. Maintained proper body alignment while shifting weight to move client and drawsheet or pullsheet to desired position.

	S	U	NP	Comments

7. Realigned client in proper body alignment. —— —— —— _____

  a. Positioned client in supported Fowler's position: —— —— —— _____

    • Elevated head of bed 45 to 60 degrees. —— —— —— _____

    • Rested client's head against mattress or placed small pillow underneath client's head. —— —— —— _____

    • Placed pillows appropriately to support client's hands and arms correctly. —— —— —— _____

    • Placed pillow at lower back. —— —— —— _____

    • Placed small pillow under thighs. —— —— —— _____

    • Placed small pillow or roll under ankles. —— —— —— _____

    • Placed footboard at bottom of client's feet. —— —— —— _____

  b. Positioned hemiplegic client in supported Fowler's position: —— —— —— _____

    • Elevated head of bed 45 to 60 degrees. —— —— —— _____

    • Sat client up as straight as possible. —— —— —— _____

    • Positioned client's head with chin slightly forward. —— —— —— _____

    • Supported involved arm and hand. —— —— —— _____

    • Positioned flaccid hand in normal resting position. —— —— —— _____

    • Positioned affected hand with wrist in neutral or slightly extended position. —— —— —— _____

    • Flexed client's knees and hips by using pillow. —— —— —— _____

    • Supported client's feet in dorsiflexed position. —— —— —— _____

  c. Positioned client in supine position: —— —— —— _____

    • Placed client on back with bed flat. —— —— —— _____

    • Placed small pillow or rolled towel under small of back. —— —— —— _____

    • Placed pillow under upper shoulders, neck, and head. —— —— —— _____

    • Placed trochanter rolls along hips and upper thighs. —— —— —— _____

    • Placed small pillow or roll under ankle. —— —— —— _____

    • Placed foot support to maintain feet in dorsiflexion. —— —— —— _____

	S	U	NP	Comments
• Placed pillows under pronated forearms.	___	___	___	_____
• Placed handrolls to maintain hands in functional position.	___	___	___	_____
d. Positioned hemiplegic client in supine position:	___	___	___	_____
• Placed client's head on flat bed.	___	___	___	_____
• Placed folded towel or pillow under shoulder of affected side.	___	___	___	_____
• Placed affected arm properly.	___	___	___	_____
• Placed affected hand properly.	___	___	___	_____
• Placed folded towel under hip of involved side.	___	___	___	_____
• Flexed affected knee 30 degrees.	___	___	___	_____
• Supported client's feet with soft pillows.	___	___	___	_____
e. Positioned client in prone position:	___	___	___	_____
• Placed client on abdomen with bed flat.	___	___	___	_____
• Turned client's head to one side; supported it with a small pillow.	___	___	___	_____
• Placed small pillow under client's abdomen.	___	___	___	_____
• Supported client's arms, flexed them at shoulders on pillows.	___	___	___	_____
• Placed pillow under client's lower legs to elevate toes off bed.	___	___	___	_____
f. Positioned hemiplegic client in prone position:	___	___	___	_____
• Moved client toward unaffected side.	___	___	___	_____
• Rolled client onto side.	___	___	___	_____
• Placed pillow on client's abdomen.	___	___	___	_____
• Rolled client onto abdomen.	___	___	___	_____
• Turned head toward involved side.	___	___	___	_____
• Positioned involved arm properly.	___	___	___	_____
• Flexed client's knees and placed pillows correctly.	___	___	___	_____
• Maintained client's feet at right angles.	___	___	___	_____
g. Positioned client in lateral (side-lying) position:	___	___	___	_____
• Lowered head of bed to comfortable level.	___	___	___	_____
• Positioned client on one side of bed.	___	___	___	_____
• Turned client onto one side.	___	___	___	_____

	S	U	NP	Comments
• Placed pillow under client's head and neck.	—	—	—	_____
• Brought client's shoulder blade forward.	—	—	—	_____
• Positioned client's arms in slightly flexed position.	—	—	—	_____
• Placed pillow behind client's back.	—	—	—	_____
• Placed pillow under client's upper leg.	—	—	—	_____
• Placed sandbag parallel to plantar surface of client's foot.	—	—	—	_____
h. Positioned client in Sims' (semiprone) position:	—	—	—	_____
• Lowered head of bed completely.	—	—	—	_____
• Placed client in supine position.	—	—	—	_____
• Positioned client in lateral position partially lying on abdomen.	—	—	—	_____
• Placed pillow under client's head.	—	—	—	_____
• Placed pillow under client's flexed upper arm to support arm level with shoulder.	—	—	—	_____
• Placed pillow under client's flexed upper leg to support leg level with hip.	—	—	—	_____
• Placed sandbags parallel to plantar surface of client's feet to maintain feet in dorsiflexion.	—	—	—	_____
i. Logrolled the client:	—	—	—	_____
• Placed pillow between client's knees.	—	—	—	_____
• Crossed client's arms over chest.	—	—	—	_____
• Positioned two nurses on side to which client was to be turned. Positioned another nurse on other side of bed.	—	—	—	_____
• Fanfolded or rolled drawsheet or pullsheet.	—	—	—	_____
• Moved the client in a smooth, continuous motion on the count of 3.	—	—	—	_____
• Placed pillows along length of client for support.	—	—	—	_____
• Leaned client back in one smooth motion toward pillows.	—	—	—	_____
8. Washed hands.	—	—	—	_____

EVALUATION

	S	U	NP	Comments
1. Observed client's body alignment and level of comfort.	—	—	—	_____
2. Measured joint ROM.	—	—	—	_____

	S	U	NP	Comments
3. Assessed for contractures or breakdown in skin integrity.	___	___	___	_____
4. Identified unexpected outcomes.	___	___	___	_____

RECORDING AND REPORTING

	S	U	NP	Comments
1. Recorded procedure, including condition of skin, joint movement, and client's ability to assist with repositioning.	___	___	___	_____
2. Reported observations at change of shift.	___	___	___	_____

Student _____ Date _____

Instructor _____ Date _____

PERFORMANCE CHECKLIST 28-1 **PERFORMING RANGE-OF-MOTION EXERCISES**

	S	U	NP	Comments
ASSESSMENT				
1. Reviewed client's medical history and obtained physician's order, if needed.	___	___	___	_____
2. Performed baseline assessment of joint function.	___	___	___	_____
3. Determined client's or caregiver's understanding of exercises.	___	___	___	_____
NURSING DIAGNOSIS				
1. Developed appropriate nursing diagnoses based on assessment data.	___	___	___	_____
PLANNING				
1. Identified expected outcomes.	___	___	___	_____
2. Explained procedure and reason for performing ROM exercises.	___	___	___	_____
3. Positioned client appropriately.	___	___	___	_____
IMPLEMENTATION				
1. Washed hands.	___	___	___	_____
2. Exposed only limbs to be exercised.	___	___	___	_____
3. Raised bed to comfortable position and stood on side of bed of joints to be exercised.	___	___	___	_____
4. Performed exercises slowly and gently.	___	___	___	_____
5. Supported joint while performing exercise.	___	___	___	_____
6. Performed appropriate exercises:	___	___	___	_____
a. Flexion, extension, hyperextension, rotation, abduction, adduction, circumduction, supination, pronation, opposition, inversion, and eversion	___	___	___	_____
7. Followed appropriate sequence of exercises:	___	U	NP	_____
a. Neck, shoulder, elbow, forearm, wrist, fingers, thumb, hip, knee, ankle, and foot	___	___	___	_____
8. Discontinued exercises if client complained of discomfort, if resistance was met, or if a spasm occurred.	___	___	___	_____
9. Repeated each movement 5 times.	___	___	___	_____

	S	U	NP	Comments
10. Repositioned client after procedure.	——	——	——	_____
11. Washed hands.	——	——	——	_____

EVALUATION

1. Assessed client's response and assistance required.	——	——	——	_____
2. Asked for client's feedback.	——	——	——	_____
3. Observed range of motion as compared with baseline.	——	——	——	_____
4. Asked client to independently perform exercises.	——	——	——	_____
5. Identified unexpected outcomes.	——	——	——	_____

RECORDING AND REPORTING

1. Documented ROM, joint assessment, and client's tolerance of procedure.	——	——	——	_____
2. Notified nurse in charge or physician if any joint abnormalities were noted.	——	——	——	_____

Student _____ Date _____

Instructor _____ Date _____

PERFORMANCE CHECKLIST 28-2 **PERFORMING ISOMETRIC EXERCISES**

	S	U	NP	Comments
ASSESSMENT				
1. Reviewed client's chart for contraindications.	___	___	___	_____
2. Performed baseline assessment of vital signs.	___	___	___	_____
3. Assessed client's baseline muscle strength.	___	___	___	_____
4. Assessed client's nutritional status.	___	___	___	_____
5. Assessed client's or caregiver's understanding of exercises.	___	___	___	_____
NURSING DIAGNOSIS				
1. Developed appropriate nursing diagnoses based on assessment data.	___	___	___	_____
PLANNING				
1. Identified expected outcomes.	___	___	___	_____
2. Explained procedure and demonstrated exercises.	___	___	___	_____
3. Assisted client to comfortable position.	___	___	___	_____
IMPLEMENTATION				
1. Provided privacy.	___	___	___	_____
2. Instructed client to perform exercises as prescribed:	___	___	___	_____
a. Gradually increase repetitions; exercise muscle groups for walking 4 times per day until ambulatory.	___	___	___	_____
b. Tighten each muscle group for 8 seconds, then completely relax for several seconds.	___	___	___	_____
c. Repeat 8 to 10 times for each muscle group.	___	___	___	_____
d. Exhale during exertion.	___	___	___	_____
3. Had client perform each isometric exercise correctly:	___	___	___	_____
a. Quadriceps	___	___	___	_____
b. Gluteal muscle	___	___	___	_____
c. Abdominal muscle	___	___	___	_____
d. Foot	___	___	___	_____
e. Hand grip	___	___	___	_____

	S	U	NP	Comments
f. Biceps	——	——	——	_____
g. Triceps	——	——	——	_____
4. Had client perform each isometric exercise correctly:	——	——	——	_____
a. Triceps	——	——	——	_____
b. Quadriceps	——	——	——	_____

EVALUATION

	S	U	NP	Comments
1. Observed client's ability to perform exercises.	——	——	——	_____
2. Determined client's level of energy, muscular strength, and comfort.	——	——	——	_____
3. Obtained vital signs.	——	——	——	_____
4. Identified unexpected outcomes.	——	——	——	_____

RECORDING AND REPORTING

	S	U	NP	Comments
1. Recorded performance of isometric exercises and objective and subjective information about muscle strength.	——	——	——	_____
2. Reported client's tolerance of exercises to nurse in charge or physician.	——	——	——	_____

Student _____   Date _____

Instructor _____   Date _____

PERFORMANCE CHECKLIST 28-3 **APPLYING ELASTIC STOCKINGS**

	S	U	NP	Comments
ASSESSMENT				
1. Assessed need for application of elastic stockings.	___	___	___	_____
2. Observed for contraindications to use of elastic stockings.	___	___	___	_____
3. Obtained physician's order.	___	___	___	_____
4. Assessed client's or caregiver's understanding of application and care of elastic stockings.	___	___	___	_____
5. Assessed and documented condition of client's skin and circulation to the legs.	___	___	___	_____
NURSING DIAGNOSIS				
1. Developed appropriate nursing diagnoses based on assessment data.	___	___	___	_____
PLANNING				
1. Identified expected outcomes.	___	___	___	_____
2. Explained procedure and reasons for applying stockings.	___	___	___	_____
3. Measured client's legs to determine proper size of stockings.	___	___	___	_____
IMPLEMENTATION				
1. Washed hands.	___	___	___	_____
2. Elevated bed to comfortable level.	___	___	___	_____
3. Positioned client in supine position.	___	___	___	_____
4. Cleansed client's legs and applied talcum powder to client's legs and feet.	___	___	___	_____
5. Applied stockings correctly; properly positioned and smoothed them.	___	___	___	_____
6. Repositioned client after procedure, and washed hands.	___	___	___	_____
7. Removed stockings at least once per shift.	___	___	___	_____
EVALUATION				
1. Inspected stockings for fit.	___	___	___	_____
2. Observed circulatory status of lower extremities.	___	___	___	_____
3. Observed client or caregiver applying stockings.	___	___	___	_____

	S	U	NP	Comments
4. Determined client's response to procedure.	___	___	___	_____
5. Identified unexpected outcomes.	___	___	___	_____

RECORDING AND REPORTING

	S	U	NP	Comments
1. Recorded pertinent information about stocking application and removal, condition of skin, and circulatory status.	___	___	___	_____
2. Reported signs of skin irritation or thrombophlebitis to physician.	___	___	___	_____

Student _____   Date _____

Instructor _____   Date _____

PERFORMANCE CHECKLIST 28-4 **APPLYING PNEUMATIC COMPRESSION DEVICE**

	S	U	NP	Comments

ASSESSMENT

1. Assessed client for risk factors that indicate need for compression device.

2. Observed for signs, symptoms, or conditions that would contraindicate use of compression device.

3. Checked medical order.

4. Assessed client's and caregiver's understanding of sequential pneumatic compression (SPC) stockings.

5. Assessed skin condition and circulation of lower extremities.

NURSING DIAGNOSIS

1. Developed appropriate nursing diagnoses based on assessment data.

PLANNING

1. Identified expected outcomes.

2. Explained procedure to client.

3. Measured client's legs to determine proper stocking size.

IMPLEMENTATION

1. Washed hands.

2. Placed client in supine position with head of bed elevated.

3. Removed SPC stockings from package and unfolded and flattened them.

4. Arranged SPC stockings under client's legs according to the position indicated on the inside of the stocking.

5. Wrapped SPC stockings securely around client's legs.

6. Checked for proper fit.

7. Attached SPC stockings' connector to plug on mechanical unit.

8. Turned machine on.

9. Monitored functioning of SPC stockings through one full cycle of inflation and deflation.

	S	U	NP	Comments
10. Repositioned client in comfortable position.	___	___	___	_____
11. Washed hands.	___	___	___	_____

EVALUATION

1. Inspected SPC stockings for kinks or twisting of tubing.	___	___	___	_____
2. Observed skin condition and circulatory status of client's lower extremities.	___	___	___	_____
3. Identified unexpected outcomes.	___	___	___	_____

RECORDING AND REPORTING

1. Recorded SPC stocking application, length and size of stockings, and time of use and removal.	___	___	___	_____
2. Recorded skin condition, circulatory status, and thigh circumference, if indicated.	___	___	___	_____
3. Reported unexpected outcomes to the nurse in charge or physician.	___	___	___	_____

Student _____   Date _____

Instructor _____   Date _____

PERFORMANCE CHECKLIST 28-5   **CHANGING CLIENT'S POSITION TO MINIMIZE OCCURRENCE OF ORTHOSTATIC HYPOTENSION**

	S	U	NP	Comments
ASSESSMENT				
1. Reviewed client's chart.	—	—	—	_____
2. Obtained set of baseline vital signs.	—	—	—	_____
3. Assessed client's environment for potential safety hazards.	—	—	—	_____
NURSING DIAGNOSIS				
1. Developed appropriate nursing diagnoses based on assessment data.	—	—	—	_____
PLANNING				
1. Identified expected outcomes.	—	—	—	_____
2. Explained procedure and reasons for getting client out of bed.	—	—	—	_____
3. Assessed whether another staff member was needed to help with procedure.	—	—	—	_____
4. Explained to client the importance of reporting symptoms of hypotension.	—	—	—	_____
5. Explained to client or caregiver the importance of adequate hydration.	—	—	—	_____
IMPLEMENTATION				
1. Washed hands.	—	—	—	_____
2. Placed bed in low position.	—	—	—	_____
3. Raised head of bed slowly to high-Fowler's position, and obtained blood pressure.	—	—	—	_____
4. Assessed client for signs of orthostatic hypotension.	—	—	—	_____
5. Assisted client to sit on side of bed and continued to assess for signs of orthostatic hypotension.	—	—	—	_____
6. Assisted client to ambulate or sit in chair.	—	—	—	_____
7. Washed hands.	—	—	—	_____
EVALUATION				
1. Assessed client for orthostatic hypotension.	—	—	—	_____

	S	U	NP	Comments

2. Rechecked client's blood pressure while the client was sitting the first few times.

3. Identified unexpected outcomes.

RECORDING AND REPORTING

1. Recorded blood pressures, client's tolerance of procedure, assessment of ambulation, and need for assistance.

2. Reported immediately if client sustained injury or was unable to tolerate procedure.

Student _____   Date _____

Instructor _____   Date _____

PERFORMANCE CHECKLIST 28-6   **ASSISTING WITH AMBULATION**

	S	U	NP	Comments

ASSESSMENT

1. Reviewed client's chart.

2. Assessed client's physical readiness.

3. Assessed client's or caregiver's understanding of ambulatory technique.

4. Determined optimal time for ambulation.

5. Assessed degree of assistance needed.

NURSING DIAGNOSIS

1. Developed appropriate nursing diagnoses based on assessment data.

PLANNING

1. Identified expected outcomes.

2. Prepared client appropriately.

3. Determined appropriate height of ambulation device.

4. Checked for rubber tips on ambulation device.

5. Made sure that walking surface was clean, dry, well-lighted, and unobstructed.

IMPLEMENTATION
Assisted Ambulation With One Nurse

1. Washed hands.

2. Reviewed ways to minimize orthostatic hypotension.

3. Applied safety belt if necessary, assisted client to standing position, and observed balance.

4. Positioned self on client's stronger side and had client take a few steps. Positioned self on client's weaker side if assistance device used.

5. Supported client at waist. Grasped walking belt, if used.

6. Took a few steps forward with client and assessed for strength and balance.

	S	U	NP	Comments

7. Allowed client to return to bed or chair if weak or dizzy.

8. Used appropriate procedure if client began to fall.

Assisted Ambulation With Two Nurses

1. Followed Steps 1 and 2 of "Assisted Ambulation With One Nurse."

2. Nurses stood on each side of client.

3. Placed arms around client's waist.

4. Stepped in unison with client.

5. Increased distance gradually.

6. Followed Steps 7 and 8 of "Assisted Ambulation With One Nurse."

Ambulation With Assistive Devices

1. Assisted client with crutch walking, using appropriate gait.

2. Assisted client in climbing stairs with crutches.

3. Assisted client in descending stairs with crutches.

4. Assisted client in ambulating with walker.

5. Assisted client in ambulating with cane.

EVALUATION

1. Assessed client's response to ambulation, including vital signs and energy level.

2. Assessed subjective response from client about experience.

3. Assessed gait and body alignment.

4. Observed client's ability to perform self-care activities.

5. Identified unexpected outcomes.

RECORDING AND REPORTING

1. Recorded type of gait client used; amount of assistance required; distance walked; and client's tolerance of activity.

2. Immediately reported any injury sustained during procedure, any alteration in vital signs, or an inability to ambulate.

Student _____ Date _____

Instructor _____ Date _____

PERFORMANCE CHECKLIST 29-1 **ASSISTING WITH CAST APPLICATION**

	S	U	NP	Comments
ASSESSMENT				
1. Assessed client's health status.	___	___	___	_____
2. Assessed client's understanding of cast application.	___	___	___	_____
3. Assessed condition of tissues to be casted.	___	___	___	_____
4. Determined client's pain status.	___	___	___	_____
5. Determined extent to which client may use casted extremity.	___	___	___	_____
NURSING DIAGNOSIS				
1. Developed appropriate nursing diagnoses based on assessment data.	___	___	___	_____
PLANNING				
1. Identified expected outcomes.	___	___	___	_____
2. Instructed client, parent, or other assistants as needed.	___	___	___	_____
3. Administered analgesic or muscle relaxant 20 to 30 minutes before cast application, if indicated.	___	___	___	_____
IMPLEMENTATION				
1. Washed hands and applied gloves.	___	___	___	_____
2. Positioned client appropriately.	___	___	___	_____
3. Prepared skin before casting. Explained that warmth may be felt during application.	___	___	___	_____
4. Assisted with cast application.	___	___	___	_____
5. Supplied dampened rolls of plaster or synthetic cast roll.	___	___	___	_____
6. Supported body part(s) during application of cast and tape.	___	___	___	_____
7. Supplied stabilization material.	___	___	___	_____
8. Assisted with "finishing" of the cast.	___	___	___	_____
9. Supplied scissors to trim plaster around edges.	___	___	___	_____
10. Facilitated drying of cast.	___	___	___	_____
11. Positioned casted extremity appropriately; handled cast only with palms until dry.	___	___	___	_____

	S	U	NP	Comments
12. Covered or reclothed client, assisted with transfer; accompanied client to room; and assisted with transfer to bed, if necessary.	——	——	——	_____
13. Cleaned equipment. Removed gloves and washed hands.	——	——	——	_____
14. Explained procedures of exposure for fast drying.	——	——	——	_____
15. Had client turn every 2 to 3 hours.	——	——	——	_____
16. Informed client to notify personnel of alteration in sensation or mobility.	——	——	——	_____
17. Covered cast for client bathing.	——	——	——	_____

EVALUATION

	S	U	NP	Comments
1. Observed client for signs of "cast syndrome."	——	——	——	_____
2. Assessed neurovascular status.	——	——	——	_____
3. Observed for edema distal to cast.	——	——	——	_____
4. Assessed temperature of tissues.	——	——	——	_____
5. Compared tissue with unaffected areas.	——	——	——	_____
6. Inspected skin condition around cast edges.	——	——	——	_____
7. Determined client's mobility.	——	——	——	_____
8. Assessed client's subjective response.	——	——	——	_____
9. Smelled the cast edges.	——	——	——	_____
10. Observed client performing cast care.	——	——	——	_____
11. Identified unexpected outcomes.	——	——	——	_____

RECORDING AND REPORTING

	S	U	NP	Comments
1. Recorded application of cast, condition of skin, and circulation.	——	——	——	_____
2. Reported abnormal or untoward progression of findings obtained from assessments.	——	——	——	_____

Student _____   Date _____

Instructor _____   Date _____

PERFORMANCE CHECKLIST 29-2 **ASSISTING WITH CAST REMOVAL**

	S	U	NP	Comments
ASSESSMENT				
1. Assessed client's understanding of upcoming cast removal.	___	___	___	_____
2. Assessed client's readiness for cast removal.	___	___	___	_____
3. Asked client if itching or irritation under cast is felt.	___	___	___	_____
NURSING DIAGNOSIS				
1. Developed appropriate nursing diagnoses based on assessment data.	___	___	___	_____
PLANNING				
1. Identified expected outcomes.	___	___	___	_____
2. Explained procedure to client and detailed physical sensations to expect.	___	___	___	_____
IMPLEMENTATION				
1. Applied gloves if indicated and assisted with cast removal.	___	___	___	_____
2. Inspected underlying tissues.	___	___	___	_____
3. Applied enzyme wash to intact skin.	___	___	___	_____
4. Cleansed tissues with water and patted dry.	___	___	___	_____
5. Applied lotion to skin.	___	___	___	_____
6. Put joints and muscles through ROM exercises.	___	___	___	_____
7. Assisted in transfer of client for return to room or for discharge.	___	___	___	_____
8. Cleaned or disposed of equipment appropriately.	___	___	___	_____
EVALUATION				
1. Inspected underlying skin.	___	___	___	_____
2. Observed client's behavior.	___	___	___	_____
3. Asked client to explain and demonstrate exercises.	___	___	___	_____
4. Had client explain and perform skin care.	___	___	___	_____
5. Identified unexpected outcomes.	___	___	___	_____

	S	U	NP	Comments

RECORDING AND REPORTING

1. Recorded cast removal, condition of tissues under cast, and person removing cast.   ___ ___ ___ _____

2. Reported unexpected outcomes to nurse in charge or physician.   ___ ___ ___ _____

Student _____   Date _____

Instructor _____   Date _____

PERFORMANCE CHECKLIST 29-3 **ASSISTING WITH APPLICATION OF SKIN TRACTION**

	S	U	NP	Comments
ASSESSMENT				
1. Assessed client's health status.	—	—	—	_____
2. Assessed specific tissues to be placed in traction.	—	—	—	_____
3. Assessed client's understanding of reason for traction.	—	—	—	_____
4. Assessed client's level of pain.	—	—	—	_____
5. Assessed client's neurovascular status.	—	—	—	_____
NURSING DIAGNOSIS				
1. Developed appropriate nursing diagnoses based on assessment data.	—	—	—	_____
PLANNING				
1. Identified expected outcomes.	—	—	—	_____
2. Explained procedure to client.	—	—	—	_____
IMPLEMENTATION				
1. Administered analgesic or muscle relaxant in advance.	—	—	—	_____
2. Prepared client and area of body to be placed in traction.	—	—	—	_____
3. Positioned client as requested by physician.	—	—	—	_____
4. Assisted with application of specific traction equipment.	—	—	—	_____
5. Assisted with attachment of bars, ropes, and pulleys.	—	—	—	_____
6. Attached and gently lowered traction weights.	—	—	—	_____
7. Assessed client's body alignment in traction.	—	—	—	_____
8. Assessed client's initial response to traction.	—	—	—	_____
9. Elevated side rails.	—	—	—	_____
10. Assessed neurovascular status within 15 minutes after application, then every 1 to 2 hours for 24 hours.	—	—	—	_____
11. Returned unused materials to storage area.	—	—	—	_____
12. Washed hands.	—	—	—	_____

	S	U	NP	Comments

EVALUATION

1. Observed client's participation in self-care. ___ ___ ___ _____

2. Observed entire traction setup. ___ ___ ___ _____

3. Assessed condition of skin around traction. ___ ___ ___ _____

4. Asked if client understands mobility restrictions. ___ ___ ___ _____

5. Determined if client was having pain, spasms, or burning. ___ ___ ___ _____

6. Conducted neurovascular checks. ___ ___ ___ _____

7. Released skin traction every 4 to 8 hours, and assessed and cleansed skin. ___ ___ ___ _____

8. Identified unexpected outcomes. ___ ___ ___ _____

RECORDING AND REPORTING

1. Recorded type of traction, site, skin condition, weight applied, client's response, and findings of neurovascular and skin assessments. ___ ___ ___ _____

2. Recorded length of time client was in or out of traction. ___ ___ ___ _____

3. Reported untoward findings to physician or nurse in charge. ___ ___ ___ _____

Student _____ Date _____

Instructor _____ Date _____

PERFORMANCE CHECKLIST 29-4 **ASSISTING WITH INSERTION OF PINS, WIRES, OR NAILS FOR SKELETAL TRACTION**

	S	U	NP	Comments
ASSESSMENT				
1. Assessed client's health status.	___	___	___	_____
2. Assessed specific tissues to be placed in skeletal traction.	___	___	___	_____
3. Assessed client's understanding of traction.	___	___	___	_____
4. Assessed client's level of pain.	___	___	___	_____
5. Observed client's nonverbal behavior.	___	___	___	_____
NURSING DIAGNOSIS				
1. Developed appropriate nursing diagnoses based on assessment data.	___	___	___	_____
PLANNING				
1. Identified expected outcomes.	___	___	___	_____
IMPLEMENTATION				
Traction Setup				
1. Positioned client according to physician's order.	___	___	___	_____
2. Assisted with skin preparation and during injection of local anesthetic.	___	___	___	_____
3. Supported client's limb.	___	___	___	_____
4. Assisted with application of nails or pins.	___	___	___	_____
5. Assisted in completion of traction setup and maintenance of client's alignment.	___	___	___	_____
6. Ascertained client's initial reactions or response to traction.	___	___	___	_____
7. Elevated side rails.	___	___	___	_____
8. Returned equipment and supplies.	___	___	___	_____
9. Washed hands.	___	___	___	_____
Pin Care				
1. Washed hands and applied gloves.	___	___	___	_____
2. Removed and discarded old dressing around pins. Noted condition of tissues around pins.	___	___	___	_____
3. Prepared supplies and applied sterile or clean gloves.	___	___	___	_____

	S	U	NP	Comments
4. Cleaned pins correctly.	___	___	___	_____
5. Cleaned pin site with hydrogen peroxide and saline on a cotton-tipped applicator.	___	___	___	_____
6. Cleaned pin area with normal saline.	___	___	___	_____
7. Applied a small amount of povidone-iodine or topical antibiotic and covered pin site with sterile gauze dressing.	___	___	___	_____
8. Repeated procedure for other pin site.	___	___	___	_____
9. Discarded supplies.	___	___	___	_____
10. Removed and disposed of gloves. Washed hands.	___	___	___	_____

EVALUATION

	S	U	NP	Comments
1. Assessed traction setup and functioning.	___	___	___	_____
2. Determined client's response to traction apparatus.	___	___	___	_____
3. Determined client's need for analgesics or muscle relaxants.	___	___	___	_____
4. Inspected pin sites. Assessed for indications of infection.	___	___	___	_____
5. Performed neurovascular checks.	___	___	___	_____
6. Assessed for indicators of hypoxemia.	___	___	___	_____
7. Checked for fracture blisters.	___	___	___	_____
8. Performed motor assessment.	___	___	___	_____
9. Identified unexpected outcomes.	___	___	___	_____

RECORDING AND REPORTING

	S	U	NP	Comments
1. Recorded type of traction applied, person applying traction, site, time, weights, and client's initial response.	___	___	___	_____
2. Recorded all findings of skin and neurovascular checks.	___	___	___	_____
3. Reported untoward reactions or unexpected outcomes to nurse in charge or physician.	___	___	___	_____

Student _____   Date _____

Instructor _____   Date _____

PERFORMANCE CHECKLIST 30-1 **PLACING A CLIENT ON A SUPPORT SURFACE MATTRESS**

	S	U	NP	Comments
ASSESSMENT				
1. Determined client's risk for pressure ulcer formation using assessment tool.	___	___	___	_____
2. Inspected condition of client's skin.	___	___	___	_____
3. Assessed client's understanding of purpose of mattress.	___	___	___	_____
4. Assessed client's comfort level.	___	___	___	_____
5. Checked physician's orders.	___	___	___	_____
NURSING DIAGNOSIS				
1. Developed appropriate nursing diagnoses based on assessment data.	___	___	___	_____
PLANNING				
1. Identified expected outcomes.	___	___	___	_____
2. Explained purpose and procedure to client.	___	___	___	_____
3. Washed hands and applied gloves, as indicated. Obtained assistance as needed.	___	___	___	_____
IMPLEMENTATION				
1. Provided for client's privacy.	___	___	___	_____
2. Correctly applied support surface to bed or prepared alternate bed.	___	___	___	_____
Mattress Replacement				
a. Applied mattress to bed frame after removing hospital mattress.	___	___	___	_____
b. Applied sheet over mattress.	___	___	___	_____
Air Mattress/Overlay				
a. Applied deflated mattress over bed.	___	___	___	_____
b. Secured air mattress over corners of bed mattress.	___	___	___	_____
c. Attached connector on air mattress to inflation device and inflated mattress to proper air pressure.	___	___	___	_____
d. Applied sheet over air mattress.	___	___	___	_____
e. Checked air pump for proper cycling.	___	___	___	_____

	S	U	NP	Comments

f. Kept sharp objects away from mattress.

g. Assisted with client transfers.

Integrated Air Surface
a. Obtained and made bed.

b. Placed switch in the "Prevention" mode.

Water Mattress
a. Applied unfilled mattress flat over surface of bed mattress.

b. Secured water mattress in place.

c. Attached connector on water mattress to water source.

d. Filled mattress to recommended level.

e. Placed sheet over water mattress.

f. Kept sharp objects away from mattress.

3. Positioned client comfortably, and repositioned client routinely.

4. Removed gloves, if worn, and washed hands.

EVALUATION
1. Inspected condition of client's skin.

2. Reassessed client's risk for pressure sore formation at routine intervals.

3. Assessed client's comfort level.

4. Evaluated inflation of mattress periodically.

5. Identified unexpected outcomes.

RECORDING AND REPORTING
1. Recorded placement of mattress and condition of client's skin.

2. Reported evidence of pressure sores to nurse in charge or physician.

Student _____   Date _____

Instructor _____   Date _____

PERFORMANCE CHECKLIST 30-2 **PLACING A CLIENT ON AN AIR-SUSPENSION BED**

	S	U	NP	Comments
ASSESSMENT				
1. Identified clients who would benefit from air-suspension therapy.	—	—	—	_____
2. Reviewed client's medical orders.	—	—	—	_____
3. Assessed client for pain.	—	—	—	_____
4. Assessed condition of client's skin.	—	—	—	_____
5. Assessed client's level of consciousness.	—	—	—	_____
6. Assessed client's and family member's understanding of purpose of bed.	—	—	—	_____
7. Reviewed client's serum electrolyte levels if available.	—	—	—	_____
8. Checked if client required frequent weight measurement.	—	—	—	_____
NURSING DIAGNOSIS				
1. Developed appropriate nursing diagnoses based on assessment data.	—	—	—	_____
PLANNING				
1. Identified expected outcomes.	—	—	—	_____
2. Explained procedure and purpose of bed to client and family.	—	—	—	_____
3. Washed hands, applied gloves, and prepared necessary equipment and supplies.	—	—	—	_____
4. Reviewed bed manufacturer's instructions.	—	—	—	_____
5. Premedicated client as necessary 30 minutes before transfer.	—	—	—	_____
6. Obtained additional personnel needed to transfer client to bed.	—	—	—	_____
IMPLEMENTATION				
1. Maintained client's privacy.	—	—	—	_____
2. Explained steps of transfer.	—	—	—	_____
3. Transferred client to bed using appropriate transfer techniques.	—	—	—	_____
4. Turned bed on and regulated temperature.	—	—	—	_____

	S	U	NP	Comments

5. Positioned client and performed ROM exercises as appropriate.

6. Set bed to firm position (instaflate) when turning or positioning client in bed.

7. In emergencies, deflated bed immediately.

8. Removed gloves, if worn, and washed hands.

EVALUATION

1. Inspected condition of client's skin.

2. Asked client to rate sense of comfort.

3. Assessed client's orientation.

4. Identified unexpected outcomes.

RECORDING AND REPORTING

1. Recorded transfer of client to bed, tolerance to procedure, condition of skin and client/caregiver teaching.

2. Reported changes in condition of skin and electrolyte levels to nurse in charge or physician.

3. Reported restlessness or change in orientation.

Student _____   Date _____

Instructor _____   Date _____

PERFORMANCE CHECKLIST 30-3 **PLACING A CLIENT ON AN AIR-FLUIDIZED BED**

	S	U	NP	Comments
ASSESSMENT				
1. Performed pressure ulcer risk assessment to identify clients who would benefit from air-fluidized therapy.	—	—	—	_____
2. Reviewed client's medical orders.	—	—	—	_____
3. Assessed condition of client's skin.	—	—	—	_____
4. Assessed client's comfort level.	—	—	—	_____
5. Assessed client's level of consciousness.	—	—	—	_____
6. Assessed client's and family member's understanding of purpose of bed.	—	—	—	_____
7. Reviewed client's serum electrolyte levels in medical record.	—	—	—	_____
8. Identified clients at risk for complications of air-fluidized therapy.	—	—	—	_____
NURSING DIAGNOSIS				
1. Developed appropriate nursing diagnoses based on assessment data.	—	—	—	_____
PLANNING				
1. Identified expected outcomes.	—	—	—	_____
2. Explained procedure and purpose of bed to client and family.	—	—	—	_____
3. Reviewed instructions supplied by bed manufacturer.	—	—	—	_____
4. Premedicated client as necessary 30 minutes before transfer.	—	—	—	_____
5. Obtained any additional personnel needed to transfer client to bed.	—	—	—	_____
IMPLEMENTATION				
1. Closed client's room door or bedside curtain.	—	—	—	_____
2. Explained steps of transfer.	—	—	—	_____
3. Washed hands and applied gloves.	—	—	—	_____
4. Transferred client to bed.	—	—	—	_____
5. Turned fluidization cycle on and regulated temperature.	—	—	—	_____

	S	U	NP	Comments

6. Positioned client and performed ROM exercises as appropriate.   ___ ___ ___ _____

7. Correctly set fluidization mode for other therapies.   ___ ___ ___ _____

8. In event of emergency, defluidized bed.   ___ ___ ___ _____

9. Removed gloves, if worn, and washed hands.   ___ ___ ___ _____

EVALUATION

1. Inspected condition of client's skin while on bed, and monitored risk assessment.   ___ ___ ___ _____

2. Asked client to rate ability to sleep or rest.   ___ ___ ___ _____

3. Reviewed client's serum electrolyte levels, monitored body temperature, and noted hydration status of skin and mucous membranes.   ___ ___ ___ _____

4. Measured client's level of orientation.   ___ ___ ___ _____

5. Identified unexpected outcomes.   ___ ___ ___ _____

RECORDING AND REPORTING

1. Recorded transfer of client to bed, tolerance to procedure, and condition of skin.   ___ ___ ___ _____

2. Reported changes in condition of skin and electrolyte levels to nurse in charge or physician.   ___ ___ ___ _____

3. Reported change in orientation.   ___ ___ ___ _____

Student _____   Date _____

Instructor _____   Date _____

PERFORMANCE CHECKLIST 30-4   **PLACING A CLIENT ON A BARIATRIC BED**

	S	U	NP	Comments
ASSESSMENT				
1. Identified clients who would benefit from the bariatric bed system.	——	——	——	_____
2. Assessed condition of client's skin, particularly potential pressure sites.	——	——	——	_____
3. Determined client's and family member's understanding of purpose of bed.	——	——	——	_____
4. Reviewed client's medical orders.	——	——	——	_____
5. Determined client's need to be weighed.	——	——	——	_____
NURSING DIAGNOSIS				
1. Developed appropriate nursing diagnoses based on assessment data.	——	——	——	_____
PLANNING				
1. Identified expected outcomes.	——	——	——	_____
2. Explained procedure and purpose of bed to client and family.	——	——	——	_____
3. Reviewed instructions supplied by bed manufacturer.	——	——	——	_____
4. Premedicated client as necessary 30 minutes before transfer.	——	——	——	_____
5. Obtained additional personnel needed to transfer client to bed.	——	——	——	_____
IMPLEMENTATION				
1. Provided privacy.	——	——	——	_____
2. Explained steps of transfer.	——	——	——	_____
3. Washed hands and applied gloves as indicated before assisting client to bed using appropriate transfer techniques.	——	——	——	_____
4. Covered and positioned client, and placed hand controls within client's reach. Attached overhead frame, if needed.	——	——	——	_____
5. Removed gloves, if worn, and washed hands.	——	——	——	_____

	S	U	NP	Comments

EVALUATION

1. Inspected condition of skin. ___ ___ ___ _____

2. Asked client to rate sense of comfort and safety. ___ ___ ___ _____

3. Evaluated client's risk for injury. ___ ___ ___ _____

4. Evaluated client's ability to move in bed. ___ ___ ___ _____

5. Identified unexpected outcomes. ___ ___ ___ _____

RECORDING AND REPORTING

1. Recorded transfer of client to bed, tolerance of procedure, and condition of skin. ___ ___ ___ _____

2. Reported changes in condition of skin to nurse in charge or physician. ___ ___ ___ _____

Student _____   Date _____

Instructor _____   Date _____

PERFORMANCE CHECKLIST 30-5   **PLACING A CLIENT ON A ROTOKINETIC BED**

	S	U	NP	Comments
ASSESSMENT				
1. Assessed condition of client's skin.	—	—	—	_____
2. Reviewed medical order.	—	—	—	_____
3. Assessed client's level of comfort.	—	—	—	_____
4. Assessed client's level of orientation.	—	—	—	_____
5. Assessed client's and caregiver's understanding of use of Rotokinetic bed.	—	—	—	_____
NURSING DIAGNOSIS				
1. Developed appropriate nursing diagnoses based on assessment data.	—	—	—	_____
PLANNING				
1. Identified expected outcomes.	—	—	—	_____
2. Explained procedure to client.	—	—	—	_____
3. Reviewed manufacturer's instructions.	—	—	—	_____
4. Premedicated client 30 minutes before transfer.	—	—	—	_____
5. Obtained additional assistance to transfer client.	—	—	—	_____
IMPLEMENTATION				
1. Washed hands.	—	—	—	_____
2. Provided privacy.	—	—	—	_____
3. Placed Rotokinetic bed in horizontal position; removed all bolsters, straps, and supports. Closed posterior hatches.	—	—	—	_____
4. Unplugged electrical cord and locked hatch.	—	—	—	_____
5. Transferred client to bed; maintained client's proper body alignment.	—	—	—	_____
6. Secured thoracic panels, bolsters, head and knee packs, and safety straps.	—	—	—	_____
7. Covered client with top sheet.	—	—	—	_____
8. Plugged bed in.	—	—	—	_____
9. Had company representative set optional angle as ordered.	—	—	—	_____
10. Increased degree of rotation gradually.	—	—	—	_____

	S	U	NP	Comments
11. Provided adequate space for caregivers and family to move around bed.	——	——	——	————————
12. Stopped bed for client assessments and procedures.	——	——	——	————————
13. Informed client of expected sensations and safety measures to prevent falls.	——	——	——	————————
14. Washed hands.	——	——	——	————————

EVALUATION

	S	U	NP	Comments
1. Inspected condition of client's skin.	——	——	——	————————
2. Inspected pressure ulcers for healing.	——	——	——	————————
3. Observed body alignment and joint range of motion.	——	——	——	————————
4. Auscultated lung sounds and compared with baseline.	——	——	——	————————
5. Determined client's level of orientation.	——	——	——	————————
6. Asked if client was experiencing nausea or dizziness.	——	——	——	————————
7. Monitored client's blood pressure for orthostatic hypotension.	——	——	——	————————
8. Identified unexpected outcomes.	——	——	——	————————

RECORDING AND REPORTING

	S	U	NP	Comments
1. Described skin condition before placement on Rotokinetic bed.	——	——	——	————————
2. Recorded time of transfer to bed and degree of rotation.	——	——	——	————————
3. Documented vital signs and subjective response of client.	——	——	——	————————
4. Reported unexpected outcomes to the nurse in charge or physician.	——	——	——	————————

Student _____   Date _____

Instructor _____   Date _____

PERFORMANCE CHECKLIST 31-1   **HAND WASHING**

	S	U	NP	Comments
ASSESSMENT				
1. Inspected surface of hands and fingers for cuts or breaks.	—	—	—	_____
2. Inspected hands for heavy soiling.	—	—	—	_____
3. Assessed client's risk for or extent of infection.	—	—	—	_____
NURSING DIAGNOSIS				
1. Developed appropriate nursing diagnoses.	—	—	—	_____
PLANNING				
1. Identified expected outcomes.	—	—	—	_____
IMPLEMENTATION				
1. Removed jewelry and pushed clothing or wristwatch above wrist level.	—	—	—	_____
2. Kept fingernails short and filed.	—	—	—	_____
3. Stood at sink without touching sink with hands or uniform.	—	—	—	_____
4. Regulated water flow.	—	—	—	_____
5. Avoided splashing.	—	—	—	_____
6. Adjusted water temperature to "warm."	—	—	—	_____
7. Wet hands and wrists, keeping hands and forearms lower than elbows.	—	—	—	_____
8. Applied antiseptic liquid soap to hands.	—	—	—	_____
9. Lathered hands and applied friction to skin surfaces for 10 to 15 seconds on each hand; interlaced fingers and rubbed palms and back of hands in circular motion.	—	—	—	_____
10. Cleaned thoroughly under fingernails.	—	—	—	_____
11. Rinsed thoroughly, keeping hands below elbows.	—	—	—	_____
12. Dried hands thoroughly, wiping from fingers up to wrists and forearms.	—	—	—	_____
13. Discarded paper towel properly.	—	—	—	_____
14. Turned off water at sink with paper towel or pedal.	—	—	—	_____

	S	U	NP	Comments
EVALUATION				
1. Inspected surface of hands.	___	___	___	_____
2. Identified unexpected outcomes.	___	___	___	_____

Student _____   Date _____

Instructor _____   Date _____

PERFORMANCE CHECKLIST 31-2 **CARING FOR CLIENTS UNDER ISOLATION PRECAUTIONS**

	S	U	NP	Comments
ASSESSMENT				
1. Reviewed precautions for client's specific isolation category.	___	___	___	_____
2. Reviewed appropriate laboratory test results.	___	___	___	_____
3. Considered types of care to be delivered to client.	___	___	___	_____
4. Assessed client's emotional status.	___	___	___	_____
5. Determined client's understanding of purpose of isolation and procedures.	___	___	___	_____
6. Determined if client allergic to latex.	___	___	___	_____
NURSING DIAGNOSIS				
1. Developed appropriate nursing diagnoses based on client's isolated status.	___	___	___	_____
PLANNING				
1. Identified expected outcomes.	___	___	___	_____
2. Prepared equipment and supplies.	___	___	___	_____
IMPLEMENTATION				
1. Washed hands.	___	___	___	_____
2. Applied protective wear:	___	___	___	_____
a. Applied mask or respirator securely over nose and mouth.	___	___	___	_____
b. Applied eyewear or goggles, if needed, to fit snugly around face and eyes.	___	___	___	_____
c. Applied isolation gown correctly, and secured ties at neck and waist.	___	___	___	_____
d. Applied disposable gloves with edges overlying gown cuffs.	___	___	___	_____
3. Entered client's room. Arranged supplies and equipment.	___	___	___	_____
4. Explained purpose of isolation and necessary precautions to client, family, and visitors.	___	___	___	_____

	S	U	NP	Comments
5. Assessed vital signs:	___	___	___	_____
a. Placed clean paper towel on bedside table, with additional paper towel on top.	___	___	___	_____
b. Placed watch on towel for easy visibility.	___	___	___	_____
c. Avoided contact of equipment with infective material while assessing vital signs.	___	___	___	_____
d. Returned stethoscope to clean surface, and cleansed diaphragm/bell with alcohol as needed.	___	___	___	_____
e. Used individual or disposable thermometer.	___	___	___	_____
6. Administered medications:	___	___	___	_____
a. Gave oral medication in wrapper or cup.	___	___	___	_____
b. Properly disposed of wrapper or cup.	___	___	___	_____
c. Administered injection while wearing gloves.	___	___	___	_____
d. Discarded syringe and uncapped needle in proper receptacle.	___	___	___	_____
e. Placed reusable syringe on clean towel for removal.	___	___	___	_____
7. Administered hygiene:	___	___	___	_____
a. Prevented isolation gown from becoming wet.	___	___	___	_____
b. Assisted client in removing gown, and disposed of gown appropriately.	___	___	___	_____
c. Removed linen from bed, and disposed of linen appropriately.	___	___	___	_____
d. Provided clean linen and towels.	___	___	___	_____
e. Changed gloves, if necessary.	___	___	___	_____
8. Collected specimens:	___	___	___	_____
a. Placed specimen containers on clean paper towel in bathroom.	___	___	___	_____
b. Followed procedure for specimen collection.	___	___	___	_____
c. Transferred collected specimen to appropriate container without contaminating container's outer surface. Transferred specimens correctly into plastic bag held by second nurse standing outside of room.	___	___	___	_____
d. Checked label for accuracy. Sent specimen to laboratory.	___	___	___	_____

	S	U	NP	Comments

9. Disposed of linen and trash bags: ___ ___ ___ _____

   a. Used appropriate bags for soiled articles. ___ ___ ___ _____

   b. Tied bags securely. ___ ___ ___ _____

10. Removed all reusable equipment, and disinfected contaminated surfaces. ___ ___ ___ _____

11. Resupplied room as needed, with another caregiver handling supplies at door. ___ ___ ___ _____

12. Left isolation room: ___ ___ ___ _____

   a. Removed gloves by turning them inside out, avoiding contact with contaminated surfaces. Untied and removed mask. Disposed of mask. ___ ___ ___ _____

   b. Untied neck strings of gown. Allowed gown to fall from shoulders. ___ ___ ___ _____

   e. Pulled gown off correctly and discarded in receptacle. ___ ___ ___ _____

   d. Removed eyewear or goggles. ___ ___ ___ _____

   e. Washed hands thoroughly. ___ ___ ___ _____

   f. Picked up wristwatch and stethoscope before leaving room and recorded vital signs. ___ ___ ___ _____

   g. Determined client's needs before leaving room. ___ ___ ___ _____

   h. Left room and closed door. ___ ___ ___ _____

EVALUATION

1. While in room, determined if client had had an opportunity to discuss health problems, course of treatment, and related concerns. ___ ___ ___ _____

2. Identified unexpected outcomes. ___ ___ ___ _____

RECORDING AND REPORTING

1. Documented client's response to social isolation and client education. ___ ___ ___ _____

Student _____ Date _____

Instructor _____ Date _____

PERFORMANCE CHECKLIST 32-1 APPLYING AND REMOVING CAP, MASK, AND PROTECTIVE EYEWEAR

	S	U	NP	Comments
ASSESSMENT				
1. Determined need to apply cap or mask.	___	___	___	_____
2. Considered risk of transmitting infection to client.	___	___	___	_____
NURSING DIAGNOSIS				
1. Developed appropriate nursing diagnoses based on assessment data.	___	___	___	_____
PLANNING				
1. Identified expected outcomes.	___	___	___	_____
2. Prepared equipment.	___	___	___	_____
IMPLEMENTATION				
Donning Cap				
1. Combed long hair back and arranged on crown of head.	___	___	___	_____
2. Secured hair in place.	___	___	___	_____
3. Applied cap over all of hair.	___	___	___	_____
4. Applied hood over head to cover facial hair, if indicated.	___	___	___	_____
Donning Mask				
1. Located top edge of mask.	___	___	___	_____
2. Held mask by top two ties with top edge of mask above nose.	___	___	___	_____
3. Tied top strings at top of back of head properly.	___	___	___	_____
4. Tied two lower strings snugly around neck with mask under chin.	___	___	___	_____
5. Pinched upper metal bank around bridge of nose.	___	___	___	_____
Applying Protective Eyewear				
1. Applied protective eyewear or goggles comfortably and checked vision.	___	___	___	_____
2. Checked that eyewear fit snugly around forehead and face.	___	___	___	_____
Disposing of Cap and Mask and Removing Eyewear				
1. Removed gloves first, if worn.	___	___	___	_____
2. Untied bottom strings of mask.	___	___	___	_____

	S	U	NP	Comments
3. Untied top strings of mask; removed and discarded mask.	——	——	——	—————————
4. Removed eyewear without placing hands on soiled lens.	——	——	——	—————————
5. Grasped outer surface of cap and lifted from head.	——	——	——	—————————
6. Discarded cap and mask in receptacle, and washed hands.	——	——	——	—————————

EVALUATION

1. Assessed the client for signs of infection.	——	——	——	—————————
2. Identified unexpected outcomes.	——	——	——	—————————

RECORDING AND REPORTING

1. Recorded procedure performed and client's status.	——	——	——	—————————

Student _____   Date _____

Instructor _____   Date _____

PERFORMANCE CHECKLIST 32-2 **PREPARING A STERILE FIELD**

	S	U	NP	Comments
ASSESSMENT				
1. Verified that procedure required sterile technique.	___	___	___	_____
2. Checked integrity of sterile packages.	___	___	___	_____
3. Determined client's comfort, oxygen, and elimination needs before procedure.	___	___	___	_____
4. Anticipated number and variety of supplies needed.	___	___	___	_____
NURSING DIAGNOSIS				
1. Developed appropriate nursing diagnoses based on assessment data.	___	___	___	_____
PLANNING				
1. Identified expected outcomes.	___	___	___	_____
2. Completed all priority tasks before beginning procedure.	___	___	___	_____
3. Prepared equipment at bedside.	___	___	___	_____
4. Asked visitors to step out. Discouraged movement by staff.	___	___	___	_____
5. Positioned client comfortably.	___	___	___	_____
6. Explained purpose of procedure and sterile technique.	___	___	___	_____
IMPLEMENTATION				
1. Applied cap, mask, protective eyewear, and gown, as needed.	___	___	___	_____
2. Selected clean, dry work surface above waist level.	___	___	___	_____
3. Washed hands.	___	___	___	_____
Preparing Sterile Work Surface				
1. Placed sterile kit or package on clean work surface above waist level.	___	___	___	_____
2. Opened sterile kit; pulled paper wrapper off and away from body. Continued to open the side flaps and, lastly, the innermost flap.	___	___	___	_____
3. Used opened kit or package as sterile field.	___	___	___	_____

	S	U	NP	Comments

Preparing a Sterile Drape

1. Placed sterile drape pack on flat, dry surface, and opened with sterile technique. ___ ___ ___ _____

2. Donned sterile gloves and sterile gown, if indicated. ___ ___ ___ _____

3. Using fingertips, picked up folded top edge of sterile drape. ___ ___ ___ _____

4. Lifted drape from outer cover and let it unfold without touching any object; discarded outer cover. ___ ___ ___ _____

5. With nondominant hand, grasped adjacent corner of drape; held drape straight up and away from body. ___ ___ ___ _____

6. Held drape and positioned its bottom half over work surface. ___ ___ ___ _____

7. Allowed top half of drape to be placed over work surface last. ___ ___ ___ _____

Adding Sterile Items

1. Grasped outside wrapper of sterile package in nondominant hand and opened sterile item. ___ ___ ___ _____

2. Peeled wrapper onto the nondominant hand. ___ ___ ___ _____

3. Placed item onto sterile field without reaching over sterile field. ___ ___ ___ _____

4. Disposed of outer wrapper. ___ ___ ___ _____

Pouring Sterile Solutions

1. Verified contents and expiration date of solution. ___ ___ ___ _____

2. Removed seal and cap from bottle in an upward motion. ___ ___ ___ _____

3. Poured solution slowly, holding edge of bottle well above and away from edge and inside of sterile container. ___ ___ ___ _____

EVALUATION

1. Identified break in sterile technique. ___ ___ ___ _____

2. Observed client for signs of local infection. ___ ___ ___ _____

3. Identified unexpected outcomes. ___ ___ ___ _____

RECORDING AND REPORTING

1. Recorded area and description of treatment site. ___ ___ ___ _____

Student _____   Date _____

Instructor _____   Date _____

PERFORMANCE CHECKLIST 32-3   **OPEN GLOVING**

	S	U	NP	Comments
ASSESSMENT				
1. Considered procedure to be performed and consulted institutional policy on use of gloves.	__	__	__	_____
2. Considered client's risk for infection.	__	__	__	_____
3. Examined condition of glove package.	__	__	__	_____
4. Inspected condition of hands.	__	__	__	_____
5. Determined if client allergic to latex.	__	__	__	_____
NURSING DIAGNOSIS				
1. Developed appropriate nursing diagnoses based on assessment data.	__	__	__	_____
PLANNING				
1. Identified expected outcomes.	__	__	__	_____
2. Selected correct size and type of gloves.	__	__	__	_____
3. Placed glove package near work area.	__	__	__	_____
IMPLEMENTATION				
Glove Application				
1. Washed hands thoroughly.	__	__	__	_____
2. Removed outer glove wrapper.	__	__	__	_____
3. Opened inner package, keeping gloves on wrapper's inside surface, and laid package on surface at waist level.	__	__	__	_____
4. Applied powder to hands as desired.	__	__	__	_____
5. Identified right and left glove.	__	__	__	_____
6. With nondominant hand, grasped inside edge of cuff of glove for dominant hand.	__	__	__	_____
7. Carefully pulled glove over dominant hand with thumb and fingers in proper spaces.	__	__	__	_____
8. With gloved dominant hand, slipped fingers under cuff of second glove.	__	__	__	_____
9. Pulled glove over nondominant hand without contaminating gloved dominant hand.	__	__	__	_____
10. Interlocked fingers of gloved hands to ensure proper fit.	__	__	__	_____

	S	U	NP	Comments

Glove Disposal

1. Grasped outside of one cuff with other gloved hand.   ___ ___ ___ _____

2. Pulled glove off, turning it inside out. Discarded in receptacle.   ___ ___ ___ _____

3. Slid fingers of ungloved hand underneath cuff of gloved hand and pulled remaining glove off; discarded glove in receptacle.   ___ ___ ___ _____

4. Washed hands.   ___ ___ ___ _____

EVALUATION

1. Assessed client for signs of infection.   ___ ___ ___ _____

2. Identified unexpected outcomes.   ___ ___ ___ _____

RECORDING AND REPORTING

1. Recorded procedure performed and client's response and status.   ___ ___ ___ _____

Student _____ Date _____

Instructor _____ Date _____

PERFORMANCE CHECKLIST 33-1 **PREPARING THE CLIENT FOR SURGERY**

	S	U	NP	Comments
ASSESSMENT				
1. Determined client's ability to answer questions.	—	—	—	_____
2. Obtained nursing history.	—	—	—	_____
3. Performed physical examination.	—	—	—	_____
4. Identified risk factors.	—	—	—	_____
5. Assessed client's and family member's expectations of surgery.	—	—	—	_____
6. Assessed client's preoperative orders.	—	—	—	_____
NURSING DIAGNOSIS				
1. Developed appropriate nursing diagnoses based on assessment data.	—	—	—	_____
PLANNING				
1. Identified expected outcomes.	—	—	—	_____
2. Prepared client's chart, and assembled necessary equipment.	—	—	—	_____
3. Explained procedures and allowed client, family members, or significant others to ask questions.	—	—	—	_____
IMPLEMENTATION				
1. Oriented client to room or presurgical area.	—	—	—	_____
2. Assisted client with informed consent.	—	—	—	_____
3. Checked medical record, and completed preoperative checklist.	—	—	—	_____
4. Provided preoperative teaching.	—	—	—	_____
5. Instructed client about the need and rationale for NPO for 4 to 8 hours before surgery.	—	—	—	_____
6. Confirmed that preoperative orders were completed.	—	—	—	_____
7. Provided for hygiene.	—	—	—	_____
8. Provided privacy and instructed client to remove clothes and put on gown and cap.	—	—	—	_____
9. Instructed client to remove hair appliances, jewelry, and makeup.	—	—	—	_____
10. Assisted client to remove prostheses. Inventoried and stored valuables per agency policy.	—	—	—	_____

	S	U	NP	Comments
11. Applied antiembolism stockings as ordered.	___	___	___	_____
12. Assessed client's vital signs immediately before going to operating room.	___	___	___	_____
13. Assisted client to void before receiving preoperative medication.	___	___	___	_____
14. Administered preoperative medications as ordered.	___	___	___	_____
15. Placed client on bed rest with side rails up and call light within reach.	___	___	___	_____

EVALUATION

	S	U	NP	Comments
1. Confirmed client's level of knowledge about surgical procedure.	___	___	___	_____
2. Compared assessment data with client's baseline and expected normals.	___	___	___	_____
3. Had client repeat preoperative instructions and demonstrate postoperative exercises.	___	___	___	_____
4. Assessed client for signs and symptoms of anxiety.	___	___	___	_____
5. Identified unexpected outcomes.	___	___	___	_____

RECORDING AND REPORTING

	S	U	NP	Comments
1. Documented all preoperative preparations.	___	___	___	_____
2. Documented client condition on transfer to operating room.	___	___	___	_____
3. Reported abnormal findings, lack of signed consent form, or failure to maintain NPO status.	___	___	___	_____
4. Recorded and reported client's cultural practices or religious beliefs that may necessitate modification of the care plan.	___	___	___	_____

Student _____   Date _____

Instructor _____   Date _____

PERFORMANCE CHECKLIST 33-2 **DEMONSTRATING POSTOPERATIVE EXERCISES**

	S	U	NP	Comments
ASSESSMENT				
1. Assessed client's risk for postoperative respiratory complications.	___	___	___	_____
2. Assessed client's ability to cough and deep breathe.	___	___	___	_____
3. Assessed client's risk for postoperative thrombus formation.	___	___	___	_____
4. Assessed client's ability to move independently in bed.	___	___	___	_____
5. Assessed client's willingness and ability to learn exercises.	___	___	___	_____
6. Assessed family members' willingness to learn and to support client.	___	___	___	_____
7. Assessed client's medical orders.	___	___	___	_____
NURSING DIAGNOSIS				
1. Developed appropriate nursing diagnoses based on assessment data.	___	___	___	_____
PLANNING				
1. Identified expected outcomes.	___	___	___	_____
2. Prepared necessary equipment.	___	___	___	_____
3. Prepared room for teaching.	___	___	___	_____
IMPLEMENTATION				
Teaching Diaphragmatic Breathing				
1. Assisted client to comfortable sitting or standing position.	___	___	___	_____
2. Stood or sat facing client.	___	___	___	_____
3. Correctly placed hands on anterior rib cage.	___	___	___	_____
4. Instructed client to take slow deep breaths.	___	___	___	_____
5. Avoided using chest and shoulders while inhaling.	___	___	___	_____
6. Held slow, deep breath for a count of 3 and exhaled.	___	___	___	_____
7. Repeated breathing exercise three to five times.	___	___	___	_____
8. Had client practice the exercise.	___	___	___	_____

	S	U	NP	Comments

Teaching Controlled Coughing

1. Explained to client the importance of an upright position.

2. Demonstrated two slow, deep breaths, inhaling through the nose and exhaling through the mouth.

3. Inhaled, held breath to count of 3, and coughed.

4. Cautioned client against just clearing throat.

5. For client with an abdominal or thoracic incision, taught client to place pillow over incisional area and to place hands on top of pillow.

6. Had client continue to practice coughing exercises while splinting an imaginary incision.

7. Instructed client to examine characteristics of sputum.

Teaching Turning

1. Instructed client to assume a supine position on the right side of the bed.

2. Instructed client to place right hand over incisional area to splint it.

3. Instructed client to keep right leg straight and flex left knee up and over right leg.

4. Had client grab right side rail with left hand and pull toward and roll onto right side.

5. Instructed client to turn every 2 hours while awake.

Teaching Leg Exercises

1. Had client assume supine position and demonstrated passive range-of-motion exercises.

2. Rotated each ankle.

3. Alternated dorsiflexion and plantar flexion of both feet.

4. Had client flex and extend knees.

5. Had client alternately raise each leg straight up from bed, keeping legs straight.

6. Had client continue to practice exercises at least every 2 hours.

EVALUATION

1. Observed client's ability to perform all four exercises independently.

2. Observed family members' ability to coach client.

	S	U	NP	Comments
3. Assessed client's chest excursion.	—	—	—	_____
4. Auscultated client's lungs.	—	—	—	_____
5. Assessed for Homans' sign.	—	—	—	_____
6. Identified unexpected outcomes.	—	—	—	_____

RECORDING AND REPORTING

	S	U	NP	Comments
1. Recorded those exercises that had been demonstrated to client and whether client could perform exercises independently.	—	—	—	_____
2. Recorded physical assessment findings.	—	—	—	_____
3. Reported any problems with client performance of exercises to the next shift.	—	—	—	_____

Student _____ Date _____

Instructor _____ Date _____

PERFORMANCE CHECKLIST 33-3 **PREPARING THE SURGICAL SITE**

	S	U	NP	Comments
ASSESSMENT				
1. Inspected general condition of skin.	—	—	—	_____
2. Assessed for allergy to iodine or shellfish.	—	—	—	_____
3. Reviewed physician's order for area to be shaved.	—	—	—	_____
4. Assessed for bleeding tendency.	—	—	—	_____
5. Assessed client's understanding and acceptance of hair removal.	—	—	—	_____
NURSING DIAGNOSIS				
1. Developed appropriate nursing diagnoses based on assessment data.	—	—	—	_____
PLANNING				
1. Identified expected outcomes.	—	—	—	_____
2. Prepared needed equipment at bedside.	—	—	—	_____
3. Explained procedure and rationale for shaving a larger surface area.	—	—	—	_____
IMPLEMENTATION				
1. Washed hands.	—	—	—	_____
2. Closed room doors and bed curtains for privacy; raised bed to high position, and positioned lamp.	—	—	—	_____
3. Positioned client with surgical site accessible.	—	—	—	_____
4. Applied disposable gloves.	—	—	—	_____
5. Depilatory hair removal:	—	—	—	_____
a. Applied depilatory cream to area.	—	—	—	_____
b. Waited required time and wiped off cream.	—	—	—	_____
c. Washed and rinsed skin.	—	—	—	_____
6. Hair clipping:	—	—	—	_____
a. Lightly dried area to be clipped with towel.	—	—	—	_____
b. Held clippers in dominant hand and clipped hair about 1 cm (½ inch) above skin in direction of growth.	—	—	—	_____

	S	U	NP	Comments

c. Lightly brushed off cut hair with towel. ___ ___ ___ _____

d. Cleansed areas over body crevices with antiseptic solution. ___ ___ ___ _____

7. Wet shave: ___ ___ ___ _____

   a. Placed towel or waterproof pad under area to be shaved. ___ ___ ___ _____

   b. Draped client correctly with bath blanket. ___ ___ ___ _____

   c. Adjusted lamp. ___ ___ ___ _____

   d. Lathered skin with gauze sponges dipped in antiseptic soap. ___ ___ ___ _____

   e. Correctly shaved a small area at a time, holding razor at a 45-degree angle. ___ ___ ___ _____

   f. Rinsed razor as soap and hair accumulated on the blade; changed and discarded blades as they became dull. ___ ___ ___ _____

   g. Rearranged bath blanket as each portion of the shave was completed. ___ ___ ___ _____

   h. Used washcloth and warm water to rinse away hair and soap solution; changed water as necessary. ___ ___ ___ _____

   i. Cleansed areas over body crevices with antiseptic solution. ___ ___ ___ _____

   j. Dried body crevices. ___ ___ ___ _____

   k. Discarded waterproof towel or pad. ___ ___ ___ _____

   l. Observed skin closely for nicks or cuts. ___ ___ ___ _____

8. Told client when procedure was completed. ___ ___ ___ _____

9. Cleaned and disposed of equipment properly. Disposed of gloves. ___ ___ ___ _____

10. Washed hands. ___ ___ ___ _____

EVALUATION

1. Inspected condition of the skin. ___ ___ ___ _____

2. Evaluated client's response to procedure. ___ ___ ___ _____

3. Identified unexpected outcomes. ___ ___ ___ _____

RECORDING AND REPORTING

1. Recorded procedure, area clipped or shaved, and condition of skin. ___ ___ ___ _____

2. Reported any skin alterations to physician. ___ ___ ___ _____

Student _____ Date _____

Instructor _____ Date _____

PERFORMANCE CHECKLIST 33-4 **PERFORMING POSTOPERATIVE CARE OF THE SURGICAL CLIENT**

	S	U	NP	Comments

ASSESSMENT
Immediate Recovery Period

1. Determined client's condition during operative procedure.

2. Obtained report from surgeon and anesthesiologist.

3. Considered surgery performed.

4. Performed thorough client assessment.

Convalescent Period

1. Received phone report from nurse in RR/PACU.

2. Obtained detailed report from nurse at time of client's transfer to division.

3. Reviewed client's medical record.

4. Reviewed surgeon's postoperative orders.

NURSING DIAGNOSIS

1. Developed appropriate nursing diagnoses based on assessment data.

PLANNING

1. Identified expected outcomes.

2. Prepared equipment at bedside.

3. Explained procedures to client.

IMPLEMENTATION
Immediate Recovery Period

1. Washed hands.

2. Checked equipment setup.

3. Immediately after client entered RR/PACU, attached oxygen equipment and drainage tubes, and checked IV flow rates.

4. Assessed vital signs and continued monitoring as needed. Provided warm blankets.

5. Maintained patent airway with proper client positioning and suctioning, and encouraged deep breathing and coughing.

	S	U	NP	Comments
6. Called client by name, and oriented client to surroundings.	——	——	——	——————————
7. Assessed circulatory perfusion.	——	——	——	——————————
8. Inspected surgical dressing and drains for bright red blood.	——	——	——	——————————
9. Inspected area of surgical wound.	——	——	——	——————————
10. Inspected condition of dressing.	——	——	——	——————————
11. Reinforced dressing as needed.	——	——	——	——————————
12. Inspected condition and contents of drainage tubes.	——	——	——	——————————
13. Observed patency and intactness of urinary catheter and volume and character of urine.	——	——	——	——————————
14. If nasogastric tube was present, irrigated as ordered.	——	——	——	——————————
15. Monitored IV fluid infusion.	——	——	——	——————————
16. Provided client mouth care.	——	——	——	——————————
17. Assessed client's pain and administered analgesia as ordered.	——	——	——	——————————
18. Encouraged leg exercises.	——	——	——	——————————
19. Explained to client status of recovery.	——	——	——	——————————
20. Contacted physician for order to transfer stabilized client.	——	——	——	——————————
21. Measured I&O.	——	——	——	——————————

Convalescent Period

1. Checked equipment setup.	——	——	——	——————————
2. Transferred client to bed.	——	——	——	——————————
3. Connected any existing oxygen tubing, and regulated IV infusion.	——	——	——	——————————
4. Assessed vital signs routinely, as ordered.	——	——	——	——————————
5. Maintained airway correctly.	——	——	——	——————————
6. Ensured patency and intactness of all drainage tubes.	——	——	——	——————————
7. Inspected condition of dressing or wound.	——	——	——	——————————
8. Assessed client for bladder distention.	——	——	——	——————————
9. Measured sources of fluid intake and output.	——	——	——	——————————
10. Positioned client for comfort.	——	——	——	——————————

	S	U	NP	Comments

11. Encouraged continuation of leg exercises.   ___ ___ ___ _____

12. Applied elastic stockings or pneumatic compression cuffs.   ___ ___ ___ _____

13. Explained to client nature of observations, and allowed family into room.   ___ ___ ___ _____

14. Explained activities and purpose of room equipment to family.   ___ ___ ___ _____

15. Administered analgesia appropriately.   ___ ___ ___ _____

16. Provided oral hygiene.   ___ ___ ___ _____

17. Maintained support measures for functioning body systems.   ___ ___ ___ _____

18. Increased client's involvement in decision making.   ___ ___ ___ _____

19. Taught client and family signs and symptoms of complications.   ___ ___ ___ _____

20. Included family in discussion about discharge.   ___ ___ ___ _____

21. Prepared for referral to home health or convalescent care.   ___ ___ ___ _____

EVALUATION

1. Compared assessment findings with client's baseline and expected range.   ___ ___ ___ _____

2. Evaluated pain relief measures.   ___ ___ ___ _____

3. Monitored changes in surgical wound.   ___ ___ ___ _____

4. Monitored lung sounds.   ___ ___ ___ _____

5. Auscultated client's bowel sounds.   ___ ___ ___ _____

6. Monitored I&O.   ___ ___ ___ _____

7. Discussed client's feelings about recovery.   ___ ___ ___ _____

8. Routinely conducted needed physical assessments.   ___ ___ ___ _____

9. Identified unexpected outcomes.   ___ ___ ___ _____

RECORDING AND REPORTING

1. Recorded client's arrival at recovery room or nursing division, assessments made, and nursing care initiated.   ___ ___ ___ _____

2. Recorded vital signs and I&O on flowsheets.   ___ ___ ___ _____

3. Reported abnormal assessment findings and signs of complications to nurse in charge or physician.   ___ ___ ___ _____

Student _____   Date _____

Instructor _____   Date _____

PERFORMANCE CHECKLIST 34-1   **SURGICAL HAND WASHING**

	S	U	NP	Comments

ASSESSMENT

1. Checked institutional policy for length of time for hand washing.

2. Assessed condition of nails for length and presence of polish.

3. Inspected condition of hands.

4. Checked that clothing top was secured.

NURSING DIAGNOSIS

1. Developed appropriate nursing diagnoses based on assessment data.

PLANNING

1. Identified expected outcomes.

2. Prepared needed equipment.

3. Removed all jewelry.

4. Made sure uniform was fitted or tucked at waist, with sleeves above elbows.

IMPLEMENTATION

1. Applied appropriate surgical attire.

2. Turned on water with knee or foot controls. Wet hands and arms under lukewarm water and lathered with detergent to 2 inches above elbows.

3. Rinsed hands and arms thoroughly under running water, keeping hands above elbows.

4. Cleaned under surface of nails with hands under running water.

5. Wet brush and applied antimicrobial soap. Scrubbed nails of one hand with 15 strokes. Scrubbed palm, each side of thumb, and posterior side of hand with 10 strokes each. Divided arm into three sections and scrubbed each 10 times. Repeated sequence for other arm.

6. Discarded brush and rinsed hands and arm thoroughly; turned off water with foot or knee pedal.

7. Used sterile towel to dry one hand thoroughly, moving from fingers to elbow.

	S	U	NP	Comments
8. Repeated drying method for other hand, using different area of towel or new sterile towel.	___	___	___	_____

EVALUATION

	S	U	NP	Comments
1. Observed client for signs of localized wound infection.	___	___	___	_____
2. Identified unexpected outcomes.	___	___	___	_____

RECORDING AND REPORTING

	S	U	NP	Comments
1. Recorded area and description of surgical site postoperatively.	___	___	___	_____

Student _____   Date _____

Instructor _____   Date _____

PERFORMANCE CHECKLIST 34-2   **DONNING A STERILE GOWN AND GLOVES (CLOSED GLOVING)**

	S	U	NP	Comments
ASSESSMENT				
1. Inspected condition of hands.	—	—	—	_____
2. Checked fingernails.	—	—	—	_____
3. Chose proper type and size of glove and gown.	—	—	—	_____
NURSING DIAGNOSIS				
1. Developed appropriate nursing diagnoses based on assessment data.	—	—	—	_____
PLANNING				
1. Identified expected outcomes.	—	—	—	_____
2. Prepared equipment.	—	—	—	_____
IMPLEMENTATION				
Gowning				
1. Applied surgical attire before entering operating room.	—	—	—	_____
2. Performed surgical hand scrub. Kept hands above waist.	—	—	—	_____
3. Asked circulating nurse to assist by opening sterile gown pack.	—	—	—	_____
4. Had circulating nurse prepare sterile glove package.	—	—	—	_____
5. Grasped gown appropriately and lifted from sterile package.	—	—	—	_____
6. Lifted gown and stepped away from table.	—	—	—	_____
7. Located neckband and grasped gown appropriately.	—	—	—	_____
8. Properly allowed gown to unfold.	—	—	—	_____
9. Inserted arms into gown and had circulating nurse bring gown over shoulders.	—	—	—	_____
10. Secured gown appropriately with assistance of circulating nurse.	—	—	—	_____

	S	U	NP	Comments

Closed Gloving

11. Opened inner sterile glove package correctly.   ___ ___ ___ _____

12. Picked up glove for dominant hand with non-dominant hand.   ___ ___ ___ _____

13. Placed glove on dominant palm correctly.   ___ ___ ___ _____

14. Had glove cuff turned over end of dominant hand correctly.   ___ ___ ___ _____

15. Carefully extended fingers into glove.   ___ ___ ___ _____

16. Gloved nondominant hand in same manner.   ___ ___ ___ _____

17. Made sure fingers were fully extended into both gloves.   ___ ___ ___ _____

18. With wrap-around sterile gown, released fasteners on front of gown.   ___ ___ ___ _____

19. Had gown flap wrapped and tied appropriately.   ___ ___ ___ _____

EVALUATION

1. Observed for break in sterile technique.   ___ ___ ___ _____

2. Identified unexpected outcomes.   ___ ___ ___ _____

RECORDING AND REPORTING

1. Recorded area and description of surgical site postoperatively.   ___ ___ ___ _____

2. Documented that no breach in sterile technique was observed or reported.   ___ ___ ___ _____

Student _____   Date _____

Instructor _____   Date _____

PERFORMANCE CHECKLIST 35-1   **PERFORMING WOUND IRRIGATION**

	S	U	NP	Comments
ASSESSMENT				
1. Reviewed client's medical record for physician's order.	—	—	—	_____
2. Checked recent records of wound progress.	—	—	—	_____
3. Assessed pain or comfort levels, and identified symptoms of anxiety.	—	—	—	_____
4. Identified history of allergies.	—	—	—	_____
NURSING DIAGNOSIS				
1. Developed appropriate nursing diagnoses based on assessment data.	—	—	—	_____
PLANNING				
1. Identified expected outcomes.	—	—	—	_____
2. Explained procedure.	—	—	—	_____
3. Administered premedication.	—	—	—	_____
4. Positioned client.	—	—	—	_____
IMPLEMENTATION				
1. Warmed irrigant.	—	—	—	_____
2. Washed hands.	—	—	—	_____
3. Prepared waterproof bag.	—	—	—	_____
4. Provided privacy.	—	—	—	_____
5. Applied gown and goggles, if needed.	—	—	—	_____
6. Put on clean gloves; removed and discarded soiled dressing.	—	—	—	_____
7. Prepared equipment and opened sterile supplies.	—	—	—	_____
8. Applied sterile gloves.	—	—	—	_____
9. Irrigated wound with wide opening:	—	—	—	_____
a. Used 19-gauge angiocatheter on syringe.	—	—	—	_____
b. Flushed wound until return was clear.	—	—	—	_____
10. Irrigated deep wound with small opening:	—	—	—	_____
a. Attached soft angiocatheter to syringe.	—	—	—	_____
b. Lubricated and inserted tip of catheter 1 cm (½ inch).	—	—	—	_____

	S	U	NP	Comments
c. Using slow pressure, flushed wound.	___	___	___	_____
d. Pinched off catheter, removed, refilled syringe, and continued to flush until return was clear.	___	___	___	_____
11. Cleansed wound with hand-held shower:	___	___	___	_____
a. Seated client in shower/tub.	___	___	___	_____
b. Adjusted water temperature to warm.	___	___	___	_____
c. Held shower approximately 12 inches from client.	___	___	___	_____
12. Cleansed wound with whirlpool.	___	___	___	_____
a. Adjusted water temperature.	___	___	___	_____
b. Placed client or client's extremity in whirlpool.	___	___	___	_____
c. Maintained treatment for prescribed time.	___	___	___	_____
13. Obtained necessary cultures.	___	___	___	_____
14. Dried wound edges with sterile gauze.	___	___	___	_____
15. Applied sterile dressing.	___	___	___	_____
16. Assisted client to comfortable position.	___	___	___	_____
17. Disposed of used equipment.	___	___	___	_____
18. Removed gloves, gowns, and goggles. Washed hands.	___	___	___	_____

EVALUATION

	S	U	NP	Comments
1. Inspected dressing periodically.	___	___	___	_____
2. Assessed type of tissue in the wound bed.	___	___	___	_____
3. Evaluated skin integrity.	___	___	___	_____
4. Observed client for signs of discomfort.	___	___	___	_____
5. Observed for retained irrigant.	___	___	___	_____
6. Identified unexpected outcomes.	___	___	___	_____

RECORDING AND REPORTING

	S	U	NP	Comments
1. Reported any evidence of fresh bleeding, increase in pain, retention of irrigant, or signs of shock to physician.	___	___	___	_____
2. Reported outcomes at change of shift.	___	___	___	_____
3. Recorded wound irrigation and client's response.	___	___	___	_____

Student _____   Date _____

Instructor _____   Date _____

PERFORMANCE CHECKLIST 35-2 **PERFORMING SUTURE AND STAPLE REMOVAL**

	S	U	NP	Comments
ASSESSMENT				
1. Identified client and reviewed physician's order.	—	—	—	_____
2. Observed healing status of wound.	—	—	—	_____
3. Assessed client for history of allergies.	—	—	—	_____
NURSING DIAGNOSIS				
1. Developed appropriate nursing diagnoses related to suture or staple removal.	—	—	—	_____
PLANNING				
1. Identified expected outcomes.	—	—	—	_____
2. Explained procedure to client.	—	—	—	_____
IMPLEMENTATION				
1. Provided privacy.	—	—	—	_____
2. Positioned client.	—	—	—	_____
3. Adjusted light on suture line.	—	—	—	_____
4. Washed hands.	—	—	—	_____
5. Prepared refuse bag.	—	—	—	_____
6. Prepared sterile field.	—	—	—	_____
7. Applied clean gloves and removed dressing; discarded dressing and gloves.	—	—	—	_____
8. Inspected wound.	—	—	—	_____
9. Applied sterile gloves.	—	—	—	_____
10. Cleaned sutures or staples and incision with antiseptic swabs.	—	—	—	_____
11. Removed staples:	—	—	—	_____
a. Applied staple extractor correctly.	—	—	—	_____
b. Carefully controlled staple extractor.	—	—	—	_____
c. Moved staple away from skin surface.	—	—	—	_____
d. Released handles of staple extractor, allowing staple to fall into refuse bag.	—	—	—	_____
e. Repeated Steps a-d until all staples removed.	—	—	—	_____

	S	U	NP	Comments
12. Removed intermittent sutures:	—	—	—	_____
a. Placed sterile gauze and grasped scissors and forceps correctly.	—	—	—	_____
b. Snipped sutures close to skin surface at end distal to knot.	—	—	—	_____
c. Grasped knotted end with forceps and removed suture.	—	—	—	_____
d. Repeated Steps a-c until all sutures removed.	—	—	—	_____
e. Observed healing level.	—	—	—	_____
13. Removed continuous sutures:	—	—	—	_____
a. Placed sterile gauze and grasped scissors and forceps correctly.	—	—	—	_____
b. Snipped first suture correctly.	—	—	—	_____
c. Snipped second suture on same side.	—	—	—	_____
d. Grasped knotted end and removed first line of spiral in continuous smooth action. Placed removed suture on gauze compress.	—	—	—	_____
e. Repeated Steps a-d until entire line removed.	—	—	—	_____
14. Inspected incision site. Placed supportive butterfly closure at areas of separation.	—	—	—	_____
15. Cleaned suture line and applied light dressing.	—	—	—	_____
16. Noted number of sutures or staples removed.	—	—	—	_____
17. Discarded contaminated supplies, and removed and disposed of gloves.	—	—	—	_____
18. Routed reusable items for sterilization and washed hands.	—	—	—	_____

EVALUATION

	S	U	NP	Comments
1. Assessed site of suture or staple removal.	—	—	—	_____
2. Determined if client had pain along incision.	—	—	—	_____
3. Identified unexpected outcomes.	—	—	—	_____

RECORDING AND REPORTING

	S	U	NP	Comments
1. Notified physician of abnormal findings immediately.	—	—	—	_____
2. Reported procedure at change of shift.	—	—	—	_____
3. Recorded number of sutures or staples removed, wound appearance, and client's response.	—	—	—	_____

Student _____   Date _____

Instructor _____   Date _____

PERFORMANCE CHECKLIST 35-3   **PERFORMING DRAINAGE EVACUATION**

	S	U	NP	Comments
ASSESSMENT				
1. Identified presence of closed wound drain and drainage system.	—	—	—	_____
2. Identified number of wound drainage tubes.	—	—	—	_____
3. Verified physician's order to determine if suction is needed.	—	—	—	_____
4. Inspected system for straight tube or Y-tube arrangement.	—	—	—	_____
5. Inspected system for proper functioning.	—	—	—	_____
6. Secured drainage reservoirs.	—	—	—	_____
7. Identified type of drainage container.	—	—	—	_____
NURSING DIAGNOSIS				
1. Developed appropriate nursing diagnoses based on assessment data.	—	—	—	_____
PLANNING				
1. Identified expected outcomes.	—	—	—	_____
2. Explained procedure to client.	—	—	—	_____
IMPLEMENTATION				
1. Provided privacy.	—	—	—	_____
2. Washed hands and applied gloves.	—	—	—	_____
3. Placed open sterile laboratory specimen and graduated container on bed.	—	—	—	_____
4. Maintained asepsis while opening and emptying evacuator; followed correct procedure for either Hemovac or Jackson-Pratt evacuator.	—	—	—	_____
5. Noted characteristics of drainage.	—	—	—	_____
6. Placed and secured drainage reservoirs to prevent pull on insertion sites.	—	—	—	_____
7. Routed labeled specimen to laboratory.	—	—	—	_____
8. Discarded soiled supplies, and washed hands.	—	—	—	_____
9. Changed dressing and inspected skin.	—	—	—	_____
10. Discarded contaminated materials, and washed hands.	—	—	—	_____

	S	U	NP	Comments

EVALUATION

1. Evaluated for presence of drainage.

2. Inspected wound for drainage.

3. Measured drainage.

4. Assessed client's comfort level.

5. Identified unexpected outcomes.

RECORDING AND REPORTING

1. Reported abnormal findings to physician immediately.

2. Reported procedure and findings at change of shift.

3. Recorded procedure and results and completed an I&O report.

Student _____ Date _____

Instructor _____ Date _____

PERFORMANCE CHECKLIST 36-1 **APPLYING A DRY DRESSING**

	S	U	NP	Comments
ASSESSMENT				
1. Accurately assessed size of wound.	___	___	___	_____
2. Assessed location of wound.	___	___	___	_____
3. Assessed client's comfort.	___	___	___	_____
4. Assessed client's knowledge about dressing.	___	___	___	_____
5. Assessed appropriateness of client and family participation.	___	___	___	_____
6. Checked physician's orders.	___	___	___	_____
7. Identified clients at risk for wound healing problems.	___	___	___	_____
NURSING DIAGNOSIS				
1. Developed appropriate nursing diagnoses based on assessment data.	___	___	___	_____
PLANNING				
1. Identified expected outcomes.	___	___	___	_____
2. Explained procedure to client.	___	___	___	_____
3. Assessed need for pain medication.	___	___	___	_____
IMPLEMENTATION				
1. Provided privacy. Washed hands. Applied gown, goggles, and mask, if indicated.	___	___	___	_____
2. Positioned client in comfortable manner.	___	___	___	_____
3. Properly placed disposable bag. Put on clean disposable gloves.	___	___	___	_____
4. Removed tape.	___	___	___	_____
5. Removed dressing properly.	___	___	___	_____
6. Observed drainage on dressing. Described appearance of wound to client.	___	___	___	_____
7. Properly disposed of dressing. Removed and disposed of gloves properly.	___	___	___	_____
8. Opened sterile supplies properly.	___	___	___	_____
9. Poured cleansing solution over gauze.	___	___	___	_____
10. Put on gloves.	___	___	___	_____

	S	U	NP	Comments
11. Inspected wound.	___	___	___	_____
12. Cleansed wound.	___	___	___	_____
13. Dried wound.	___	___	___	_____
14. Applied antiseptic ointment as ordered.	___	___	___	_____
15. Applied dressing; cut to fit around drains, if necessary.	___	___	___	_____
16. Secured dressing.	___	___	___	_____
17. Removed and disposed of gloves properly. Disposed of all supplies. Removed gown, mask, and goggles, if worn.	___	___	___	_____
18. Positioned client comfortably.	___	___	___	_____
19. Washed hands.	___	___	___	_____

EVALUATION

	S	U	NP	Comments
1. Assessed condition of wound.	___	___	___	_____
2. Asked client if discomfort noted during procedure.	___	___	___	_____
3. Inspected condition of dressing.	___	___	___	_____
4. Asked client to describe steps and techniques of dressing change.	___	___	___	_____
5. Identified unexpected outcomes.	___	___	___	_____

RECORDING AND REPORTING

	S	U	NP	Comments
1. Recorded and reported dressing change and wound appearance.	___	___	___	_____
2. Wrote date and time of dressing change on tape.	___	___	___	_____
3. Reported unexpected outcomes to nurse in charge or physician.	___	___	___	_____

Student _____   Date _____

Instructor _____   Date _____

PERFORMANCE CHECKLIST 36-2 **APPLYING A WET-TO-DRY DRESSING**

	S	U	NP	Comments
ASSESSMENT				
1. Assessed location and size of wound. (See skill 36-1.)	___	___	___	_____
NURSING DIAGNOSIS				
1. Developed appropriate nursing diagnoses based on assessment data.	___	___	___	_____
PLANNING				
1. Identified expected outcomes.	___	___	___	_____
2. Explained procedure to client.	___	___	___	_____
3. Positioned client for privacy and wound access.	___	___	___	_____
4. Administered analgesic 30 minutes before dressing change.	___	___	___	_____
IMPLEMENTATION				
1. Provided privacy, and exposed wound site.	___	___	___	_____
2. Placed disposable bag correctly.	___	___	___	_____
3. Placed disposable pad under wound site.	___	___	___	_____
4. Washed hands. Put on mask, goggles, and gown, if indicated. Put on disposable gloves. Removed tape.	___	___	___	_____
5. Removed dressing.	___	___	___	_____
6. Observed drainage and condition of wound.	___	___	___	_____
7. Disposed of dressings properly.	___	___	___	_____
8. Removed and disposed of gloves.	___	___	___	_____
9. Prepared sterile dressing supplies.	___	___	___	_____
10. Poured sterile solution, and added gauze.	___	___	___	_____
11. Applied sterile gloves.	___	___	___	_____
12. Inspected wound.	___	___	___	_____
13. Cleansed wound.	___	___	___	_____
14. Applied moistened gauze or "packing strip."	___	___	___	_____
15. Loosely packed dead spaces.	___	___	___	_____
16. Applied dry sterile gauze fluffs.	___	___	___	_____

	S	U	NP	Comments
17. Covered dressing with abdominal pad, surgipad, or thick gauze.	___	___	___	_____
18. Applied tape or Montgomery ties.	___	___	___	_____
19. Removed and disposed of gloves. Removed mask, gown, and goggles.	___	___	___	_____
20. Positioned client comfortably.	___	___	___	_____
21. Washed hands.	___	___	___	_____

EVALUATION

	S	U	NP	Comments
1. Assessed client's comfort level.	___	___	___	_____
2. Observed wound for healing.	___	___	___	_____
3. Monitored status of dressing.	___	___	___	_____
4. Asked client to describe wound care method.	___	___	___	_____
5. Identified unexpected outcomes.	___	___	___	_____

RECORDING AND REPORTING

	S	U	NP	Comments
1. Reported unexpected outcomes to physician.	___	___	___	_____
2. Reported wound appearance and drainage at shift change.	___	___	___	_____
3. Recorded data about wound, drainage, and client's tolerance of procedure.	___	___	___	_____
4. Wrote date and time of dressing change on tape.	___	___	___	_____

Student _____   Date _____

Instructor _____   Date _____

PERFORMANCE CHECKLIST 36-3   **APPLYING A PRESSURE BANDAGE**

	S	U	NP	Comments

ASSESSMENT

1. Identified clients at risk for unexpected bleeding.   ___ ___ ___   _____

Phase I

1. Identified client with sudden hemorrhage, and applied direct pressure.   ___ ___ ___   _____

2. Sought assistance.   ___ ___ ___   _____

Phase II

1. Rapidly observed bleeding site and size.   ___ ___ ___   _____

2. Observed area underneath client.   ___ ___ ___   _____

3. Rapidly assessed vital signs and client appearance.   ___ ___ ___   _____

NURSING DIAGNOSIS

1. Developed appropriate nursing diagnoses based on assessment data.   ___ ___ ___   _____

PLANNING

1. Identified expected outcomes.   ___ ___ ___   _____

IMPLEMENTATION

1. Washed hands and provided privacy as client's condition permitted. Applied clean gloves.   ___ ___ ___   _____

2. Pressed on site of bleeding.   ___ ___ ___   _____

3. Unwrapped roller bandage. Cut lengths of tape.   ___ ___ ___   _____

4. Applied bandage quickly and correctly; maintained pressure and secured with tape.   ___ ___ ___   _____

5. Removed gloves and washed hands.   ___ ___ ___   _____

EVALUATION

1. Assessed client's response to treatment.   ___ ___ ___   _____

2. Identified unexpected outcomes.   ___ ___ ___   _____

RECORDING AND REPORTING

1. Immediately reported client's status to physician.   ___ ___ ___   _____

2. Recorded and implemented physician's verbal orders.   ___ ___ ___   _____

3. Made between-shift report of emergency situation.   ___ ___ ___   _____

4. Recorded findings and care administered.   ___ ___ ___   _____

Student _____   Date _____

Instructor _____   Date _____

PERFORMANCE CHECKLIST 36-4 **APPLYING A TRANSPARENT DRESSING**

	S	U	NP	Comments
ASSESSMENT				
1. Assessed size and location of wound.	___	___	___	_____
2. Reviewed physician's orders.	___	___	___	_____
3. Assessed client's level of comfort.	___	___	___	_____
4. Assessed client's knowledge level.	___	___	___	_____
5. Assessed client's risk for wound healing problems.	___	___	___	_____
NURSING DIAGNOSIS				
1. Developed appropriate nursing diagnoses based on assessment data.	___	___	___	_____
PLANNING				
1. Identified expected outcomes.	___	___	___	_____
2. Explained procedure to client.	___	___	___	_____
3. Positioned client appropriately.	___	___	___	_____
IMPLEMENTATION				
1. Provided privacy, and exposed wound site.	___	___	___	_____
2. Placed waterproof bag properly.	___	___	___	_____
3. Washed hands and put on disposable gloves. Put on gown, mask, and goggles.	___	___	___	_____
4. Removed old dressing.	___	___	___	_____
5. Disposed of soiled dressing properly, and removed and disposed of gloves properly.	___	___	___	_____
6. Prepared sterile dressing supplies.	___	___	___	_____
7. Poured solution, and soaked 4 × 4s.	___	___	___	_____
8. Put on sterile gloves (per agency policy).	___	___	___	_____
9. Cleansed wound.	___	___	___	_____
10. Dried area.	___	___	___	_____
11. Inspected wound.	___	___	___	_____
12. Applied transparent dressing.	___	___	___	_____
13. Removed and disposed of gown, mask, goggles, and gloves correctly.	___	___	___	_____

	S	U	NP	Comments
14. Positioned client comfortably.	——	——	——	_____
15. Disposed of dressing materials properly, and washed hands.	——	——	——	_____

EVALUATION

1. Inspected condition of wound.	——	——	——	_____
2. Evaluated client for pain.	——	——	——	_____
3. Identified unexpected outcomes.	——	——	——	_____

RECORDING AND REPORTING

1. Reported unexpected outcomes.	——	——	——	_____
2. Documented findings and dressing change.	——	——	——	_____
3. Wrote date and time of change on a sticker and placed on dressing.	——	——	——	_____

Student _____   Date _____

Instructor _____   Date _____

PERFORMANCE CHECKLIST 36-5 **APPLYING A HYDROCOLLOID OR HYDROGEL DRESSING**

	S	U	NP	Comments
ASSESSMENT				
1. Assessed location and size of wound.	___	___	___	_____
2. Determined type of hydrocolloid or hydrogel dressing to be used.	___	___	___	_____
3. Reviewed orders.	___	___	___	_____
4. Assessed client's comfort level.	___	___	___	_____
5. Assessed client's knowledge of purpose of dressing.	___	___	___	_____
NURSING DIAGNOSIS				
1. Developed appropriate nursing diagnoses based on assessment data.	___	___	___	_____
PLANNING				
1. Identified expected outcomes.	___	___	___	_____
2. Explained procedure to client.	___	___	___	_____
3. Positioned client properly.	___	___	___	_____
IMPLEMENTATION				
1. Maintained client's privacy.	___	___	___	_____
2. Exposed wound and draped client.	___	___	___	_____
3. Placed cuffed disposable waterproof bag within reach.	___	___	___	_____
4. Washed hands and applied clean disposable gloves. Donned gown, mask, and goggles, if indicated.	___	___	___	_____
5. Removed old dressing.	___	___	___	_____
6. Disposed of soiled dressing in waterproof bag. Removed disposable gloves properly.	___	___	___	_____
7. Prepared sterile dressing supplies.	___	___	___	_____
8. Poured saline or prescribed solution over 4 × 4s in basin.	___	___	___	_____
9. Applied clean or sterile gloves.	___	___	___	_____
10. Cleansed area with soaked 4 × 4s; swabbed exudate from wound.	___	___	___	_____
11. Dried area.	___	___	___	_____

	S	U	NP	Comments
12. Inspected wound.	___	___	___	_____
13. Applied hydrogel or hydrocolloid dressing according to manufacturer's directions.	___	___	___	_____
14. Removed gloves properly. Removed gown, mask, and goggles, if worn.	___	___	___	_____
15. Assisted client to comfortable position.	___	___	___	_____
16. Discarded soiled dressing materials properly. Washed hands.	___	___	___	_____

EVALUATION

1. Inspected condition of wound and characteristics of wound drainage.	___	___	___	_____
2. Evaluated client's comfort level.	___	___	___	_____
3. Asked client to describe wound care.	___	___	___	_____
4. Identified unexpected outcomes.	___	___	___	_____

RECORDING AND REPORTING

1. Reported and recorded unusual observations.	___	___	___	_____
2. Recorded characteristics of wound and drainage.	___	___	___	_____
3. Wrote date, time, and initials on dressing.	___	___	___	_____

Student _____ Date _____

Instructor _____ Date _____

PERFORMANCE CHECKLIST 36-6   APPLYING A FOAM DRESSING

	S	U	NP	Comments
ASSESSMENT				
1. Assessed location and size of wound.	___	___	___	_____
2. Assessed client's level of comfort.	___	___	___	_____
3. Reviewed physician's orders.	___	___	___	_____
4. Assessed client's knowledge of purpose of dressing.	___	___	___	_____
5. Assessed client's risk for wound healing problems.	___	___	___	_____
NURSING DIAGNOSIS				
1. Developed appropriate nursing diagnoses based on assessment data.	___	___	___	_____
PLANNING				
1. Identified expected outcomes.	___	___	___	_____
2. Explained procedure to client.	___	___	___	_____
3. Positioned client correctly.	___	___	___	_____
IMPLEMENTATION				
1. Provided privacy.	___	___	___	_____
2. Exposed wound site and draped client.	___	___	___	_____
3. Properly placed disposable bag.	___	___	___	_____
4. Washed hands and put on clean disposable gloves. Donned gown, goggles, and mask, if necessary.	___	___	___	_____
5. Removed old dressing.	___	___	___	_____
6. Disposed of soiled dressing. Removed and disposed of gloves properly.	___	___	___	_____
7. Prepared sterile supplies.	___	___	___	_____
8. Poured solution over gauze.	___	___	___	_____
9. Put on gloves.	___	___	___	_____
10. Cleansed area.	___	___	___	_____
11. Removed excess wound moisture, and dried skin around wound.	___	___	___	_____
12. Inspected and measured wound.	___	___	___	_____

	S	U	NP	Comments

13. Applied foam dressing according to manufacturer's directions. ___ ___ ___ _____

14. Removed and disposed of gloves properly. ___ ___ ___ _____

15. Positioned client comfortably. ___ ___ ___ _____

16. Disposed of materials properly. ___ ___ ___ _____

17. Washed hands. ___ ___ ___ _____

EVALUATION

1. Inspected wound. ___ ___ ___ _____

2. Evaluated client's level of comfort. ___ ___ ___ _____

3. Asked client to describe wound care. ___ ___ ___ _____

4. Identified unexpected outcomes. ___ ___ ___ _____

RECORDING AND REPORTING

1. Reported and recorded unusual observations. ___ ___ ___ _____

2. Recorded characteristics of wound and drainage. ___ ___ ___ _____

3. Graphed wound surface area or volume of wound. ___ ___ ___ _____

4. Wrote time, date, and initials on new dressing or tape. ___ ___ ___ _____

Student _____   Date _____

Instructor _____   Date _____

PERFORMANCE CHECKLIST 36-7 **APPLYING ABSORPTION AND ALGINATE DRESSINGS**

	S	U	NP	Comments
ASSESSMENT				
1. Assessed location and size of wound to be dressed.	___	___	___	_____
2. Reviewed physician's orders.	___	___	___	_____
3. Assessed client's level of comfort.	___	___	___	_____
4. Assessed client's knowledge of purpose of dressing.	___	___	___	_____
NURSING DIAGNOSIS				
1. Developed appropriate nursing diagnoses based on assessment data.	___	___	___	_____
PLANNING				
1. Identified expected outcomes.	___	___	___	_____
2. Explained procedure to client.	___	___	___	_____
3. Positioned client correctly.	___	___	___	_____
IMPLEMENTATION				
1. Provided privacy.	___	___	___	_____
2. Exposed wound site and draped client.	___	___	___	_____
3. Prepared disposable bag correctly.	___	___	___	_____
4. Washed hands and put on clean disposable gloves. Donned, gown, goggles, and mask, if necessary.	___	___	___	_____
5. Removed and disposed of old dressing. Removed gloves.	___	___	___	_____
6. Prepared sterile dressing supplies.	___	___	___	_____
7. Poured solution over 4 × 4s.	___	___	___	_____
8. Put on sterile gloves (if required), and cleansed wound area.	___	___	___	_____
9. Inspected and measured wound.	___	___	___	_____
10. Applied absorption or alginate dressing according to manufacturer's directions.	___	___	___	_____
11. Removed gloves correctly and discarded.	___	___	___	_____

	S	U	NP	Comments
12. Assisted client to comfortable position.	___	___	___	_____
13. Discarded soiled materials correctly, and washed hands.	___	___	___	_____

EVALUATION

1. Inspected conditions of wound on ongoing basis.	___	___	___	_____
2. Noted length of time before dressing needed to be changed.	___	___	___	_____
3. Identified unexpected outcomes.	___	___	___	_____

RECORDING AND REPORTING

1. Reported unusual observations immediately.	___	___	___	_____
2. Recorded wound characteristics and measurements.	___	___	___	_____
3. Graphed wound surface area or volume.	___	___	___	_____
4. Wrote date, time, and initials on dressing or tape.	___	___	___	_____

Student _____ Date _____

Instructor _____ Date _____

PERFORMANCE CHECKLIST 37-1 **APPLYING GAUZE AND ELASTIC BANDAGES**

	S	U	NP	Comments
ASSESSMENT				
1. Reviewed client's medical record for order for application of elastic bandage.	___	___	___	_____
2. Observed client's skin integrity in area to be bandaged.	___	___	___	_____
3. Inspected surgical dressing. Observed cleanliness of dressing.	___	___	___	_____
4. Observed client's circulatory status.	___	___	___	_____
5. Assessed client's comfort level.	___	___	___	_____
6. Determined size of bandage needed.	___	___	___	_____
7. Identified client's and family member's knowledge level.	___	___	___	_____
NURSING DIAGNOSIS				
1. Developed appropriate nursing diagnoses based on assessment data.	___	___	___	_____
PLANNING				
1. Identified expected outcomes.	___	___	___	_____
2. Explained procedure to client.	___	___	___	_____
3. Taught skill to client and/or caregiver.	___	___	___	_____
IMPLEMENTATION				
1. Washed hands and applied gloves.	___	___	___	_____
2. Provided privacy.	___	___	___	_____
3. Assisted client to comfortable position.	___	___	___	_____
4. Held elastic bandage correctly.	___	___	___	_____
5. Applied bandage from distal point toward proximal boundary.	___	___	___	_____
6. Slightly stretched bandage as it was unrolled.	___	___	___	_____
7. Overlapped turns.	___	___	___	_____
8. Secured bandage with clips or tape.	___	___	___	_____
9. Removed gloves and washed hands.	___	___	___	_____
10. Removed and reapplied bandage once every 8 hours or per orders.	___	___	___	_____

	S	U	NP	Comments

EVALUATION

1. Checked circulation to the limb after application of bandage. ___ ___ ___ _____

2. Assessed regularly for condition of bandage and client comfort. ___ ___ ___ _____

3. Had client demonstrate bandage application. ___ ___ ___ _____

4. Identified unexpected outcomes. ___ ___ ___ _____

RECORDING AND REPORTING

1. Correctly documented treatment and client's response. ___ ___ ___ _____

2. Reported changes in neurological or circulatory status to nurse in charge or physician. ___ ___ ___ _____

Student _____   Date _____

Instructor _____   Date _____

PERFORMANCE CHECKLIST 37-2 **APPLYING AN ABDOMINAL BINDER AND A BREAST BINDER**

	S	U	NP	Comments
ASSESSMENT				
1. Identified signs and symptoms of impaired respirations.	___	___	___	_____
2. Determined if client is allergic to tape.	___	___	___	_____
3. Identified level of skin integrity.	___	___	___	_____
4. Inspected any surgical dressing.	___	___	___	_____
5. Identified client's comfort level.	___	___	___	_____
6. Gathered necessary data about size of binder based on assessment.	___	___	___	_____
NURSING DIAGNOSIS				
1. Developed appropriate nursing diagnoses based on assessment data.	___	___	___	_____
PLANNING				
1. Identified expected outcomes.	___	___	___	_____
2. Explained procedure to client.	___	___	___	_____
3. Taught skill to client and/or caregiver.	___	___	___	_____
IMPLEMENTATION				
1. Washed hands and applied gloves.	___	___	___	_____
2. Provided privacy.	___	___	___	_____
Abdominal Binder				
1. Applied abdominal binder correctly:	___	___	___	_____
a. Positioned client and assisted client to roll onto side.	___	___	___	_____
b. Fanfolded binder toward midline.	___	___	___	_____
c. Placed binder ends under client.	___	___	___	_____
d. Instructed client to roll over ends.	___	___	___	_____
e. Smoothed ends on far side of bed.	___	___	___	_____
f. Assisted client to supine position.	___	___	___	_____
g. Adjusted binder.	___	___	___	_____
h. Closed binder correctly.	___	___	___	_____
i. Assessed adequacy of breathing and coughing.	___	___	___	_____

	S	U	NP	Comments
j. Assessed client's comfort level.	___	___	___	_____
k. Adjusted binder as necessary.	___	___	___	_____

Breast Binder

1. Applied breast binder correctly:	___	___	___	_____
a. Assisted client to supine position.	___	___	___	_____
b. Assisted client in placing arms through binder.	___	___	___	_____
c. Applied padding as necessary.	___	___	___	_____
d. Secured binder with Velcro or pins.	___	___	___	_____
e. Adjusted binder.	___	___	___	_____
f. Instructed client in self-care.	___	___	___	_____
2. Removed gloves and washed hands.	___	___	___	_____

EVALUATION

1. Observed skin integrity.	___	___	___	_____
2. Noted client's comfort level.	___	___	___	_____
3. Assessed client's ability to cough and deep breathe.	___	___	___	_____
4. Identified client's need for assistance with daily activities.	___	___	___	_____
5. Identified unexpected outcomes.	___	___	___	_____

RECORDING AND REPORTING

1. Reported ineffective lung expansion immediately to physician.	___	___	___	_____
2. Reported skin irritation at between-shift report.	___	___	___	_____
3. Recorded application of binder and client assessment.	___	___	___	_____

Student _____   Date _____

Instructor _____   Date _____

PERFORMANCE CHECKLIST 38-1 **APPLYING A MOIST HOT COMPRESS TO AN OPEN WOUND**

	S	U	NP	Comments
ASSESSMENT				
1. Checked physician's orders for compress application.	—	—	—	_____
2. Inspected condition of exposed skin and wound.	—	—	—	_____
3. Assessed client's level of sensation.	—	—	—	_____
4. Checked medical record for contraindications to therapy.	—	—	—	_____
5. Assessed client's understanding of application.	—	—	—	_____
NURSING DIAGNOSIS				
1. Developed appropriate nursing diagnoses based on assessment data.	—	—	—	_____
PLANNING				
1. Identified expected outcomes.	—	—	—	_____
2. Prepared necessary equipment and supplies.	—	—	—	_____
3. Explained procedure and expected types of sensations to client.	—	—	—	_____
IMPLEMENTATION				
1. Provided privacy; assisted client to comfortable position; and placed waterproof pad under area to be treated.	—	—	—	_____
2. Draped client.	—	—	—	_____
3. Washed hands.	—	—	—	_____
4. Assembled equipment correctly, and immersed compresses in solution. Warmed solution if using portable heating source.	—	—	—	_____
5. Adjusted temperature of aquathermia pad.	—	—	—	_____
6. Applied disposable gloves, and removed soiled dressing. Disposed of soiled gloves and dressing.	—	—	—	_____
7. Assessed condition of wound and surrounding skin.	—	—	—	_____
8. Applied sterile gloves.	—	—	—	_____
9. Removed excess moisture from compress; applied gauze lightly to wound; noted client's response; and checked for redness.	—	—	—	_____

	S	U	NP	Comments

10. Packed wound snugly and covered all wound surfaces completely.   ___ ___ ___ _____

11. Covered moist compress with dry sterile dressing and bath towel. Removed gloves.   ___ ___ ___ _____

12. Changed compress every 5 minutes or as ordered using sterile technique.   ___ ___ ___ _____

13. Optionally applied aquathermia pad over towel.   ___ ___ ___ _____

14. Asked if client felt discomfort.   ___ ___ ___ _____

15. Applied gloves. Removed pad, towel, and compress after 30 minutes, and replaced dry sterile dressing as ordered.   ___ ___ ___ _____

16. Assisted client to preferred comfortable position.   ___ ___ ___ _____

17. Disposed of soiled compress, dressings, and supplies; washed hands.   ___ ___ ___ _____

EVALUATION

1. Inspected condition of skin and wound.   ___ ___ ___ _____

2. Asked client if burning sensation was felt.   ___ ___ ___ _____

3. Had client explain and demonstrate application.   ___ ___ ___ _____

4. Identified unexpected outcomes.   ___ ___ ___ _____

RECORDING AND REPORTING

1. Recorded type, location, and duration of application.   ___ ___ ___ _____

2. Described condition of wound and skin, and recorded client's response.   ___ ___ ___ _____

3. Described instruction given and client's ability to perform procedure.   ___ ___ ___ _____

4. Reported unusual findings to nurse in charge or physician.   ___ ___ ___ _____

Student _____ Date _____

Instructor _____ Date _____

PERFORMANCE CHECKLIST 38-2　**ASSISTING WITH WARM SOAKS AND SITZ BATHS**

	S	U	NP	Comments
ASSESSMENT				
1. Checked physician's order for procedure.	___	___	___	_____
2. Determined client's risk for reduced sensation.	___	___	___	_____
3. Determined if client has systemic conditions contraindicating soaks or baths.	___	___	___	_____
4. Assessed and documented client's blood pressure and pulse.	___	___	___	_____
5. Assessed and documented condition of body part being immersed.	___	___	___	_____
6. Determined client's ability to position self.	___	___	___	_____
7. Assessed client's level of comfort.	___	___	___	_____
8. Assessed client's understanding of therapy.	___	___	___	_____
NURSING DIAGNOSIS				
1. Developed appropriate nursing diagnoses based on assessment data.	___	___	___	_____
PLANNING				
1. Identified expected outcomes.	___	___	___	_____
2. Prepared necessary equipment and supplies.	___	___	___	_____
3. Explained procedure to client.	___	___	___	_____
IMPLEMENTATION				
1. Provided privacy, and washed hands. Applied gloves, if indicated.	___	___	___	_____
2. Filled basin; checked temperature of soak or bath solution.	___	___	___	_____
3. Positioned client comfortably for soak.	___	___	___	_____
4. Assisted client while immersing client in tub or basin.	___	___	___	_____
5. Covered client with bath blanket or towel.	___	___	___	_____
6. Maintained constant temperature during procedure.	___	___	___	_____
7. Kept large sheet or blanket over basin or container.	___	___	___	_____
8. Assisted client from bath or soak, and dried body part thoroughly.	___	___	___	_____

	S	U	NP	Comments
9. Assisted client to chair or bed after procedure.	___	___	___	_____
10. Disposed of soiled equipment and cleansed basin or tub. Disposed of gloves (if worn) and washed hands.	___	___	___	_____

EVALUATION

	S	U	NP	Comments
1. Inspected condition of body part that was immersed.	___	___	___	_____
2. Assessed client's response to therapy.	___	___	___	_____
3. Assessed vital signs if client complained of dizziness or lightheadedness.	___	___	___	_____
4. Asked client to demonstrate use of soak or sitz bath.	___	___	___	_____
5. Identified unexpected outcomes.	___	___	___	_____

RECORDING AND REPORTING

	S	U	NP	Comments
1. Recorded procedure. Described condition of body part immersed and client's response.	___	___	___	_____
2. Reported client complaints and unusual observations to appropriate personnel.	___	___	___	_____
3. Described instruction given and client's ability to perform procedure.	___	___	___	_____

Student _____   Date _____

Instructor _____   Date _____

PERFORMANCE CHECKLIST 38-3 **APPLYING AQUATHERMIA AND HEATING PADS**

	S	U	NP	Comments

ASSESSMENT

1. Reviewed physician's order for heat therapy. — — —

2. Assessed and documented condition of client's skin. — — —

3. Assessed and documented level of discomfort and range of motion. — — —

4. Assessed skin for sensitivity to temperature, touch, and pain. — — —

5. Checked condition of electrical cords for safety hazards. — — —

6. Assessed client's and family's knowledge of procedure. — — —

NURSING DIAGNOSIS

1. Developed appropriate nursing diagnoses based on assessment data. — — —

PLANNING

1. Identified expected outcomes. — — —

2. Prepared necessary equipment and supplies. — — —

3. Explained procedure and safety precautions to client. — — —

IMPLEMENTATION

1. Provided privacy, and washed hands. — — —

2. Positioned client comfortably and exposed area to be treated. — — —

3. Insulated surface of pad from client's skin with towel or pillowcase. — — —

4. Placed pad over area to be treated; secured pad as needed. — — —

5. Checked temperature setting of pad. — — —

6. Monitored condition of skin and client's response every 5 minutes. — — —

7. Removed pad after desired interval. — — —

8. Assisted client to comfortable position; disposed of soiled linen; and washed hands. — — —

	S	U	NP	Comments

EVALUATION

1. Inspected condition of skin exposed to heat. ___ ___ ___ _____

2. Determined level of client's discomfort. ___ ___ ___ _____

3. Noted client's ability to move strained muscle. ___ ___ ___ _____

4. Observed client applying pad. ___ ___ ___ _____

5. Identified unexpected outcomes. ___ ___ ___ _____

RECORDING AND REPORTING

1. Recorded procedure and client's response. ___ ___ ___ _____

2. Described instruction given and client's ability to perform procedure. ___ ___ ___ _____

3. Reported unusual changes in condition of client's skin. ___ ___ ___ _____

Student _____   Date _____

Instructor _____   Date _____

PERFORMANCE CHECKLIST 38-4   **APPLYING COLD APPLICATIONS**

	S	U	NP	Comments
ASSESSMENT				
1. Reviewed physician's order.	—	—	—	_____
2. Inspected and documented condition of injured or affected part.	—	—	—	_____
3. Considered time in which injury occurred.	—	—	—	_____
4. Asked client to describe pain, and documented character of pain.	—	—	—	_____
5. Assessed area for sensitivity to temperature, touch, and pain.	—	—	—	_____
6. Assessed client's understanding of procedure.	—	—	—	_____
NURSING DIAGNOSIS				
1. Developed appropriate nursing diagnoses based on assessment data.	—	—	—	_____
PLANNING				
1. Identified expected outcomes.	—	—	—	_____
2. Prepared necessary equipment and supplies.	—	—	—	_____
3. Explained procedure to client.	—	—	—	_____
IMPLEMENTATION				
1. Provided privacy.	—	—	—	_____
2. Washed hands.	—	—	—	_____
3. Positioned client comfortably, with affected body part aligned properly and only the area to be treated exposed.	—	—	—	_____
4. Placed towel or pad under area to be treated.	—	—	—	_____
5. Applied disposable gloves.	—	—	—	_____
6. Checked temperature of solution and submerged compress. Wrung out excess moisture and applied compress to affected area.	—	—	—	_____
7. Wrapped electronically controlled cooling pad around affected part, set temperature, and secured in place.	—	—	—	_____
8. Prepared ice bag or collar, wiped dry, and applied and secured over affected area.	—	—	—	_____

	S	U	NP	Comments

9. Prepared ice pack and applied over affected area. Covered bag with towel or pillowcase. ___ ___ ___ _____

10. Removed and disposed of gloves. ___ ___ ___ _____

11. Inspected condition of skin every 5 minutes during application. ___ ___ ___ _____

12. Applied clean gloves; removed cooling application after 15 to 20 minutes (or as ordered) and dried area. ___ ___ ___ _____

13. Assisted client to comfortable position. ___ ___ ___ _____

14. Emptied and stored basin; disposed of used linens and gloves; and washed hands. ___ ___ ___ _____

EVALUATION

1. Inspected condition of skin. ___ ___ ___ _____

2. Palpated affected area gently. ___ ___ ___ _____

3. Measured client's level of comfort. ___ ___ ___ _____

4. Asked client to demonstrate cold application and explain risks of treatment. ___ ___ ___ _____

5. Identified unexpected outcomes. ___ ___ ___ _____

RECORDING AND REPORTING

1. Recorded procedure and client's response. ___ ___ ___ _____

2. Described instruction given and client's ability to perform procedure. ___ ___ ___ _____

3. Reported undesirable skin changes to nurse in charge or physician. ___ ___ ___ _____

Student _____   Date _____

Instructor _____   Date _____

PERFORMANCE CHECKLIST 38-5 **CARING FOR CLIENTS REQUIRING HYPOTHERMIA OR HYPERTHERMIA BLANKETS**

	S	U	NP	Comments
ASSESSMENT				
1. Verified physician's orders, and rechecked client's current body temperature.	—	—	—	_____
2. Obtained vital signs and assessed neurologic and mental status and peripheral circulation.	—	—	—	_____
3. Verified that less intensive measures were not effective in returning body temperature to normal.	—	—	—	_____
4. Assessed client's skin on bony prominences and other susceptible areas before therapy.	—	—	—	_____
NURSING DIAGNOSIS				
1. Developed appropriate nursing diagnoses based on assessment data.	—	—	—	_____
PLANNING				
1. Identified expected outcomes.	—	—	—	_____
2. Explained procedure to client.	—	—	—	_____
3. Prepared client for procedure.	—	—	—	_____
4. Prepared blanket per agency policy and manufacturer's instructions.	—	—	—	_____
IMPLEMENTATION				
1. Washed hands and applied gloves.	—	—	—	_____
2. Obtained baseline vital signs.	—	—	—	_____
3. Applied lanolin/cold cream to client's skin.	—	—	—	_____
4. Placed blanket on client's mattress and set on desired temperature.	—	—	—	_____
5. Observed that the "cool" or "warm" light was on.	—	—	—	_____
6. Verified that pad temperature limits were correctly set.	—	—	—	_____
7. Placed sheet or thin blanket over the thermal blanket.	—	—	—	_____
8. Placed client on blanket. Wrapped client's hands and feet in towels before application of hypothermia blanket.	—	—	—	_____
9. Lubricated rectal probe and inserted into client's rectum.	—	—	—	_____

	S	U	NP	Comments
10. Properly positioned client.	___	___	___	_____
11. Double-checked fluid thermometer on blanket control panel.	___	___	___	_____
12. Removed gloves and washed hands.	___	___	___	_____

EVALUATION

1. Monitored client's vital signs at appropriate time intervals.	___	___	___	_____
2. Verified accuracy of rectal probe and automatic temperature control device.	___	___	___	_____
3. Observed the skin for injuries or changes.	___	___	___	_____
4. Observed client for signs of shivering.	___	___	___	_____
5. Determined client's level of comfort.	___	___	___	_____
6. Identified unexpected outcomes.	___	___	___	_____

RECORDING AND REPORTING

1. Recorded baseline data, time that therapy was initiated, temperature control setting, and client's response to therapy.	___	___	___	_____
2. Reported any unexpected outcomes to nurse in charge or physician.	___	___	___	_____

Student _____   Date _____

Instructor _____   Date _____

PERFORMANCE CHECKLIST 39-1   MODIFYING SAFETY RISKS IN THE HOME ENVIRONMENT

	S	U	NP	Comments
ASSESSMENT				
1. Reviewed previous findings and/or conducted sensory and neuromuscular assessments.	—	—	—	_____
2. Determined client's history of falls or other injuries in the home.	—	—	—	_____
3. Had client with near or actual fall maintain a diary.	—	—	—	_____
4. Reviewed risk factors for accidents in the home.	—	—	—	_____
5. Determined if client had fear of falling.	—	—	—	_____
6. Conducted a complete home safety assessment.	—	—	—	_____
7. Assessed client's financial resources.	—	—	—	_____
8. Assess client's and family's willingness to make changes.	—	—	—	_____
NURSING DIAGNOSIS				
1. Developed appropriate nursing diagnoses based on assessment data.	—	—	—	_____
PLANNING				
1. Identified expected outcomes.	—	—	—	_____
2. Prioritized with client and family the greatest environmental risks to safety.	—	—	—	_____
3. Recommended calling a reliable contractor if major home repairs required.	—	—	—	_____
IMPLEMENTATION				
1. Took steps to reduce physical hazards that predispose to falls.	—	—	—	_____
2. Had client use padding or clothing to cushion bony prominences.	—	—	—	_____
3. Made modifications to promote safe practice of activities of daily living.	—	—	—	_____
4. Took steps to eliminate fire hazards.	—	—	—	_____
5. Took steps to reduce chances of injury from burns.	—	—	—	_____
6. Took steps to prevent carbon monoxide exposure.	—	—	—	_____

	S	U	NP	Comments

EVALUATION

1. Had client and family member(s) identify potential safety risks. ____ ____ ____ _____

2. Asked client to discuss plans for modifications and observed changes made on subsequent visits. ____ ____ ____ _____

3. During follow-up visit or call, asked if client experienced any injuries or falls. ____ ____ ____ _____

4. Identified unexpected outcomes. ____ ____ ____ _____

RECORDING AND REPORTING

1. Retained copy of home safety assessment in client's home health record. ____ ____ ____ _____

2. Recorded any instruction given, client's response, and changes made in the home environment. ____ ____ ____ _____

Student _____   Date _____

Instructor _____   Date _____

PERFORMANCE CHECKLIST 39-2   **ADAPTING THE HOME SETTING FOR CLIENTS WITH COGNITIVE DEFICITS**

	S	U	NP	Comments
ASSESSMENT				
1. Conducted assessment during short session while maintaining sensitivity to client's needs or disabilities.	—	—	—	_____
2. Met with client and family in conducive environment.	—	—	—	_____
3. Asked client to describe level of health and self-care abilities.	—	—	—	_____
4. Asked how client is doing with home management.	—	—	—	_____
5. Assessed medications taken by client.	—	—	—	_____
6. Determined if client has family member or friend who assists with self-care or home management.	—	—	—	_____
7. Observed client's appearance and behavior during discussion.	—	—	—	_____
8. Observed immediate home environment.	—	—	—	_____
9. Completed a mini-mental exam if cognitive or mental status change is suspected.	—	—	—	_____
NURSING DIAGNOSIS				
1. Developed appropriate nursing diagnoses based on assessment data.	—	—	—	_____
PLANNING				
1. Identified expected outcomes.	—	—	—	_____
2. Referred family to homemaker services and/or respite care if client has difficulty with self-care skills.	—	—	—	_____
3. Consulted with physician and/or occupational therapist if client has a physical disability that affects fine motor skills.	—	—	—	_____
4. Considered client's level of cognitive impairment before implementing strategies.	—	—	—	_____
5. Determined best time of day for specific approaches.	—	—	—	_____

	S	U	NP	Comments

IMPLEMENTATION

1. Created methods to assist client to remember task performance.

2. Found ways to consolidate tasks to simple steps if client has difficulty completing tasks.

3. Assisted client and caregiver to determine a routine schedule for self-care activities and home management.

4. Instructed caregiver to focus on client's abilities rather than his or her disabilities.

5. Had caregiver assist with setting up tasks that the client can complete.

6. Discussed options for scheduling multiple medications with client, caregiver, and physician/primary care provider.

7. Instructed caregiver about use of simple and direct communication.

8. Kept clocks, calendars, and personal mementos situated throughout the house.

9. Had caregiver routinely orient client.

10. Encouraged regular naps or rest periods throughout the day.

11. Had caregiver encourage and support frequent visits by family and significant others.

EVALUATION

1. Asked client to review daily home management activities during follow-up visit.

2. Reviewed schedule for medication administration.

3. Asked caregiver to describe ways to increase client's success in self-care and home management activities.

4. Had caregiver show schedules of daily routines and specific approaches used.

5. Identified unexpected outcomes.

RECORDING AND REPORTING

1. Recorded assessment of client's cognitive and mental status, interventions, and client's and caregiver's responses.

2. Reported to physician any changes in client's behavior that reflected a possible decline in cognitive or mental status.

Student _____   Date _____

Instructor _____   Date _____

PERFORMANCE CHECKLIST 39-3   **MEDICATION AND MEDICAL DEVICE SAFETY**

	S	U	NP	Comments

ASSESSMENT

1. Assessed client's sensory, musculoskeletal, and neurological function.   — — — _____

2. Assessed abilities of caregiver to assist the client.   — — — _____

3. Assessed medication regimen.   — — — _____

4. Asked client to identify where medications are kept in the home. Looked at each container.   — — — _____

5. Had client describe daily schedule for drug administration.   — — — _____

6. Asked client to identify where self-injection supplies are kept and disposed of, if applicable.   — — — _____

7. Asked client to identify where glucose monitor and supplies are stored and where lancets are disposed of, if applicable.   — — — _____

8. Asked to identify where dressings are stored and disposed of, if applicable.   — — — _____

NURSING DIAGNOSIS

1. Developed appropriate nursing diagnoses based on assessment data.   — — — _____

PLANNING

1. Identified expected outcomes.   — — — _____

IMPLEMENTATION

1. Instructed client and caregiver about principles to follow to ensure that medications are safe to use.   — — — _____

2. Recommended approaches to facilitate preparation of medications.   — — — _____

3. Recommended approaches to ensure medications and supplies properly stored.   — — — _____

4. Reviewed with client and caregiver proper techniques for disposal of sharps and other medical supplies.   — — — _____

EVALUATION

1. Had client or caregiver describe steps to take to ensure that medications are safe to use.   — — — _____

2. Observed client preparing and administering a medication dose.   — — — _____

	S	U	NP	Comments
3. Observed home setting for location of medications and supplies.	——	——	——	_____
4. Had client describe disposal of sharps and other medical supplies.	——	——	——	_____
5. Performed pill counts at regular intervals.	——	——	——	_____
6. Identified unexpected outcomes.	——	——	——	_____

RECORDING AND REPORTING

	S	U	NP	Comments
1. Recorded recommendations provided to client and caregiver and their responses.	——	——	——	_____

Student _____ Date _____

Instructor _____ Date _____

PERFORMANCE CHECKLIST 40-1 **TEACHING CLIENTS TO MEASURE BODY TEMPERATURE, BLOOD PRESSURE, AND PULSE**

TEACHING CLIENTS TO MEASURE BODY TEMPERATURE

	S	U	NP	Comments

ASSESSMENT
1. Assessed client's ability to hold and read thermometer.
2. Assessed client's knowledge about temperature ranges, fever, and type of thermometer to use.
3. Observed client's technique for measuring temperature if client has had prior experience.

NURSING DIAGNOSIS
1. Developed appropriate nursing diagnoses based on assessment data.

PLANNING
1. Identified expected outcomes.
2. Selected setting in home for client to measure temperature.
3. Instructed client and/or caregiver about positioning technique.

IMPLEMENTATION
1. Demonstrated steps and stated rationale for preparation and insertion of thermometer.
2. Assisted client in performance of each step.
3. Discussed normal temperature ranges.
4. Discussed factors that influence temperature.
5. Discussed common symptoms of fever.
6. Discussed signs and symptoms of hypothermia.
7. Discussed importance of notifying physician with regard to measures to control fever.
8. Created written guidelines for reference.

EVALUATION
1. Had client measure body temperature and demonstrate ability to read thermometer without assistance.

	S	U	NP	Comments

2. Observed client cleaning and storing equipment.

3. Had client discuss and identify knowledge related to temperature measurement.

4. Had client describe signs and symptoms of fever and hypothermia and methods for control.

5. Identified unexpected outcomes.

RECORDING AND REPORTING

1. Recorded information taught and client's response.

2. Instructed client to maintain a written record of temperature readings.

TEACHING CLIENTS TO MEASURE BLOOD PRESSURE

ASSESSMENT

1. Assessed client's ability to manipulate equipment and determine reading.

2. Assessed client's knowledge of blood pressure (BP) ranges and symptoms and common causes of hypotension and hypertension.

3. Assessed client's knowledge of the significance of the BP measurement and its variations.

4. Asked for demonstration of technique if client had previous experience.

5. Determined best site for BP measurement.

6. Selected quiet place for BP measurement.

NURSING DIAGNOSIS

1. Developed appropriate nursing diagnoses based on assessment data.

PLANNING

1. Identified expected outcomes.

2. Encouraged client to perform BP measurements on a regular schedule.

3. Encouraged client to avoid activities that increase BP before measurement.

4. Had client perform measurement in a comfortable position and environment.

5. Explained procedure to client and had client rest 5 minutes before measurement.

6. Had client describe symptoms that would indicate the need to measure the BP.

	S	U	NP	Comments

IMPLEMENTATION

1. Discussed the best sites for BP measurement.

2. Demonstrated steps for skill performance.

3. Described the sounds of measurement and relationship of gauge to BP reading.

4. Had client manipulate all equipment.

5. Had client perform skill on nurse, family member, or caregiver.

6. Had client demonstrate technique on self.

7. Identified that teaching of skill may be accomplished slowly until client comfort is gained.

8. Had client perform skill under observation and record reading with nurse verification.

9. Used appropriate written and/or pictorial instructions.

EVALUATION

1. Observed client demonstrating technique for BP measurement on at least three different occasions.

2. Asked client if BP reading was within normal range.

3. Asked client to describe the rationale for BP monitoring and medications.

4. Identified unexpected outcomes.

RECORDING AND REPORTING

1. Recorded teaching and client responses in home care record.

2. Recorded BP in home care record and client's documentation system.

3. Reported abnormal readings to physician.

TEACHING CLIENTS TO MEASURE PULSE

ASSESSMENT

1. Identified client's knowledge of purpose of assessing pulse, and assessed client's level of interest in performing skill.

2. Assessed client's ability to feel pulsation by having client palpate his or her own or a nurse's artery.

3. Asked client to demonstrate technique for assessing pulse.

	S	U	NP	Comments

NURSING DIAGNOSIS

1. Identified appropriate nursing diagnoses based on client's learning capabilities and needs.

PLANNING

1. Identified expected outcomes.

2. Selected setting in home for assessing pulse.

IMPLEMENTATION

1. Discussed with client best sites for assessing pulse.

2. Cautioned client against massaging neck while attempting to locate carotid pulse; also cautioned against attempting to locate both carotid arteries at the same time (if applicable).

3. Demonstrated steps for palpating the pulse.

4. Had client perform each step.

5. Discussed information relating to pulse range, the purpose of monitoring the pulse, and the best time to monitor the pulse.

6. Discussed importance of notifying physician and/or withholding medication when pulse alterations occur.

EVALUATION

1. Observed client or family member independently assessing pulse.

2. Had learner take radial pulse at the same time as the nurse.

3. Had client discuss reasons for assessing pulse and the normal pulse rate range.

4. Asked client to reiterate instructions about withholding medication according to pulse rate.

5. Asked client to state time of day and activity level in relation to pulse measurement and medication dosage.

6. Identified unexpected outcomes.

RECORDING AND REPORTING

1. Recorded teaching and client's response in home care record.

2. Had client maintain written record of pulse measurement and medication administration.

Student _____   Date _____

Instructor _____   Date _____

PERFORMANCE CHECKLIST 40-2   **USING HOME OXYGEN EQUIPMENT**

	S	U	NP	Comments
ASSESSMENT				
1. Determined client's or family's ability to use oxygen equipment correctly in hospital and in the home.	___	___	___	_____
2. Assessed client's home environment for electrical power if compressor is to be used.	___	___	___	_____
3. Assessed client's or family's ability to observe for signs and symptoms of hypoxia.	___	___	___	_____
4. Observed client's or family's use of prescribed oxygen therapy.	___	___	___	_____
5. Determined appropriate resource in the community for equipment and assistance.	___	___	___	_____
6. Determined back-up system in the event of power failure.	___	___	___	_____
NURSING DIAGNOSIS				
1. Developed appropriate nursing diagnoses based on assessment data.	___	___	___	_____
PLANNING				
1. Identified expected outcomes.	___	___	___	_____
2. Explained procedure to client and family.	___	___	___	_____
IMPLEMENTATION				
1. Washed hands.	___	___	___	_____
2. Demonstrated steps for preparation and completion of oxygen therapy.	___	___	___	_____
3. Prepared liberator and stroller for use.	___	___	___	_____
4. Instructed client or family through each step.	___	___	___	_____
5. Discussed signs and symptoms of hypoxia and infection, and instructed client or family about when to notify physician.	___	___	___	_____
6. Discussed emergency plan.	___	___	___	_____
7. Washed hands.	___	___	___	_____
8. Recorded teaching plan and documented client's learning.	___	___	___	_____

	S	U	NP	Comments

EVALUATION

1. Evaluated client's or family's ability to use oxygen at home. ___ ___ ___ _____

2. Asked client and family to identify problems with oxygen use. ___ ___ ___ _____

3. Had client and family state safety guidelines and emergency plans. ___ ___ ___ _____

4. Identified unexpected outcomes. ___ ___ ___ _____

RECORDING AND REPORTING

1. Recorded teaching plan in the care plan. ___ ___ ___ _____

2. Recorded learning progress. ___ ___ ___ _____

3. Communicated learning activity and progress with other staff. ___ ___ ___ _____

Student _____　　Date _____

Instructor _____　　Date _____

PERFORMANCE CHECKLIST 40-3　**TEACHING HOME TRACHEOSTOMY CARE AND SUCTIONING**

	S	U	NP	Comments
ASSESSMENT				
1. Assessed client's ability to perform tracheostomy care and suctioning.	—	—	—	_____
2. Assessed client's or family's recognition of physical signs and symptoms that indicate need to perform home tracheostomy care and suctioning.	—	—	—	_____
3. Assessed client's or family's recognition of factors that normally influence airway functioning.	—	—	—	_____
4. Assessed client's understanding of and ability to perform tracheostomy care and suctioning.	—	—	—	_____
5. Observed client or family member perform tracheostomy care and suctioning.	—	—	—	_____
NURSING DIAGNOSIS				
1. Developed appropriate nursing diagnoses based on assessment data.	—	—	—	_____
PLANNING				
1. Identified expected outcomes.	—	—	—	_____
2. Selected setting in home for tracheostomy tube care.	—	—	—	_____
3. Demonstrated with client proper position for procedure.	—	—	—	_____
IMPLEMENTATION				
Demonstrated steps for tracheostomy tube suctioning				
1. Verified physician's order.	—	—	—	_____
2. Washed hands.	—	—	—	_____
3. Prepared suction equipment according to manufacturer's directions.	—	—	—	_____
4. Positioned client in semi-Fowler's position.	—	—	—	_____
5. Filled basin with ½ cup water or normal saline. Applied gloves.	—	—	—	_____
6. Connected suction catheter to suction apparatus and ensured proper functioning.	—	—	—	_____
7. Removed oxygen or humidity source, if applicable. Inserted catheter into tracheobronchial tree correctly.	—	—	—	_____

	S	U	NP	Comments

8. Applied intermittent suction correctly while withdrawing catheter. Reapplied oxygen or humidity source.   ___ ___ ___ _____

9. Rinsed secretions from catheter correctly. Repeated Steps 6-8 as needed.   ___ ___ ___ _____

10. Suctioned nasal and oral pharynx, if needed.   ___ ___ ___ _____

11. Rinsed catheter properly.   ___ ___ ___ _____

12. Had client take two to three deep breaths.   ___ ___ ___ _____

13. Disconnected suction catheter; coiled and disposed of catheter properly.   ___ ___ ___ _____

Trachestomy Care

1. Prepared equipment and site for cleaning inner cannula.   ___ ___ ___ _____

2. Prepared solutions of hydrogen peroxide, normal saline/water, and 4 × 4 gauze pads.   ___ ___ ___ _____

3. Removed old tracheostomy bib or dressing and discarded.   ___ ___ ___ _____

4. Removed and discarded gloves.   ___ ___ ___ _____

5. Applied clean gloves.   ___ ___ ___ _____

6. Cleansed site around stoma with presoaked 4 × 4s and damp applicators.   ___ ___ ___ _____

7. Dried exposed outer cannula and skin.   ___ ___ ___ _____

8. Cleaned inner cannula with nylon brush or pipe cleaners.   ___ ___ ___ _____

9. Examined patency of cannula and repeated procedure as needed. Replaced inner cannula.   ___ ___ ___ _____

10. Changed old tracheostomy ties.   ___ ___ ___ _____

11. Applied fresh dressing.   ___ ___ ___ _____

12. Cleaned and stored reusable supplies.   ___ ___ ___ _____

13. Removed and discarded gloves.   ___ ___ ___ _____

14. Disinfected reusable supplies at least weekly.   ___ ___ ___ _____

15. Had client or family member perform each step with guidance from nurse.   ___ ___ ___ _____

16. Discussed signs and symptoms of infection or inflammation and the importance of notifying the physician of these conditions.   ___ ___ ___ _____

	S	U	NP	Comments

EVALUATION

1. Observed client or caregiver demonstrating trache-ostomy tube care and suctioning independently. ___ ___ ___ _____

2. Had client or caregiver state signs of stomal or respiratory infection. ___ ___ ___ _____

3. Identified unexpected outcomes. ___ ___ ___ _____

RECORDING AND REPORTING

1. Recorded teaching and client's response in home care record. ___ ___ ___ _____

2. Developed a system of recording performance of care by client or family member. ___ ___ ___ _____

Student _____ Date _____

Instructor _____ Date _____

PERFORMANCE CHECKLIST 40-4 **HELPING CLIENTS WITH SELF-MEDICATION**

	S	U	NP	Comments
ASSESSMENT				
1. Assessed client's cognitive, sensory, and motor function.	___	___	___	_____
2. Assessed client's resources for obtaining medications.	___	___	___	_____
3. Assessed client's readiness to learn.	___	___	___	_____
4. Assessed client's knowledge of drug therapy and drug interactions.	___	___	___	_____
5. Assessed family member's knowledge of client's drug therapy.	___	___	___	_____
6. Assessed client's beliefs about drug therapy.	___	___	___	_____
7. Checked type and number of drugs prescribed.	___	___	___	_____
NURSING DIAGNOSIS				
1. Developed appropriate nursing diagnoses based on assessment data.	___	___	___	_____
PLANNING				
1. Identified expected outcomes.	___	___	___	_____
2. Prepared environment for teaching session.	___	___	___	_____
3. Provided useful teaching materials that complemented client's learning capacity.	___	___	___	_____
4. Had client wear glasses or hearing aid during teaching session, if appropriate.	___	___	___	_____
5. Consulted with physician about medications prescribed.	___	___	___	_____
6. Included family in teaching program.	___	___	___	_____
IMPLEMENTATION				
1. Presented information in a clear, concise manner.	___	___	___	_____
2. Offered frequent opportunities for client to ask questions.	___	___	___	_____
3. Presented content pertaining to drug information, drug safety, and illness prevention.	___	___	___	_____
4. Taught sessions that were short and frequent.	___	___	___	_____
5. Provided special learning aids for dosage schedule routine.	___	___	___	_____

	S	U	NP	Comments

6. Assisted client with practicing preparation of medications. ___ ___ ___ _____

7. Arranged with pharmacy to have large-print labels for medication bottles. ___ ___ ___ _____

8. Arranged for pharmacy to deliver prescriptions as needed and to provide containers client can open independently. ___ ___ ___ _____

EVALUATION

1. Had client or family member independently prepare dosages of all medications. ___ ___ ___ _____

2. Had client or family member explain content presented in teaching session. ___ ___ ___ _____

3. Identified client's problem-solving initiatives. ___ ___ ___ _____

4. Offered additional opportunity for client to ask questions. ___ ___ ___ _____

5. Identified unexpected outcomes. ___ ___ ___ _____

RECORDING AND REPORTING

1. Documented instruction. ___ ___ ___ _____

2. Developed a system of recording medication administration by client or family member. ___ ___ ___ _____

Student _____   Date _____

Instructor _____   Date _____

PERFORMANCE CHECKLIST 40-5 **ENTERAL NUTRITION IN THE HOME**

	S	U	NP	Comments
ASSESSMENT				
1. Assessed client's health status for ability to manage home feedings.	___	___	___	_____
2. Assessed client or caregiver's abilities and resources.	___	___	___	_____
3. Assessed environmental conditions in the client's home.	___	___	___	_____
4. Assessed client or caregiver's understanding of the purpose of enteral nutrition.	___	___	___	_____
5. Assessed client or caregiver's understanding of the storage, management, and acquisition of supplies.	___	___	___	_____
6. Assessed client or caregiver's ability to administer feedings.	___	___	___	_____
NURSING DIAGNOSIS				
1. Developed appropriate nursing diagnoses based on assessment data.	___	___	___	_____
PLANNING				
1. Identified expected outcomes.	___	___	___	_____
IMPLEMENTATION				
1. Washed hands.	___	___	___	_____
2. Discussed client or caregiver's understanding of enteral feeding and nutritional health.	___	___	___	_____
3. Demonstrated identification of placement of nasal tubes.	___	___	___	_____
4. Observed client or caregiver demonstrating determination of tube placement.	___	___	___	_____
5. Observed client or caregiver aspirating gastric contents.	___	___	___	_____
6. Observed client or caregiver preparing and administering feeding and cleaning and storing supplies.	___	___	___	_____
7. Observed client or caregiver administering medication and flushing tube.	___	___	___	_____
8. Discussed and observed use of infusion pump, if indicated.	___	___	___	_____

	S	U	NP	Comments

9. Discussed measures to stabilize the feeding tube and to protect skin integrity.

10. Discussed measures to prevent tube occlusion and aspiration.

11. Discussed whom to contact for equipment or supplies or in case of equipment failure.

12. Discussed emergency plan in the event of aspiration.

13. Discussed whom to contact and when for signs of diarrhea, constipation, or weight loss.

14. Washed hands.

EVALUATION

1. Asked client to state purpose of home enteral nutrition therapy.

2. Observed client or caregiver performing technique.

3. Asked client or caregiver to state measures to prevent complications.

4. Asked client about community contacts for supplies, equipment, and emergency care.

5. Identified unexpected outcomes.

RECORDING AND REPORTING

1. Documented teaching and client's response in home care record.

2. Documented specifics of enteral feeding plan.

3. Reviewed home documentation by client or caregiver of enteral feeding and client status.

Student _____   Date _____

Instructor _____   Date _____

PERFORMANCE CHECKLIST 41-1 **COLLECTING A MIDSTREAM (CLEAN-VOIDED) URINE SPECIMEN**

	S	U	NP	Comments
ASSESSMENT				
1. Assessed client's level of understanding of test.	___	___	___	_____
2. Assessed client's ability to use toilet facilities independently.	___	___	___	_____
3. Referred to medical record for history of urinary infection.	___	___	___	_____
4. Assessed client's risk for urinary tract infection.	___	___	___	_____
5. Assessed signs and symptoms of urinary tract infection.	___	___	___	_____
6. Referred to agency policy for specimen collection procedure.	___	___	___	_____
NURSING DIAGNOSIS				
1. Developed appropriate nursing diagnoses based on assessment data.	___	___	___	_____
PLANNING				
1. Identified expected outcomes.	___	___	___	_____
2. Offered client fluids before specimen collection.	___	___	___	_____
3. Explained procedure to client.	___	___	___	_____
IMPLEMENTATION				
1. Identified client. Washed hands.	___	___	___	_____
2. Provided privacy.	___	___	___	_____
3. Assisted client as needed with perineal care.	___	___	___	_____
4. Assisted bedridden client onto bedpan.	___	___	___	_____
5. Opened sterile collection kit correctly.	___	___	___	_____
6. Applied sterile gloves.	___	___	___	_____
7. Prepared sterile collection kit with specimen container.	___	___	___	_____
8. Opened specimen container correctly.	___	___	___	_____
9. Assisted or allowed client to cleanse perineum.	___	___	___	_____
10. Removed specimen container before flow of urine stopped.	___	___	___	_____
11. Secured specimen container top tightly.	___	___	___	_____

	S	U	NP	Comments
12. Cleaned urine from outer surface of specimen container.	___	___	___	_____
13. Disposed of soiled supplies. Removed and discarded gloves. Washed hands.	___	___	___	_____
14. Labeled specimen and attached laboratory requisition.	___	___	___	_____
15. Sent specimen to laboratory within 15 to 20 minutes or refrigerated specimen.	___	___	___	_____

EVALUATION

	S	U	NP	Comments
1. Observed specimen for contaminants.	___	___	___	_____
2. Assessed client's urine culture and sensitivity report.	___	___	___	_____
3. Asked client to describe procedure.	___	___	___	_____
4. Identified unexpected outcomes.	___	___	___	_____

RECORDING AND REPORTING

	S	U	NP	Comments
1. Recorded date and time specimen was collected.	___	___	___	_____
2. Recorded characteristics of urine and signs and symptoms of infection.	___	___	___	_____
3. Notified nurse in charge or physician of significant abnormalities.	___	___	___	_____

Student _____   Date _____

Instructor _____   Date _____

PERFORMANCE CHECKLIST 41-2   **COLLECTING A TIMED URINE SPECIMEN**

	S	U	NP	Comments

ASSESSMENT

1. Determined purpose and time period for specimen.

2. Assessed if test required fluid or dietary requirements or medication administration.

3. Determined if client is taking correct diet.

4. Assessed client's ability to collect specimen independently.

5. Assessed client's or family's understanding of purpose of test and reason for timed collection.

6. Referred to agency policy for specimen collection procedure.

NURSING DIAGNOSIS

1. Developed appropriate nursing diagnoses based on assessment data.

PLANNING

1. Identified expected outcomes.

2. Instructed client to drink 2 to 4 glasses of fluids $\frac{1}{2}$ hour before test began.

3. Instructed client and/or family to save all urine during time period; to notify nurse when client voids; to keep feces and toilet tissue out of specimens; to begin and end test with voiding; and to begin test at a precise time.

IMPLEMENTATION

1. Provided privacy.

2. Wore gloves when handling urine.

3. Discarded first random urine specimen obtained and noted time for beginning of test.

4. Provided client with required liquid or medication (as appropriate).

5. Placed signs in client's room indicating time collections occurred.

6. Measured volume of urine voided if client I&O is being monitored.

	S	U	NP	Comments
7. Placed all voided urine into collection bottle.	___	___	___	_____
8. Kept urine refrigerated during collection period, if appropriate.	___	___	___	_____
9. Discarded gloves after each collection, and washed hands.	___	___	___	_____
10. One hour before end of collection, instructed client to drink fluids.	___	___	___	_____
11. Encouraged client to void during last 15 minutes before end of collection period.	___	___	___	_____
12. Sent specimen to laboratory at end of collection period with appropriate requisition.	___	___	___	_____
13. Removed room signs after specimen collected.	___	___	___	_____

EVALUATION

	S	U	NP	Comments
1. Intermittently assessed client's compliance with saving all urine during collection period.	___	___	___	_____
2. Inspected urine for contaminants.	___	___	___	_____
3. Compared results of client's urinalysis with normal laboratory values.	___	___	___	_____
4. Identified unexpected outcomes.	___	___	___	_____

RECORDING AND REPORTING

	S	U	NP	Comments
1. Recorded starting time of urine collection.	___	___	___	_____
2. Recorded pertinent data at end of test.	___	___	___	_____
3. Reported abnormal results to nurse in charge or physician.	___	___	___	_____

Student _____   Date _____

Instructor _____   Date _____

PERFORMANCE CHECKLIST 41-3 **COLLECTING A STERILE URINE SPECIMEN FROM AN INDWELLING CATHETER**

	S	U	NP	Comments
ASSESSMENT				
1. Assessed client's or family's understanding of need for specimen.	___	___	___	_____
2. Assessed client for signs and symptoms of urinary tract infection.	___	___	___	_____
3. Checked catheter for presence of sampling port.	___	___	___	_____
NURSING DIAGNOSIS				
1. Developed appropriate nursing diagnoses based on assessment data.	___	___	___	_____
PLANNING				
1. Identified expected outcomes.	___	___	___	_____
2. Explained reason for clamping catheter before specimen collection.	___	___	___	_____
3. Explained procedure to client.	___	___	___	_____
IMPLEMENTATION				
1. Washed hands.	___	___	___	_____
2. Clamped drainage tubing near catheter for 30 minutes.	___	___	___	_____
3. Informed client when ready to collect specimen.	___	___	___	_____
4. Washed hands and applied gloves.	___	___	___	_____
5. Positioned client for easy access to catheter.	___	___	___	_____
6. Cleansed entry port with disinfectant swab.	___	___	___	_____
7. Inserted needle at 45-degree angle into catheter just above attachment to drainage tube or into sampling port.	___	___	___	_____
8. Collected appropriate amount of urine.	___	___	___	_____
9. Transferred urine into proper container.	___	___	___	_____
10. Placed lid tightly on container.	___	___	___	_____
11. Unclamped catheter and allowed urine to flow into drainage bag.	___	___	___	_____
12. Disposed of soiled supplies. Removed and discarded gloves. Washed hands.	___	___	___	_____

	S	U	NP	Comments
13. Securely attached label to container, and affixed requisition.	——	——	——	————————
14. Sent specimen immediately to laboratory or placed it in refrigerator.	——	——	——	————————

EVALUATION

	S	U	NP	Comments
1. Compared client's laboratory results with normal laboratory values.	——	——	——	————————
2. Observed characteristics of urine.	——	——	——	————————
3. Observed urinary drainage system.	——	——	——	————————
4. Identified unexpected outcomes.	——	——	——	————————

RECORDING AND REPORTING

	S	U	NP	Comments
1. Recorded collection procedure time and date and appearance of urine.	——	——	——	————————
2. Reported unexpected outcomes to nurse in charge or physician.	——	——	——	————————

Student _____   Date _____

Instructor _____   Date _____

PERFORMANCE CHECKLIST 41-4 **MEASURING SPECIFIC GRAVITY OF URINE**

	S	U	NP	Comments

ASSESSMENT

1. Assessed client's or family's understanding of need to test specific gravity.   ___ ___ ___ _____

2. Determined client's ability to collect specimen.   ___ ___ ___ _____

3. Assessed client's hydration status.   ___ ___ ___ _____

4. Assessed client's medical history.   ___ ___ ___ _____

NURSING DIAGNOSIS

1. Developed appropriate nursing diagnoses based on assessment data.   ___ ___ ___ _____

PLANNING

1. Identified expected outcomes.   ___ ___ ___ _____

2. Explained purpose of test to client and how specimen would be obtained.   ___ ___ ___ _____

IMPLEMENTATION

1. Washed hands and applied disposable gloves.   ___ ___ ___ _____

2. Poured specimen into glass cylinder until $\frac{2}{3}$ to $\frac{3}{4}$ full.   ___ ___ ___ _____

3. Placed urinometer into glass cylinder and twirled stem.   ___ ___ ___ _____

4. Read calibrated scale at urine level and noted reading.   ___ ___ ___ _____

5. Discarded urine and cleaned equipment in cool water.   ___ ___ ___ _____

6. Removed and discarded gloves and washed hands.   ___ ___ ___ _____

EVALUATION

1. Observed specimen for contaminants.   ___ ___ ___ _____

2. Compared client's specific gravity with normal values.   ___ ___ ___ _____

3. Identified unexpected outcomes.   ___ ___ ___ _____

RECORDING AND REPORTING

1. Recorded specific gravity reading and noted character of urine.   ___ ___ ___ _____

	S	U	NP	Comments
2. Recorded urine volume in I&O when appropriate.	___	___	___	_____
3. Reported abnormal values.	___	___	___	_____

Student _____ Date _____

Instructor _____ Date _____

PERFORMANCE CHECKLIST 41-5 **MEASURING CHEMICAL PROPERTIES OF URINE: GLUCOSE, KETONES, PROTEIN, BLOOD, AND pH**

	S	U	NP	Comments
ASSESSMENT				
1. Determined why physician requested test.	—	—	—	_____
2. Assessed client's need to learn urine testing procedure.	—	—	—	_____
3. Assessed type of reagent test to use.	—	—	—	_____
4. Assessed client's knowledge of and compliance with obtaining a double-voided specimen.	—	—	—	_____
5. Assessed medications client received for possible effects on reagent chemicals.	—	—	—	_____
6. Assessed for signs and symptoms of diabetes mellitus.	—	—	—	_____
7. Assessed client's ability to perform urine test.	—	—	—	_____
NURSING DIAGNOSIS				
1. Developed appropriate nursing diagnoses based on assessment data.	—	—	—	_____
PLANNING				
1. Identified expected outcomes.	—	—	—	_____
2. Offered client fluids to drink before specimen collection.	—	—	—	_____
3. Explained procedure to client and family.	—	—	—	_____
IMPLEMENTATION				
1. Obtained double-voided urine specimen.	—	—	—	_____
2. Applied gloves.	—	—	—	_____
3. Performed glucose reagent tablet test correctly.	—	—	—	_____
4. Performed glucose ketone reagent strip test correctly.	—	—	—	_____
5. Performed ketone tablet test correctly.	—	—	—	_____
6. Used Multistix reagent test strip correctly.	—	—	—	_____
7. Washed hands after removing and discarding gloves.	—	—	—	_____
8. Discussed test results with client.	—	—	—	_____

	S	U	NP	Comments

EVALUATION

1. Compared test results with normal chemical levels. ___ ___ ___ _____

2. Observed urine for contaminants. ___ ___ ___ _____

3. Had client demonstrate testing and reading of results. ___ ___ ___ _____

4. Identified unexpected outcomes. ___ ___ ___ _____

RECORDING AND REPORTING

1. Recorded test results. ___ ___ ___ _____

2. Had client in home setting record results on flowsheet. ___ ___ ___ _____

3. Reported abnormal findings. ___ ___ ___ _____

Student _____   Date _____

Instructor _____   Date _____

PERFORMANCE CHECKLIST 41-6   **MEASURING OCCULT BLOOD IN STOOL**

	S	U	NP	Comments
ASSESSMENT				
1. Assessed client's or family's understanding of need for stool test.	—	—	—	_____
2. Assessed client's ability to cooperate and collect specimen.	—	—	—	_____
3. Assessed medical history for evidence of bleeding or gastrointestinal disorder.	—	—	—	_____
4. Determined type of medications client receives and their potential for causing bleeding.	—	—	—	_____
5. Checked physician's orders for medication or dietary restrictions before test.	—	—	—	_____
NURSING DIAGNOSIS				
1. Developed appropriate nursing diagnoses based on assessment data.	—	—	—	_____
PLANNING				
1. Identified expected outcomes.	—	—	—	_____
2. Explained purpose of test and method by which client can assist.	—	—	—	_____
3. Initiated medication and dietary restrictions as ordered.	—	—	—	_____
IMPLEMENTATION				
1. Washed hands and applied disposable gloves.	—	—	—	_____
2. Obtained uncontaminated stool specimen.	—	—	—	_____
3. With tip of wooden applicator, obtained small amount of feces.	—	—	—	_____
4. Performed Hemoccult slide test.	—	—	—	_____
5. Performed test using Hematest tablets.	—	—	—	_____
6. Wrapped wooden applicator in paper towel and discarded.	—	—	—	_____
7. Removed gloves and washed hands.	—	—	—	_____
EVALUATION				
1. Noted color changes in guaiac paper.	—	—	—	_____
2. Noted character of stool.	—	—	—	_____

	S	U	NP	Comments
3. Asked client to explain collection procedure.	___	___	___	_____
4. Identified unexpected outcomes.	___	___	___	_____

RECORDING AND REPORTING

1. Recorded test results.	___	___	___	_____
2. Recorded unusual stool characteristics.	___	___	___	_____
3. Reported positive test results to nurse in charge or physician.	___	___	___	_____

Student _____ Date _____

Instructor _____ Date _____

PERFORMANCE CHECKLIST 41-7 **COLLECTING NOSE AND THROAT SPECIMENS FOR CULTURE**

	S	U	NP	Comments
ASSESSMENT				
1. Assessed client's understanding of procedure and ability to cooperate.	—	—	—	_____
2. Assessed condition of nasal mucosa and sinuses.	—	—	—	_____
3. Assessed client for symptoms of upper respiratory or sinus infection.	—	—	—	_____
4. Assessed condition of posterior pharynx.	—	—	—	_____
5. Assessed client for systemic signs of infection.	—	—	—	_____
6. Reviewed physician's orders for type of culture needed.	—	—	—	_____
NURSING DIAGNOSIS				
1. Developed appropriate nursing diagnoses based on assessment data.	—	—	—	_____
PLANNING				
1. Identified expected outcomes.	—	—	—	_____
2. Planned to do culture before mealtime or at least 1 hour after client had eaten.	—	—	—	_____
3. Explained purpose of specimens and how client could assist.	—	—	—	_____
4. Explained common sensations felt during collection.	—	—	—	_____
IMPLEMENTATION				
1. Washed hands and applied gloves.	—	—	—	_____
2. Assisted client to sit in bed or chair.	—	—	—	_____
3. Placed swab and tube in accessible location.	—	—	—	_____
4. Collected throat culture:	—	—	NP	_____
a. Had client tilt head back.	—	—	—	_____
b. Asked client to open mouth and say "ah."	—	—	—	_____
c. Swabbed tonsilar area from side to side without touching lips, teeth, gums, or cheeks.	—	—	—	_____

	S	U	NP	Comments
5. Collected nasal culture:	——	——	——	————————
a. Encouraged client to blow nose.	——	——	——	————————
b. Checked patency of nostrils.	——	——	——	————————
c. Had client tilt head back.	——	——	——	————————
d. Inserted speculum and swab.	——	——	——	————————
e. Rotated swab; avoided touching outside of nose when removing.	——	——	——	————————
f. Offered client a tissue.	——	——	——	————————
6. Collected nasopharyngeal culture:	——	——	——	————————
a. Followed steps for nasal culture.	——	——	——	————————
b. Used special swab with flexible wire.	——	——	——	————————
7. Placed swab into collection tube, crushed ampule, and pushed tip into liquid.	——	——	——	————————
8. Removed and discarded gloves. Washed hands.	——	——	——	————————
9. Securely attached label to culture tube and affixed requisition.	——	——	——	————————
10. Sent specimen immediately to lab or refrigerated specimen.	——	——	——	————————

EVALUATION

	S	U	NP	Comments
1. Checked laboratory record for test results.	——	——	——	————————
2. Inspected client's nose for evidence of bleeding.	——	——	——	————————
3. Identified unexpected outcomes.	——	——	——	————————

RECORDING AND REPORTING

	S	U	NP	Comments
1. Recorded specimen collection.	——	——	——	————————
2. Described appearance of nasal and oral mucosa.	——	——	——	————————
3. Reported unusual test results to physician or nurse in charge.	——	——	——	————————

Student _____   Date _____

Instructor _____   Date _____

PERFORMANCE CHECKLIST 41-8 **OBTAINING VAGINAL OR URETHRAL DISCHARGE SPECIMENS**

	S	U	NP	Comments
ASSESSMENT				
1. Assessed client's understanding of need for specimen and ability to cooperate.	—	—	—	_____
2. Assessed condition of client's external genitalia.	—	—	—	_____
3. Assessed client for symptoms of urinary or vaginal infection.	—	—	—	_____
4. Collected sexual history of client, when appropriate.	—	—	—	_____
5. Referred to physician's orders for type of culture.	—	—	—	_____
NURSING DIAGNOSIS				
1. Developed appropriate nursing diagnoses based on assessment data.	—	—	—	_____
PLANNING				
1. Identified expected outcomes.	—	—	—	_____
2. Explained procedure to client.	—	—	—	_____
3. Selected area where privacy ensured.	—	—	—	_____
4. Maintained nonjudgmental attitude.	—	—	—	_____
IMPLEMENTATION				
1. Washed hands.	—	—	—	_____
2. Closed bed curtains or room door and hung "Do not enter" door sign.	—	—	—	_____
3. Assisted client to proper position and draped.	—	—	—	_____
4. Applied disposable gloves.	—	—	—	_____
5. Directed light onto perineum.	—	—	—	_____
6. Opened culture tube and held swab in dominant hand.	—	—	—	_____
7. Instructed client to breathe slowly during procedure.	—	—	—	_____
8. Obtained specimen(s) using proper procedure according to sex of client.	—	—	—	_____

	S	U	NP	Comments

Female

    a. Exposed vaginal or urethral orifice. ___ ___ ___ _____

    b. Inserted swabs 1 to 2.5 cm (½-1 inch) ___ ___ ___ _____

    c. Avoided touching labia. ___ ___ ___ _____

Male

    a. Retracted foreskin, if present. ___ ___ ___ _____

    b. Gently swabbed urinary meatus. ___ ___ ___ _____

9. Returned swab(s) to culture tube and secured top. ___ ___ ___ _____

10. Properly removed and discarded gloves. ___ ___ ___ _____

11. Squeezed ampule in bottom of tube, and pushed swab tip into medium. ___ ___ ___ _____

12. Labeled and affixed requisition to each specimen. ___ ___ ___ _____

13. Sent specimen immediately to laboratory or refrigerated specimen. ___ ___ ___ _____

14. Assisted client in returning to comfortable position; replaced gown and removed drape. ___ ___ ___ _____

15. Washed hands. ___ ___ ___ _____

EVALUATION

1. Checked laboratory results for bacterial growth. ___ ___ ___ _____

2. Noted character of discharge. ___ ___ ___ _____

3. Observed specimen for presence of feces. ___ ___ ___ _____

4. Identified unexpected outcomes. ___ ___ ___ _____

RECORDING AND REPORTING

1. Recorded type of culture and date and time sent to laboratory. ___ ___ ___ _____

2. Described character of discharge and appearance of vaginal orifice and urethra. ___ ___ ___ _____

3. Reported laboratory test results. ___ ___ ___ _____

Student _____   Date _____

Instructor _____   Date _____

PERFORMANCE CHECKLIST 41-9 **COLLECTING SPUTUM SPECIMENS**

	S	U	NP	Comments
ASSESSMENT				
1. Reviewed physician's orders for specimen collection.	—	—	—	_____
2. Assessed client's understanding of procedure.	—	—	—	_____
3. Assessed client's ability to cough and expectorate.	—	—	—	_____
4. Checked when client last ate.	—	—	—	_____
5. Determined if client required assistance in producing specimen.	—	—	—	_____
6. Assessed client's respiratory status.	—	—	—	_____
NURSING DIAGNOSIS				
1. Developed appropriate nursing diagnoses based on assessment data.	—	—	—	_____
PLANNING				
1. Identified expected outcomes.	—	—	—	_____
2. Explained procedure to client.	—	—	—	_____
3. Assisted client in rinsing mouth before collecting expectorated specimen.	—	—	—	_____
IMPLEMENTATION				
1. Washed hands.	—	—	—	_____
2. Provided privacy.	—	—	—	_____
3. Positioned client correctly.	—	—	—	_____
4. Assisted client to splint painful area, if necessary.	—	—	—	_____
5. Collected expectorated specimen:	—	—	—	_____
a. Applied clean gloves.	—	—	—	_____
b. Instructed client to take three to four slow, deep breaths.	—	—	—	_____
c. Instructed client to cough after one full exhalation and expectorate into container.	—	—	—	_____
6. Collected suctioned specimen:	—	—	—	_____
a. Prepared suction equipment.	—	—	—	_____
b. Connected suction to adapter on sputum trap.	—	—	—	_____

	S	U	NP	Comments
c. Applied sterile gloves.	—	—	—	_____
d. Connected sterile suction catheter.	—	—	—	_____
e. Inserted suction catheter into nasopharynx and trachea.	—	—	—	_____
f. Suctioned 5 to 10 seconds while client coughed.	—	—	—	_____
g. Removed catheter without suctioning.	—	—	—	_____
h. Detached and disposed of suction catheter.	—	—	—	_____
7. Secured top of container or sputum trap.	—	—	—	_____
8. Cleaned outside of container with disinfectant if needed.	—	—	—	_____
9. Offered client facial tissues.	—	—	—	_____
10. Removed and disposed of gloves.	—	—	—	_____
11. Provided client's mouth care.	—	—	—	_____
12. Washed hands.	—	—	—	_____
13. Labeled specimen correctly.	—	—	—	_____
14. Placed specimen in appropriate bag or container.	—	—	—	_____
15. Sent specimen to lab or refrigerated specimen.	—	—	—	_____

EVALUATION

	S	U	NP	Comments
1. Observed client's respiratory status during procedure.	—	—	—	_____
2. Noted presence of anxiety or discomfort.	—	—	—	_____
3. Observed character of sputum.	—	—	—	_____
4. Noted laboratory results.	—	—	—	_____
5. Asked client to describe/demonstrate procedure.	—	—	—	_____
6. Identified unexpected outcomes.	—	—	—	_____

RECORDING AND REPORTING

	S	U	NP	Comments
1. Recorded method of collection, date and time sent to laboratory, and type of test ordered.	—	—	—	_____
2. Described characteristics of sputum.	—	—	—	_____
3. Described client's tolerance of procedure.	—	—	—	_____
4. Reported unusual sputum characteristics.	—	—	—	_____
5. Reported abnormal test results.	—	—	—	_____

Student _____   Date _____

Instructor _____   Date _____

PERFORMANCE CHECKLIST 41-10 **OBTAINING GASTRIC SPECIMENS**

	S	U	NP	Comments
ASSESSMENT				
1. Reviewed physician's orders before collecting specimen.	___	___	___	_____
2. Determined presence of nasogastric tube, or obtained order for inserting tube.	___	___	___	_____
3. Assessed client's understanding of procedure.	___	___	___	_____
4. Assessed medications and foods client received.	___	___	___	_____
5. Determined if any dietary or medication restrictions required before test.	___	___	___	_____
6. Assessed client for symptoms of gastrointestinal alterations.	___	___	___	_____
NURSING DIAGNOSIS				
1. Developed appropriate nursing diagnoses based on assessment data.	___	___	___	_____
PLANNING				
1. Identified expected outcomes.	___	___	___	_____
2. Instituted ordered dietary or medication restrictions.	___	___	___	_____
3. Explained procedure to client.	___	___	___	_____
IMPLEMENTATION				
1. Washed hands.	___	___	___	_____
2. Applied disposable gloves.	___	___	___	_____
3. Positioned client in high-Fowler's position.	___	___	___	_____
4. Provided privacy by closing curtains or door.	___	___	___	_____
5. Inserted nasogastric tube or verified placement of tube.	___	___	___	_____
6. Obtained specimen by attaching bulb syringe and aspirating 5 to 10 ml.	___	___	___	_____
7. Applied 1 drop of gastric sample to pH paper.	___	___	___	_____
8. Read pH results correctly after 30 seconds.	___	___	___	_____
9. Applied 1 drop of gastric sample to Gastrooccult test paper.	___	___	___	_____
10. Applied 2 drops of developer solution over sample and 1 drop to performance monitors.	___	___	___	_____

	S	U	NP	Comments
11. Read test results correctly within 60 seconds.	___	___	___	_____
12. Explained results to client.	___	___	___	_____
13. Disposed of soiled supplies correctly.	___	___	___	_____
14. Reconnected nasogastric tube to drainage or clamped as ordered; removed tube if appropriate.	___	___	___	_____
15. Removed and disposed of gloves.	___	___	___	_____
16. Returned client to comfortable position, and provided oral hygiene.	___	___	___	_____
17. Washed hands.	___	___	___	_____

EVALUATION

	S	U	NP	Comments
1. Assessed quantity and character of gastric secretions.	___	___	___	_____
2. Measured emesis for pH and blood.	___	___	___	_____
3. Compared test findings with normal expected results.	___	___	___	_____
4. Asked client to describe purpose of test.	___	___	___	_____
5. Identified unexpected outcomes.	___	___	___	_____

RECORDING AND REPORTING

	S	U	NP	Comments
1. Recorded test, source of specimen, and results.	___	___	___	_____
2. Described characteristics of gastric contents.	___	___	___	_____
3. Reported abnormal results.	___	___	___	_____

Student _____   Date _____

Instructor _____   Date _____

PERFORMANCE CHECKLIST 41-11   **OBTAINING WOUND DRAINAGE SPECIMENS**

	S	U	NP	Comments
ASSESSMENT				
1. Assessed client's understanding of purpose of culture and ability to cooperate.	—	—	—	_____
2. Assessed condition of wound using sterile gloves.	—	—	—	_____
3. Assessed client for systemic signs of infection.	—	—	—	_____
4. Determined character of pain at wound site.	—	—	—	_____
5. Reviewed physician's orders for culture.	—	—	—	_____
6. Determined schedule for dressing change.	—	—	—	_____
NURSING DIAGNOSIS				
1. Developed appropriate nursing diagnoses based on assessment data.	—	—	—	_____
PLANNING				
1. Identified expected outcomes.	—	—	—	_____
2. Determined client's need for analgesic before dressing change or specimen collection and administered correctly.	—	—	—	_____
3. Explained procedure to client.	—	—	—	_____
4. Explained that client may feel tickling sensation when wound is swabbed.	—	—	—	_____
IMPLEMENTATION				
1. Washed hands.	—	—	—	_____
2. Provided privacy.	—	—	—	_____
3. Removed and disposed of soiled dressings while wearing disposable gloves.	—	—	—	_____
4. Cleansed wound edges with antiseptic.	—	—	—	_____
5. Disposed of antiseptic swab and gloves.	—	—	—	_____
6. Opened culture tube kits and sterile dressing supplies; kept items sterile.	—	—	—	_____
7. Applied sterile gloves.	—	—	—	_____
8. Collected aerobic or anaerobic cultures. Inserted swab into wound and rotated gently.	—	—	—	_____
9. Returned swab to culture tube, crushed ampule, and pushed tip into liquid medium.	—	—	—	_____

	S	U	NP	Comments
10. Placed each specimen on appropriate label.	___	___	___	_____
11. Asked staff member to label and affix requisitions and send specimens to laboratory immediately.	___	___	___	_____
12. Cleaned wound as ordered, and applied new sterile dressing.	___	___	___	_____
13. Disposed of gloves and soiled supplies.	___	___	___	_____
14. Secured dressing.	___	___	___	_____
15. Assisted client to comfortable position.	___	___	___	_____
16. Washed hands.	___	___	___	_____

EVALUATION

1. Checked laboratory report for culture results.	___	___	___	_____
2. Assessed character of wound and wound drainage.	___	___	___	_____
3. Asked client about purpose of culture.	___	___	___	_____
4. Identified unexpected outcomes.	___	___	___	_____

RECORDING AND REPORTING

1. Recorded specimen type, source, and date and time sent to laboratory.	___	___	___	_____
2. Described appearance of wound and drainage.	___	___	___	_____
3. Reported evidence of infection to nurse in charge or physician.	___	___	___	_____

Student _____   Date _____

Instructor _____   Date _____

PERFORMANCE CHECKLIST 41-12   **COLLECTING BLOOD SPECIMENS BY VENIPUNCTURE (SYRINGE METHOD, VACUTAINER METHOD) AND BLOOD CULTURES**

	S	U	NP	Comments
ASSESSMENT				
1. Determined client's understanding of procedure.	___	___	___	_____
2. Determined if special conditions needed to be addressed before collection.	___	___	___	_____
3. Determined client's risk for venipuncture.	___	___	___	_____
4. Determined client's ability to cooperate with procedure.	___	___	___	_____
5. Identified site contraindications for venipuncture.	___	___	___	_____
6. Reviewed physician orders for type of test(s).	___	___	___	_____
NURSING DIAGNOSIS				
1. Developed appropriate nursing diagnoses based on assessment data.	___	___	___	_____
PLANNING				
1. Identified expected outcomes.	___	___	___	_____
2. Explained procedure to client.	___	___	___	_____
IMPLEMENTATION				
1. Obtained blood sample:	___	___	___	_____
a. Syringe method	___	___	___	_____
• Prepared syringe with needle securely attached.	___	___	___	_____
• Cleansed site with alcohol or other antiseptic.	___	___	___	_____
• Removed needle cover and explained expected sensation to client.	___	___	___	_____
• Pulled skin taut with thumb or forefinger 2.5 cm (1 inch) below site.	___	___	___	_____
• Held syringe and needle at 15- to 30-degree angle and slowly inserted needle into vein.	___	___	___	_____
• Held syringe securely and pulled back on plunger, watching for blood return.	___	___	___	_____
• Obtained desired amount of blood.	___	___	___	_____

	S	U	NP	Comments
b. Vacutainer method	——	——	——	_____
• Attached double-ended needle to vacuum tube.	——	——	——	_____
• Placed blood specimen tube in Vacutainer without puncturing rubber stopper.	——	——	——	_____
• Followed procedure for syringe method for venipuncture.	——	——	——	_____
• Held Vacutainer securely and advanced specimen tube onto needle in Vacutainer.	——	——	——	_____
• Noted blood flow.	——	——	——	_____
• Removed specimen tube after filled; inserted additional tubes, if necessary.	——	——	——	_____
2. Released tourniquet after sample obtained.	——	——	——	_____
3. Applied 2 × 2 gauze pad or alcohol swab over site, and withdrew needle.	——	——	——	_____
4. Applied pressure on site after needle removal.	——	——	——	_____
5. Discarded needle without recapping.	——	——	——	_____
6. Transferred specimen obtained with syringe method to tubes.	——	——	——	_____
7. Rotated all blood tubes that contained additives.	——	——	——	_____
8. Inspected puncture site for bleeding, and applied gauze or bandage.	——	——	——	_____
9. Cleansed outside of specimen tubes with antiseptic if necessary.	——	——	——	_____
10. Assisted client to comfortable position.	——	——	——	_____
11. Labeled each specimen tube and affixed requisition.	——	——	——	_____
12. Disposed of all equipment properly.	——	——	——	_____
13. Placed specimens in bag to be sent to laboratory.	——	——	——	_____
14. Removed gloves and washed hands.	——	——	——	_____
15. Sent specimens to laboratory immediately.	——	——	——	_____
16. Collected specimen for blood cultures:	——	——	——	_____
a. Cleansed site with povidone-iodine.	——	——	——	_____
b. Cleansed tips of vacuum tubes or culture bottles.	——	——	——	_____
c. Collected 10 to 15 ml venous blood by venipuncture.	——	——	——	_____

	S	U	NP	Comments
d. Discarded needle from syringe.	___	___	___	_____
e. Attached new needle for transfer of blood to specimen tube or bottle.	___	___	___	_____
f. Inoculated anaerobic specimen first.	___	___	___	_____
g. Mixed specimen gently after inoculation.	___	___	___	_____
h. Applied pressure over venipuncture site and covered with gauze or bandage.	___	___	___	_____
i. Labeled specimens, placed in bag, and sent to laboratory.	___	___	___	_____

EVALUATION

	S	U	NP	Comments
1. Reinspected venipuncture site.	___	___	___	_____
2. Determined if client remained anxious or fearful.	___	___	___	_____
3. Checked laboratory results.	___	___	___	_____
4. Asked client to explain purpose of test.	___	___	___	_____
5. Identified unexpected outcomes.	___	___	___	_____

RECORDING AND REPORTING

	S	U	NP	Comments
1. Recorded procedure.	___	___	___	_____
2. Described venipuncture site and client's response.	___	___	___	_____
3. Reported "stat" test results to physician.	___	___	___	_____
4. Reported any abnormal findings to physician.	___	___	___	_____

Student _____   Date _____

Instructor _____   Date _____

PERFORMANCE CHECKLIST 41-13 **MEASURING BLOOD GLUCOSE LEVEL AFTER SKIN PUNCTURE**

	S	U	NP	Comments
ASSESSMENT				
1. Assessed client's understanding of procedure.	___	___	___	_____
2. Determined if specific conditions needed to be met before procedure.	___	___	___	_____
3. Determined risks for performing procedure.	___	___	___	_____
4. Assessed area of skin to be used as puncture site.	___	___	___	_____
5. Reviewed physician's order.	___	___	___	_____
6. Assessed diabetic client's ability to handle skin puncture device.	___	___	___	_____
NURSING DIAGNOSIS				
1. Developed appropriate nursing diagnoses based on assessment data.	___	___	___	_____
PLANNING				
1. Identified expected outcomes.	___	___	___	_____
2. Explained procedure to client.	___	___	___	_____
IMPLEMENTATION				
1. Washed hands.	___	___	___	_____
2. Instructed client to wash hands.	___	___	___	_____
3. Positioned client comfortably.	___	___	___	_____
4. Removed reagent strip from container and tightly sealed caps.	___	___	___	_____
5. Turned glucose meter on.	___	___	___	_____
6. Inserted strip into glucose meter. Made adjustments if necessary.	___	___	___	_____
7. Removed reagent strip from meter and placed on clean, dry surface.	___	___	___	_____
8. Applied disposable gloves.	___	___	___	_____
9. Selected puncture site.	___	___	___	_____
10. Gently massaged finger to be punctured.	___	___	___	_____
11. Cleansed site with antiseptic swab and allowed to dry.	___	___	___	_____
12. Removed cover of lancet or blood-letting device.	___	___	___	_____

	S	U	NP	Comments
13. Correctly punctured finger or heel quickly.	___	___	___	_____
14. Wiped away first droplet of blood with cotton ball or as manufacturer's directions describe.	___	___	___	_____
15. Squeezed puncture site until droplet formed.	___	___	___	_____
16. Lightly transferred drop of blood to reagent strip test pad. Prepared meter and reagent strip per manufacturer's instructions.	___	___	___	_____
17. Applied pressure to skin puncture site.	___	___	___	_____
18. Noted glucose reading on display.	___	___	___	_____
19. Turned meter off and disposed of test strip and cotton balls.	___	___	___	_____
20. Removed disposable gloves and disposed of properly.	___	___	___	_____
21. Washed hands.	___	___	___	_____
22. Shared test results with client.	___	___	___	_____

EVALUATION

	S	U	NP	Comments
1. Compared glucose meter reading with normal levels.	___	___	___	_____
2. Inspected puncture site for bleeding or tissue injury.	___	___	___	_____
3. Determined if client had any questions or concerns.	___	___	___	_____
4. Asked client to describe/demonstrate procedure.	___	___	___	_____
5. Identified unexpected outcomes.	___	___	___	_____

RECORDING AND REPORTING

	S	U	NP	Comments
1. Recorded procedure, glucose level, and action taken for abnormal range.	___	___	___	_____
2. Described client's response and appearance of puncture site.	___	___	___	_____
3. Described any explanations or teaching provided for client.	___	___	___	_____
4. Reported abnormal blood glucose levels to physician.	___	___	___	_____

Student _____   Date _____

Instructor _____   Date _____

PERFORMANCE CHECKLIST 41-14   **OBTAINING AN ARTERIAL SPECIMEN FOR BLOOD GAS MEASUREMENT**

	S	U	NP	Comments
ASSESSMENT				
1. Identified need to obtain sample.	___	___	___	_____
2. Identified factors that could alter sample.	___	___	___	_____
3. Performed physical assessment of thorax and lungs.	___	___	___	_____
4. Reviewed criteria for choosing site for sample collection.	___	___	___	_____
5. Assessed arterial sites.	___	___	___	_____
6. Determined client's baseline arterial blood gases.	___	___	___	_____
7. Determined client's knowledge of procedure.	___	___	___	_____
NURSING DIAGNOSIS				
1. Developed appropriate nursing diagnoses based on assessment data.	___	___	___	_____
PLANNING				
1. Identified expected outcomes.	___	___	___	_____
2. Prepared heparinized syringe.	___	___	___	_____
3. Explained procedure to client.	___	___	___	_____
IMPLEMENTATION				
1. Washed hands and applied gloves.	___	___	___	_____
2. Selected and palpated arterial site.	___	___	___	_____
3. Stabilized artery appropriately.	___	___	___	_____
4. Cleansed area with alcohol swab.	___	___	___	_____
5. Held swab with fingers to palpate artery.	___	___	___	_____
6. Kept fingertip on artery.	___	___	___	_____
7. Correctly performed arterial stick, inserting needle at 45-degree angle.	___	___	___	_____
8. Stopped advancing needle when blood noted.	___	___	___	_____
9. If open needle used, attached syringe securely.	___	___	___	_____
10. Used swab to catch any spilled blood.	___	___	___	_____
11. Drew sample slowly.	___	___	___	_____

	S	U	NP	Comments
12. Removed needle, holding swab over site.	___	___	___	_____
13. Applied pressure over site.	___	___	___	_____
14. Maintained pressure for 3 to 5 minutes or longer, as indicated.	___	___	___	_____
15. Inspected site for to signs of bleeding.	___	___	___	_____
16. Palpated artery distal to puncture site.	___	___	___	_____
17. Expelled air bubbles from syringe.	___	___	___	_____
18. Removed and disposed of gloves and washed hands.	___	___	___	_____
19. Prepared syringe for laboratory according to agency policy using common principles such as the following:				
a. Labeled syringe properly.	___	___	___	_____
b. Placed sample on ice.	___	___	___	_____
c. Prepared laboratory requisition.	___	___	___	_____
d. Indicated client's FiO_2, use of oxygen, and temperature on requisition.	___	___	___	_____
e. Sent sample to laboratory immediately.	___	___	___	_____

EVALUATION

	S	U	NP	Comments
1. Inspected area distal to puncture site for complications.	___	___	___	_____
2. Reviewed results as soon as possible.	___	___	___	_____
3. Obtained client's respiratory rate.	___	___	___	_____
4. Identified unexpected outcomes.	___	___	___	_____

RECORDING AND REPORTING

	S	U	NP	Comments
1. Recorded puncture site and disposition of specimen to laboratory.	___	___	___	_____
2. Reported results to physician.	___	___	___	_____
3. Included FiO_2 and any ventilator settings in report.	___	___	___	_____
4. Recorded test results and condition of puncture site.	___	___	___	_____

Student _____   Date _____

Instructor _____   Date _____

PERFORMANCE CHECKLIST 42-1 **ASSISTING WITH ABDOMINAL PARACENTESIS**

	S	U	NP	Comments
ASSESSMENT				
1. Assessed for contraindications.	—	—	—	_____
2. Assessed vital signs.	—	—	—	_____
3. Assessed client's bladder for distention or determined time of last void.	—	—	—	_____
4. Determined whether client was allergic to local anesthetic or antiseptic solution.	—	—	—	_____
5. Weighed client. Assessed abdomen and correctly measured abdominal girth of client with ascites.	—	—	—	_____
6. Assessed respiratory status.	—	—	—	_____
7. Assessed client's knowledge about procedure.	—	—	—	_____
8. Checked institution's policy about written informed consent.	—	—	—	_____
NURSING DIAGNOSIS				
1. Developed appropriate nursing diagnoses based on assessment data.	—	—	—	_____
PLANNING				
1. Identified expected outcomes.	—	—	—	_____
2. Organized equipment at client's bedside.	—	—	—	_____
3. Explained procedure and had client void.	—	—	—	_____
4. Administered preprocedure medication.	—	—	—	_____
5. Assisted client to semi-Fowler's or upright position with feet supported.	—	—	—	_____
IMPLEMENTATION				
Nurse's Responsibility				
1. Washed hands.	—	—	—	_____
2. Set up sterile tray or opened sterile supplies.	—	—	—	_____
3. Prepared fluid to be used for lavage; attached to IV tubing.	—	—	—	_____
4. Assisted client through procedure.	—	—	—	_____
5. Assessed vital signs before, during, and after procedure.	—	—	—	_____
6. Apppplied gloves.	—	—	—	_____

	S	U	NP	Comments
7. Implemented fluid instillation for lavage.	___	___	___	_____
8. Opened tubing clamp to allow drainage of peritoneal lavage fluid.	___	___	___	_____
9. Collected laboratory specimens in sterile containers.	___	___	___	_____
10. Assessed client's tolerance of procedure, vital signs, pain, and sensorium.	___	___	___	_____
11. Disposed of equipment; removed gloves and washed hands.	___	___	___	_____

EVALUATION

	S	U	NP	Comments
1. Monitored vital signs every 15 minutes for 1 hour, then every 30 minutes for 2 hours.	___	___	___	_____
2. Monitored urinary status for 24 hours.	___	___	___	_____
3. Checked dressing over insertion site.	___	___	___	_____
4. Measured abdominal girth and weight.	___	___	___	_____
5. Inspected character of lavage or aspirate.	___	___	___	_____
6. Observed client for signs of discomfort.	___	___	___	_____
7. Identified unexpected outcomes.	___	___	___	_____

RECORDING AND REPORTING

	S	U	NP	Comments
1. Recorded procedure, type of dressing, presence of drainage, and client's tolerance.	___	___	___	_____
2. Recorded changes in abdominal girth and weight and characteristics of peritoneal fluid.	___	___	___	_____
3. Reported unexpected outcomes to physician.	___	___	___	_____

Student _____   Date _____

Instructor _____   Date _____

PERFORMANCE CHECKLIST 42-2 **ASSISTING WITH ANGIOGRAPHY (ARTERIOGRAPHY)**

	S	U	NP	Comments

ASSESSMENT
1. Assessed client's knowledge of procedure.

2. Assessed vital signs including peripheral pulses. Auscultated heart and lungs and obtained weight for cardiac catheterization.

3. Determined type of arteriogram to be performed.

4. Assessed need for signed informed consent.

5. Assessed time of last ingested fluid or food.

6. Determined if client allergic to iodine dye and, if so, notified appropriate physician.

7. Determined if client taking anticoagulants.

8. Assessed laboratory results.

9. Reviewed physician's orders.

NURSING DIAGNOSIS
1. Developed appropriate nursing diagnoses based on assessment data.

PLANNING
1. Identified expected outcomes.

2. Explained procedure and prepared client.

IMPLEMENTATION
Nurse's Responsibility
1. Washed hands and applied gloves.

2. If client is having cardiac catheterization, provided IV access using a large-bore cannula.

3. Measured vital signs, obtained weight, and palpated peripheral pulses.

4. Assisted client with assuming comfortable position on x-ray table.

5. Provided support throughout procedure.

6. Told client sensation that may be felt during dye injection.

7. Ensured monitoring of levels of sedation and consciousness for client receiving intravenous conscious sedation.

	S	U	NP	Comments

8. Noted tendency of client to cough when catheter placed into pulmonary artery. ___ ___ ___ _____

EVALUATION

1. Monitored vital signs and assessed peripheral pulses. Auscultated heart and lungs if cardiac catheterization performed. ___ ___ ___ _____

2. Applied pressure dressing to vascular access site. ___ ___ ___ _____

3. Maintained client on bedrest for 4 to 8 hours. ___ ___ ___ _____

4. Kept affected extremity immobilized for 6 to 8 hours. ___ ___ ___ _____

5. Emphasized need for client to lay flat for 6 to 12 hours. ___ ___ ___ _____

6. Encouraged client to drink fluids. ___ ___ ___ _____

7. Assessed for delayed reaction to dye. ___ ___ ___ _____

8. Determined level of sedation and oxygenation. ___ ___ ___ _____

9. Assessed postprocedure laboratory values. ___ ___ ___ _____

10. Observed for signs of discomfort. ___ ___ ___ _____

11. Identified unexpected outcomes. ___ ___ ___ _____

RECORDING AND REPORTING

1. Recorded type of procedure and how client tolerated procedure. ___ ___ ___ _____

2. Recorded changes in vital signs, peripheral pulses, and laboratory values. ___ ___ ___ _____

3. Followed specific postangiography orders according to agency guidelines. ___ ___ ___ _____

4. Recorded type of dressing, type and amount of drainage, and presence of pain. ___ ___ ___ _____

5. Reported unexpected outcomes to physician immediately. ___ ___ ___ _____

6. Reported pertinent data to oncoming shift. ___ ___ ___ _____

Student _____   Date _____

Instructor _____   Date _____

PERFORMANCE CHECKLIST 42-3 **ASSISTING WITH BONE MARROW ASPIRATION/BIOPSY**

	S	U	NP	Comments
ASSESSMENT				
1. Assessed client's knowledge of procedure.	___	___	___	_____
2. Assessed client's ability to assume position required for procedure.	___	___	___	_____
3. Assessed vital signs to obtain baseline data.	___	___	___	_____
4. Assessed client's coagulation status.	___	___	___	_____
5. Determined purpose of procedure.	___	___	___	_____
6. Ascertained presence of signed informed consent form.	___	___	___	_____
7. Determined whether client was allergic to antiseptic and anesthetic solutions.	___	___	___	_____
NURSING DIAGNOSIS				
1. Developed appropriate nursing diagnoses based on assessment data.	___	___	___	_____
PLANNING				
1. Identified expected outcomes.	___	___	___	_____
2. Explained steps to client.	___	___	___	_____
IMPLEMENTATION				
Nurse's Responsibility				
1. Washed hands.	___	___	___	_____
2. Set up sterile tray or opened supplies for physician.	___	___	___	_____
3. Assisted client with maintaining correct position; reassured client while explaining procedure.	___	___	___	_____
4. Assessed client's condition during procedure.	___	___	___	_____
5. Noted characteristics of bone marrow aspirate.	___	___	___	_____
EVALUATION				
1. Monitored vital signs.	___	___	___	_____
2. Inspected dressing over puncture site.	___	___	___	_____
3. Observed client's level of comfort.	___	___	___	_____
4. Identified unexpected outcomes.	___	___	___	_____

	S	U	NP	Comments

RECORDING AND REPORTING

1. Recorded procedure, location of puncture site, characteristics of aspirate, tests ordered, type of dressing, and client assessment.   ___ ___ ___ _____

2. Reported unexpected outcomes to physician.   ___ ___ ___ _____

3. Reported results of procedure to oncoming shift.   ___ ___ ___ _____

Student _____   Date _____

Instructor _____   Date _____

PERFORMANCE CHECKLIST 42-4 **ASSISTING WITH BRONCHOSCOPY**

	S	U	NP	Comments
ASSESSMENT				
1. Assessed client's knowledge about procedure.	—	—	—	_____
2. Assessed vital signs to obtain baseline data.	—	—	—	_____
3. Assessed respiratory function.	—	—	—	_____
4. Determined purpose of procedure.	—	—	—	_____
5. Assessed need for signed informed consent form.	—	—	—	_____
6. Determined whether client was allergic to local anesthetic.	—	—	—	_____
7. Assessed need for preprocedure medication.	—	—	—	_____
8. Assessed time client last ingested food.	—	—	—	_____
9. Assessed vital signs and oxygen saturation if using intravenous conscious sedation.	—	—	—	_____
NURSING DIAGNOSIS				
1. Developed appropriate nursing diagnoses based on assessment data.	—	—	—	_____
PLANNING				
1. Identified expected outcomes.	—	—	—	_____
2. Explained procedure to client.	—	—	—	_____
3. Assisted client with maintaining position.	—	—	—	_____
4. Removed and stored client's eyeglasses, contact lenses, and/or dentures.	—	—	—	_____
5. Made sure that client remained NPO 8 hours before procedure.	—	—	—	_____
IMPLEMENTATION				
Nurse's Responsibility				
1. Instructed client not to swallow local anesthetic; provided emesis basin.	—	—	—	_____
2. Assisted client through procedure with explanations.	—	—	—	_____
3. Assessed client's respiratory status during procedure.	—	—	—	_____
4. Noted characteristics of suctioned material.	—	—	—	_____

	S	U	NP	Comments
5. Wiped client's mouth and nose to remove lubricant after bronchoscope was removed.	___	___	___	_____
6. Did not allow client to eat or drink until tracheobronchial anesthesia had worn off.	___	___	___	_____

EVALUATION

1. Monitored vital signs.	___	___	___	_____
2. Observed sputum production.	___	___	___	_____
3. Observed respiratory status.	___	___	___	_____
4. Determined level of sedation.	___	___	___	_____
5. Assessed for return of gag reflex.	___	___	___	_____
6. Asked client to describe postprocedure normal and abnormal symptoms.	___	___	___	_____
7. Identified unexpected outcomes.	___	___	___	_____

RECORDING AND REPORTING

1. Recorded procedure and client assessment.	___	___	___	_____
2. Reported unexpected outcomes to physician immediately.	___	___	___	_____
3. Reported results of procedure to oncoming shift.	___	___	___	_____

Student _____   Date _____

Instructor _____   Date _____

PERFORMANCE CHECKLIST 42-5 **ASSISTING WITH ELECTROCARDIOGRAM**

	S	U	NP	Comments
ASSESSMENT				
1. Determined rationale for ECG.	—	—	—	_____
2. Determined if client had chest pain.	—	—	—	_____
3. Assessed client's knowledge about procedure.	—	—	—	_____
4. Obtained baseline vital signs.	—	—	—	_____
NURSING DIAGNOSIS				
1. Developed appropriate nursing diagnoses based on assessment data.	—	—	—	_____
PLANNING				
1. Identified expected outcomes.	—	—	—	_____
2. Provided privacy.	—	—	—	_____
3. Prepared client for procedure:	—	—	—	_____
a. Exposed client's chest and arms.	—	—	—	_____
b. Placed client in supine position.	—	—	—	_____
c. Instructed client to lie still and not cross legs.	—	—	—	_____
IMPLEMENTATION				
1. Washed hands.	—	—	—	_____
2. Cleansed and prepared client's skin.	—	—	—	_____
3. Applied electrode paste and attached leads to chest and extremities.	—	—	—	_____
4. Obtained tracing.	—	—	—	_____
5. Disconnected leads, cleansed skin, and washed hands.	—	—	—	_____
6. Delivered ECG tracing to appropriate laboratory or heart station.	—	—	—	_____
EVALUATION				
1. Assessed client's response to procedure.	—	—	—	_____
2. Measured vital signs.	—	—	—	_____
3. Identified unexpected outcomes.	—	—	—	_____

	S	U	NP	Comments

RECORDING AND REPORTING

1. Recorded procedure and baseline vital signs.   ___ ___ ___ _____

2. Reported any unexpected outcomes.   ___ ___ ___ _____

Student _____   Date _____

Instructor _____   Date _____

PERFORMANCE CHECKLIST 42-6   **ASSISTING WITH ENDOSCOPY**

	S	U	NP	Comments

ASSESSMENT

1. Assessed client's knowledge about procedure.   ___ ___ ___ _____

2. Assessed vital signs.   ___ ___ ___ _____

3. Determined presence of gastrointestinal bleeding.   ___ ___ ___ _____

4. Determined purpose of procedure.   ___ ___ ___ _____

5. Assessed need for signed informed consent form.   ___ ___ ___ _____

6. Verified that client was NPO for at least 8 hours.   ___ ___ ___ _____

7. Verified that client did not have esophageal diverticulum.   ___ ___ ___ _____

8. Reviewed physician's orders for preprocedure medication and intravenous conscious sedation (IVCS).   ___ ___ ___ _____

NURSING DIAGNOSIS

1. Developed appropriate nursing diagnoses based on assessment data.   ___ ___ ___ _____

PLANNING

1. Identified expected outcomes.   ___ ___ ___ _____

2. Prepared client for procedure.   ___ ___ ___ _____

3. Explained steps of procedure.   ___ ___ ___ _____

4. Explained purpose and effects of IVCS.   ___ ___ ___ _____

5. Administered preprocedure medication.   ___ ___ ___ _____

IMPLEMENTATION
Nurse's Responsibility

1. Washed hands and applied gloves, goggles, and mask.   ___ ___ ___ _____

2. Removed dentures and partial bridges.   ___ ___ ___ _____

3. Assisted client with maintaining proper position.   ___ ___ ___ _____

4. Ensured IV line patency for IVCS.   ___ ___ ___ _____

5. Assisted client through procedure. Anticipated needs and promoted comfort.   ___ ___ ___ _____

6. Placed tissue specimens in proper containers.   ___ ___ ___ _____

7. Suctioned if client began to vomit or accumulated saliva.   ___ ___ ___ _____

	S	U	NP	Comments

8. Maintained client's NPO status until gag reflex returned.

9. Provided oral hygiene when gag reflex returned.

10. Assisted client to comfortable position. Washed hands.

EVALUATION

1. Monitored vital signs and oxygen saturation.

2. Assessed for level of sedation.

3. Observed for discomfort.

4. Evaluated character of emesis or aspirate.

5. Assessed for return of gag reflex.

6. Asked client to state postprocedure dietary and activity limitations.

7. Identified unexpected outcomes.

RECORDING AND REPORTING

1. Recorded procedure, specimen collection, and client assessment.

2. Reported unexpected outcomes to physician.

3. Reported pertinent findings to nurse in charge.

Student _____   Date _____

Instructor _____   Date _____

PERFORMANCE CHECKLIST 42-7 **ASSISTING WITH LUMBAR PUNCTURE**

	S	U	NP	Comments

ASSESSMENT

1. Assessed client's ability to understand and follow directions.

2. Assessed client's ability to assume correct position for procedure.

3. Assessed degree of cooperativeness of client to remain in position.

4. Examined medical record for contraindications.

5. Determined whether client was allergic to medication to be used in procedure.

6. Ascertained presence of signed consent form.

7. Assessed client's knowledge about procedure.

8. Assessed client's vital signs and neurologic status of legs.

NURSING DIAGNOSIS

1. Developed appropriate nursing diagnoses based on assessment data.

PLANNING

1. Identified expected outcomes.

2. Explained procedure to client.

3. Had client empty bladder and bowels before procedure.

4. Positioned client correctly in lateral recumbent position with head and neck flexed.

IMPLEMENTATION
Nurse's Responsibility

1. Explained to client need to remain in position.

2. Held client's arms and legs in flexed position.

3. Cautioned client to not cough and to breathe slowly and deeply.

4. Explained each step that might produce discomfort.

5. Applied gloves in preparation for handling body fluids.

	S	U	NP	Comments

6. Properly labeled tubes.

7. Assisted with placement of direct pressure and bandage.

8. Removed gloves and washed hands.

9. Assisted client in assuming comfortable position.

10. Asked client to maintain supine or dorsal recumbent position.

11. Provided client with medication, if ordered.

12. Observed client's response to procedure.

13. Encouraged client to force PO fluids if not contraindicated.

EVALUATION
1. Assessed needle insertion site for drainage.

2. Assessed level of consciousness, vital signs, pupils, respiratory status, and numbness or tingling in legs.

3. Asked client to describe postprocedure positioning and activity restriction.

4. Identified unexpected outcomes.

RECORDING AND REPORTING
1. Recorded procedure, specimens obtained, and client response.

2. Recorded and reported pertinent findings to nurse in charge or physician.

Student _____   Date _____

Instructor _____   Date _____

PERFORMANCE CHECKLIST 42-8 **ASSISTING WITH MAGNETIC RESONANCE IMAGING**

	S	U	NP	Comments
ASSESSMENT				
1. Assessed client's knowledge about procedure.	—	—	—	_____
2. Assessed stability of client's medical condition.	—	—	—	_____
3. Assessed need for signed informed consent form.	—	—	—	_____
4. Assessed client's weight.	—	—	—	_____
5. Assessed client for cardiac pacemaker, aneurysm clips, or history of valve replacement (implantable metal objects).	—	—	—	_____
6. Assessed client for claustrophobia.	—	—	—	_____
7. Assessed client for pregnancy.	—	—	—	_____
8. Assessed client's ability to remain still throughout procedure.	—	—	—	_____
9. Assessed for allergies to dye and contrast medium.	—	—	—	_____
NURSING DIAGNOSIS				
1. Developed appropriate nursing diagnoses based on assessment data.	—	—	—	_____
PLANNING				
1. Identified expected outcomes.	—	—	—	_____
IMPLEMENTATION				
Nurse's Responsibility				
1. Showed client picture of magnetic resonance imaging (MRI) machine, if possible, and encouraged questions.	—	—	—	_____
2. Removed all metallic objects from client.	—	—	—	_____
3. Had client void and put on hospital gown.	—	—	—	_____
EVALUATION				
1. Evaluated client's status after procedure.	—	—	—	_____
2. Identified unexpected outcomes.	—	—	—	_____
RECORDING AND REPORTING				
1. Recorded and reported date, time, place MRI performed, whether contrast medium was used, and client's tolerance of procedure.	—	—	—	_____

Student _____   Date _____

Instructor _____   Date _____

PERFORMANCE CHECKLIST 42-9   **ASSISTING WITH THORACENTESIS**

	S	U	NP	Comments
ASSESSMENT				
1. Assessed client's knowledge about procedure.	—	—	—	_____
2. Assessed client's ability to assume correct position for procedure.	—	—	—	_____
3. Assessed vital signs.	—	—	—	_____
4. Determined presence of possible bleeding disorder.	—	—	—	_____
5. Assessed respiratory function.	—	—	—	_____
6. Determined purpose of procedure.	—	—	—	_____
7. Assessed need for signed informed consent form.	—	—	—	_____
8. Determined whether client was allergic to antiseptic or anesthetic solutions.	—	—	—	_____
9. Assessed need for preprocedure pain medication.	—	—	—	_____
NURSING DIAGNOSIS				
1. Developed appropriate nursing diagnoses based on assessment data.	—	—	—	_____
PLANNING				
1. Identified expected outcomes.	—	—	—	_____
2. Prepared client for procedure.	—	—	—	_____
3. Explained sensations that may be felt during procedure.	—	—	—	_____
4. Had client void before procedure.	—	—	—	_____
5. Assisted client to upright or side-lying position.	—	—	—	_____
IMPLEMENTATION				
Nurse's Responsibility				
1. Washed hands.	—	—	—	_____
2. Set up sterile tray or opened supplies for physician.	—	—	—	_____
3. Assisted client with maintaining correct position.	—	—	—	_____
4. Assisted client through procedure.	—	—	—	_____
5. Assessed client's pulse and respiratory status during procedure.	—	—	—	_____
6. Assisted client with assuming comfortable position in bed.	—	—	—	_____

	S	U	NP	Comments

EVALUATION

1. Noted characteristics of pleural fluid.

2. Monitored vital signs and auscultated lung sounds.

3. Monitored client for complications.

4. Noted presence of drainage on chest dressing.

5. Followed-up on postthoracentesis chest x-ray.

6. Asked client to describe postprocedure limitations and positioning.

7. Identified unexpected outcomes.

RECORDING AND REPORTING

1. Recorded procedure, laboratory tests, condition of puncture site, characteristics of fluid, and client assessment.

2. Reported unexpected outcomes to physician immediately.

3. Reported to oncoming staff.

Student _____   Date _____

Instructor _____   Date _____

PERFORMANCE CHECKLIST 43-1   **CARE OF THE BODY AFTER DEATH**

	S	U	NP	Comments

ASSESSMENT

1. Assessed for presence of family or significant others and whether they had been informed of client's death. Asked if family wished to view the body.

2. Approached next of kin for tissue donation.

3. Allowed time for family or significant others to ask questions.

4. Completed necessary organ/tissue donation forms.

5. Assessed client's religious preference or cultural heritage and determined if family wished to have minister or priest at bedside.

6. Determined general condition of body.

7. Reviewed agency policy for preparation of the body; determined if autopsy planned.

NURSING DIAGNOSIS

1. Developed appropriate nursing diagnoses based on assessment data.

PLANNING

1. Identified expected outcomes.

2. Explained to family about time period needed to prepare body for viewing.

3. If another client is in the room, explained what has happened and offered that other client the opportunity to leave the room.

4. Prepared needed equipment.

IMPLEMENTATION

1. Washed hands.

2. Applied disposable gloves and gown or protective devices, if applicable.

3. Provided privacy.

4. Correctly identified client.

5. Correctly positioned client.

6. Placed small pillow under client's head or elevated head of bed slightly.

	S	U	NP	Comments
7. Gently held client's eyelids closed for a few seconds.	—	—	—	_____
8. Inserted client's dentures into mouth.	—	—	—	_____
9. Removed all collection devices and tubes not needed for autopsy examination.	—	—	—	_____
10. Clamped or cut tubes that would remain in body and secured with tape.	—	—	—	_____
11. Removed soiled dressings and replaced with clean gauze dressings.	—	—	—	_____
12. Washed soiled body parts.	—	—	—	_____
13. Placed absorbent pad under client's buttocks.	—	—	—	_____
14. Brushed and combed client's hair.	—	—	—	_____
15. Removed all jewelry unless otherwise requested by client's family.	—	—	—	_____
16. Placed clean gown on body.	—	—	—	_____
17. Accounted for all valuables that remained in client's room.	—	—	—	_____
18. Placed client's clothing and shoes in labeled bag.	—	—	—	_____
19. Completed identification tags and placed on client according to policy.	—	—	—	_____
20. If family requested viewing, placed sheet or blanket over client with shoulders and head exposed.	—	—	—	_____
21. Remained at bedside with family and allowed time for them to view body privately.	—	—	—	_____
22. After family left, removed all linen and client's gown. Placed body in body bag or applied shroud.	—	—	—	_____
23. Secured shroud or body bag.	—	—	—	_____
24. Attached label to outside of shroud or body bag.	—	—	—	_____
25. If client had transmissible infection, applied special labeling as indicated.	—	—	—	_____
26. Arranged for transportation of body.	—	—	—	_____
27. Carefully transferred body to stretcher.	—	—	—	_____
28. Closed other client's doors and arranged for transport to be as inconspicuous as possible.	—	—	—	_____
29. Removed remaining items and linens from client's room.	—	—	—	_____
30. Washed hands.	—	—	—	_____

	S	U	NP	Comments

EVALUATION

1. Observed family's response to loss of loved one.

2. Offered family the opportunity to ask questions and express feelings.

3. Assisted family in making necessary calls to other family members and significant others.

4. Noted appearance and condition of client's skin during body preparation.

5. Identified unexpected outcomes.

RECORDING AND REPORTING

1. Recorded date and time of death and pertinent data.

2. Documented any marks, bruises, or wounds on the body.

3. Documented handling of valuables and personal belongings.